Planning Later Life

This book examines the relevance of modern medicine and healthcare in shaping the lives of elderly persons and the practices and institutions of ageing societies. Combining individual and social dimensions, *Planning Later Life* discusses the ethical, social, and political consequences of increasing life expectancies and demographic change in the context of biomedicine and public health.

By focusing on the field of biomedicine and healthcare, the authors engage readers in a dialogue on the ethical and social implications of recent trends in dementia research and care, advance healthcare planning, or the rise of anti-ageing medicine and prevention. Bringing together the largely separated debates of individualist bioethics on the one hand, and public health ethics on the other, the volume deliberately considers the entanglements of envisioning, evaluating, and controlling individual and societal futures. So far, the process of devising and exploring the various positive and negative visions and strategies related to later life has rarely been reflected systematically from a philosophical, sociological, and ethical point of view.

As such, this book will be crucial to those working and studying in the life sciences, the humanities, and the social sciences, particularly in the areas of bioethics, social work, gerontology and ageing studies, healthcare and social services, sociology, social policy, and geography and population studies.

Mark Schweda is Research Fellow at the Department for Medical Ethics and History of Medicine, University Medical Center Göttingen.

Larissa Pfaller is Research Associate at the Institute of Sociology at the University of Erlangen-Nuremberg and currently Deputy Professor at the University of Hamburg.

Kai Brauer is a sociologist and teaches empirical methods and sociology of ageing at Carinthia University of Applied Sciences (CUAS).

Frank Adloff is Professor of Sociology at the University of Hamburg.

Silke Schicktanz is a bioethicist and Professor for Cultural and Ethical Studies of Biomedicine at the Department for Medical Ethics and History of Medicine, University Medical Center Göttingen.

Routledge Advances in Health and Social Policy

For a full list of titles in this series, please visit https://www.routledge.com/Routledge-Advances-in-Health-and-Social-Policy/book-series/RAHSP

Titles in this series:

The Invisible Work of Nurses
Hospitals, Organisation and Healthcare
Davina Allen

Domestic Violence in Diverse Contexts
A Re-examination of Gender
Sarah Wendt and Lana Zannettino

Maternity Services and Policy in an International Context
Risk, Citizenship and Welfare Regimes
Edited by Patricia Kennedy and Naonori Kodate

Innovation in Social Welfare and Human Services
Rolf Rønning and Marcus Knutagård

Social Development and Social Work Perspectives on Social Protection
Edited by Julie Drolet

Moralising Poverty
The 'Undeserving' Poor in the Public Gaze
Serena Romano

Forthcoming titles:

M-Health in Developing Countries
Design and Implementation Perspectives on Using Mobiles in Healthcare
Arul Chib

Alcohol, Power and Public Health
A Comparative Study of Alcohol Policy
Shane Butler, Betsy Thom, James Nicholls and Karen Elmeland

Social Policies and Public Action
Lavinia Bifulco

Planning Later Life

Bioethics and Public Health in Ageing Societies

Edited by Mark Schweda, Larissa Pfaller, Kai Brauer, Frank Adloff, and Silke Schicktanz

Routledge
Taylor & Francis Group
LONDON AND NEW YORK

First published 2017
by Routledge

2 Park Square, Milton Park, Abingdon, Oxfordshire OX14 4RN
52 Vanderbilt Avenue, New York, NY 10017

Routledge is an imprint of the Taylor & Francis Group, an informa business

First issued in paperback 2019

British Library Cataloguing-in-Publication Data
A catalogue record for this book is available from the British Library

Library of Congress Cataloging-in-Publication Data
Names: Schweda, Mark, editor.
Title: Planning later life / edited by Mark Schweda, Larissa Pfaller, Kai Brauer, Frank Adloff, & Silke Schicktanz.
Description: Milton Park, Abingdon, Oxon ; New York, NY : Routledge, 2017. | Includes bibliographical references and index.
Identifiers: LCCN 2016058994 | ISBN 9781472481320 (hardback) | ISBN 9781315600772 (ebook)
Subjects: LCSH: Bioethics. | Longevity. | Aging—Prevention. | Medical ethics.
Classification: LCC QH332 .P57 2017 | DDC 174.2—dc23
LC record available at https://lccn.loc.gov/2016058994

ISBN: 978-1-4724-8132-0 (hbk)
ISBN: 978-0-367-35007-9 (pbk)

Typeset in Times New Roman
by Apex CoVantage, LLC

Contents

Figures and tables

Figures

Tables

Contributors

Frank Adloff is Professor of Sociology at the University of Hamburg. His research interests include social theory, political sociology, culture and affectivity, conviviality, the gift, and civil society.

Kai Brauer is a sociologist and teaches empirical methods and sociology of ageing at Carinthia University of Applied Sciences (CUAS). He is co-founder of the IARA: Institute of Applied Research on Ageing. He has studied and worked at the Free University of Berlin and at the Universities of Kassel, Erlangen, and Vechta as well as at the WZB Berlin Social Science Center.

Chris Gilleard is a Visiting Research Fellow in the Division of Psychiatry at University College London. He has co-authored a number of books theorizing the place of ageing and later life in contemporary society, including *Cultures of Ageing: Self, Citizen and the Body* (2000), *Ageing, Corporeality and Embodiment* (2013), and *Rethinking Old Age: Theorising the Fourth Age* (2015) (all with Paul Higgs).

Paul Higgs is Professor of the Sociology of Ageing at University College London. He co-authored *Cultures of Ageing: Self, Citizen and the Body* (2000), *Ageing, Corporeality and Embodiment* (2013), and *Rethinking Old Age: Theorising the Fourth Age* (2015) (all with Chris Gilleard). He is editor of *Social Theory and Health* and has published in both social gerontology and medical sociology. He is currently engaged in a number of large research projects investigating the social aspects of dementia. He is a Fellow of the Academy of Social Sciences and the Gerontological Society of America.

Søren Holm is a Danish medical doctor and philosopher. He is Professor of Bioethics at the University of Manchester School of Law's Centre for Social Ethics and Policy and holds part-time chairs in Medical Ethics at the Center for Medical Ethics at Oslo University and the Department of Health Sciences and Technology at Aalborg University. He has presided over the European Society for the Philosophy of Medicine and Health Care and is the vice-president of the International Association of Bioethics. He is a former member of the Danish Council of Ethics and of the Nuffield Council on Bioethics.

François Höpflinger is Professor for Sociology (Emeritus) at Zurich University. He was director of the institute "Ageing and Generations" in Sion, Switzerland. His research interests include sociology of ageing and gerontology, demographics, generational ties and societal generational relations, and living and working in later life. He has published on family and care, the baby-boomer generation, dependency and long-term care. He is a member of the steering committee of the Center for Gerontology at the University of Zurich.

Nancy S. Jecker is Professor of Bioethics & Humanities at the University of Washington School of Medicine and Adjunct Professor of Philosophy at the School of Law. Her research addresses age-group justice, healthcare allocation, withholding and withdrawing treatment, and ethical theory. She co-authored (with L.J. Schneiderman) *Wrong Medicine, 2nd edition* (2011/Taiwan: 2015), co-edited (with A.R. Jonsen and R.A. Pearlman) *Bioethics, 3rd edition* (2011), and has published over 100 papers in bioethics and philosophy.

Ralf J. Jox is Associate Professor for Geriatric Palliative Care at Lausanne University Hospital, Switzerland, and Assistant Professor for Medical Ethics at the University of Munich, Germany. He has published widely on palliative care, end-of-life decision making, advance directives, and surrogate decision making. He is a member of the task force "Advance Care Planning" of the European Association for Palliative Care as well as a member of the task force "Advance Care Planning" of the Swiss Federal Public Health Office.

Stephen Katz is Professor for Sociology at Trent University. He has worked on ageing, pharmaceutical expertise, sexuality, and enhancement and is currently working on the cultural aspects of ageing memory and cognitive impairment. He is author of *Disciplining Old Age: The Formation of Gerontological Knowledge* (1996) and *Cultural Ageing: Life Course, Lifestyle, and Senior Worlds* (2005).

Andreas Kruse is Professor at and Director of the Institute of Gerontology at Heidelberg University. He is a psychologist, gerontologist, and demographer, a member of the German Ethics Council, and the author of many scientific publications on ageing and old age, perspectives of gerontology, and quality of life in dementia. Among many other honors, he was awarded the Federal Cross of Merit with Ribbon of the Federal Republic of Germany.

Ruud ter Meulen is Emeritus Professor in Ethics in Medicine at the University of Bristol. He was Director and Professor in Philosophy at the Institute of Bioethics and the University of Maastricht before moving to Bristol in 2005. He was principal investigator of a range of projects funded within the various Framework Programs of the European Commission, and he presides over the European Association of Centres for Medical Ethics (EACME).

S. Jay Olshansky is a Professor in the School of Public Health at the University of Illinois at Chicago, Research Associate at the Center on Ageing at the University of Chicago and at the London School of Hygiene and Tropical Medicine, and chief scientist at Lapetus Solutions. The focus of his research has been on estimates of the upper limits to human longevity, exploring the health and public-policy implications associated with individual and population ageing; forecasts of the size, survival, and age structure of the population; pursuit of the scientific means to slow ageing in people; and global implications of the re-emergence of infectious and parasitic diseases.

Larissa Pfaller is Research Associate at the Institute of Sociology at the University of Erlangen-Nuremberg and currently Deputy Professor at the University of Hamburg. She is especially interested in qualitative methods of empirical social research, cultural sociology, and the sociology of ageing. She wrote her PhD dissertation on the usage of anti-ageing medicine.

Thomas Rentsch is Professor for Practical Philosophy and Ethics at the TU Dresden. His working fields are practical philosophy, ethics, the philosophy of religion, philosophical anthropology, the philosophy of language, and hermeneutics. Among his most recent publications are (with Andreas Kruse and Harm-Peer Zimmermann) *Gutes Leben im hohen Alter* (2012) and (also with Kruse and Zimmermann) *Altern in unserer Zeit* (2013).

Silke Schicktanz is a bioethicist and Professor for Cultural and Ethical Studies of Biomedicine at the University Medical Center Göttingen. Her research is located at the intersection of normative bioethics and socio-empirical studies of medical practice, with a strong emphasis on cross-cultural comparative work. Her recent research topics include dementia research, ageing, and predictive medicine, as well as how concepts of responsibility and autonomy link laypeople's morality and professional bioethics.

Mark Schweda is Research Fellow in the Department for Medical Ethics and History of Medicine at University Medical Center Göttingen. As a philosopher and bioethicist, his research focuses on philosophical, bioethical, and sociocultural aspects of ageing and the life course, as well as on questions of political philosophy. Among his recent publications are the edited volumes *Pro-Age oder Anti-Ageing? Altern im Fokus der modernen Medizin* (together with Silke Schicktanz, 2012) and *Popularizing Dementia. Public Expressions and Representations of Forgetfulness* (together with Aagje Swinnen, 2015).

Perla Werner is currently Professor of Community Mental Health at the University of Haifa. She has been involved in gerontological research since 1978 and has contributed to the expansion of knowledge in the area of psychosocial aspects of Alzheimer's disease and other dementing disorders. She has devoted the last decade to the study of stigma in the area of Alzheimer's disease – its conceptualization, assessment, and correlates. She served as the Head of the Department of Gerontology, as the Dean of the Faculty of Social Welfare and Health Sciences, and as the Vice Rector of the University of Haifa.

Peter J. Whitehouse is Strategic Advisor in Innovation and Visiting Scholar at Baycrest, Professor of Medicine at the University of Toronto, and Professor of

Neurology Psychiatry, Neuroscience, and Organizational Behavior at Case Western Reserve University. He is president of Intergenerational Schools International.

Hsiu-I Yang is Associate Professor of Public Health at the National Yang Ming University in Taipei, in the Division of Law and Policy. She studied in Stanford, Seattle, and Taiwan and was Associate Professor of Health Care Management at Chang Gung University. She is especially interested in patient autonomy (informed consent) and medical malpractice.

Introduction

Mark Schweda, Larissa Pfaller, and Silke Schicktanz

Medicine and healthcare have become central elements in planning human life. The second half of life, especially, often turns into a projection screen of individual and political decision-making regarding various medical and healthcare scenarios. On one hand, new diagnostic, therapeutic, and preventive options, including technological developments (such as predictive testing, ambient assisted living, and monitoring technologies) – as well as legal tools, such as advance healthcare directives and living wills – encourage the idea of self-determined and 'successful' ageing that can be prudently modeled and actively shaped. On the other hand, dealing with old age and growing populations of elderly people with chronic diseases, frailty, and dementia is often perceived as a serious problem and an increasing challenge to families, care providers, and social security systems.

Biomedical life plans for ageing

The possibility of medical planning for old age is not self-evident. It presupposes that some middle ground exists between the two extremes of a completely unpredictable future and a strictly determined course of life. Only within this obscure space of limited (in-)determinacy, of possibilities and probabilities, of chances and risks, the endeavor of conceiving and shaping future life and old age according to particular medical or public health visions and strategies makes sense. The emergence of such a scope for planning results from three crucial developments of the last 200 years: the rise in average life expectancy, the process of modernization and individualization, and the growing importance of biomedicine (for the following, see Schweda and Schicktanz 2012).

Since the 19th century, Western societies have witnessed an unprecedented increase in life expectancy. In the US, for example, life expectancy at birth has risen from 47.3 years in 1900 to 78.8 years in 2014 (National Center for Health Statistics 2016, 95). In Germany, it has increased from 46.6 years for boys and 52.5 for girls to 78.2 and 83.1 years in the same period of time (Statistisches Bundesamt 2016, 14). In the course of this development, large swathes of the population experienced, for the first time, the opportunity to plan their lives on a long-term basis. Statistically, death no longer was considered a life-long threat but became a phenomenon of old age. This shift from 'unreliable to reliable life time' also engendered a change in consciousness (Imhof 1987). While death has moved to the end of a life spanning eight decades, *statistical* life expectancy has turned into *normative* life expectancy. 'Premature' death is perceived not only as a disaster but as a *moral* problem of personal failure or social injustice. Correspondingly, ageing and old age also are not any longer seen as a piece of good fortune or divine mercy but as something we may and indeed *must* expect; a period of time that, as a standard, forms part of a complete human life cycle and a "full-size life career" (Imhof 1987). In addition, this phase has not only expanded but has also diversified. British historian Peter Laslett (1987, 1991) differentiated between a 'third age' characterized by unremitting health and activity and a 'fourth age' with beginning physical and mental impairment. Although the distinction has become a target of critical discussion (Hazan 2015; Higgs and Gilleard 2015), it still captures a fundamental change of perspective in view of later life. Old age as a whole does not anymore appear in light of imminent death, a step toward the inevitable end, marked by decay and decline. Today, when people retire, they may still expect to live a considerable number of years in good health and may hardly be limited in their capacities. Both the individual and the society have to make provisions for this "abundance of life" (Moody 1988).

At the same time, the disintegration of traditionally fixed biographies in the course of modernization (Giddens 1991a, 1991b; Inglehart and Welzel 2005) and individualization (Bauman 2001; Beck and Beck-Gernsheim 2002) also did away with many certainties, giving rise to new questions about the future and future uncertainties, opportunities, and dangers. In this vein, sociological theory highlights that today's late modern societies have to be regarded as reflexive, post-traditional ones that are obsessed with decisions and risks (Beck 1992). Traditional authoritative institutions are replaced by 'new,' pluralistic systems, such as liberal law, global markets, scientific discourses, and transnational organizations (Giddens 1991a). On one hand, this development has been celebrated as a form of 'emancipation,' an increase in personal freedom and options regarding the choice of professional careers, relationships, and religious or ideological commitments. On the other hand, modernization and individualization are experienced as an inevitable dynamic constantly forcing us to engage and decide, thus 'normativizing' and moralizing everyday life and expectations. The individual is constantly challenged to ask moral questions: "What should I do? How should I live?" A symptom of this development can be illustrated by the culture of psychotherapy and the booming popularity of 'how-to' manuals. Both try to satisfy the growing demand for guidance: Be it partnership, child rearing, career choices, or coping with illness and death – all areas of life are covered (Giddens 1991a, 70). The pervasive tension between autonomy and responsibility also becomes manifest in a project-like perspective on morality. The model of the 'planning self' is based on the assumption that individual identity cannot be understood as essential. Personality does not rest on a pre-existing substantial core but should be conceived of as a 'project' of individual self-conception and self-fashioning that is in constant need of reflections, decisions, and justifications (Taylor 1989). This 'de-essentializing' and 'reflexivization' ultimately also affect the 'gained life years.' These processes turn ageing and old age into an important part of the life project and at the same time give rise to new models and orientation guides regarding later life – expressed, for example, in gerontological discourses on 'successful ageing' (Pruchno 2015).

Finally, under late-modern conditions, science becomes responsible for measuring and projecting the newly gained scope of action and for assessing predictable and manageable risks associated with it. At the moment, (bio-)medicine seems to be dominating the concert of authoritative voices offering expert advice. Critical commentators have pointed out that new forms of medical prevention, diagnosis, and treatment bring about problematic changes in our way of perceiving and handling ageing and old age. They address the problems of an increasing '(bio-)medicalization of ageing' subjecting old age to medical jurisdiction and transforming its normal features into physiological conditions and its anomalies into pathologies to be medically treated and cured (Estes and Binney 1989; Kaufman, Shim, and Russ 2004; Larkin 2011; Zola 1991). Others criticize the concomitant emergence of new, more subtle forms of disciplinary power and (self-) control in a late modern neoliberal society (Leedham and Hendricks 2006; Powell and Biggs 2000, 2003). Some authors call this kind of future-oriented biomedical decision-making, which encompasses all areas of life, "life strategies" (Rose 2007, 128). According to their analysis, the concept of life, with its numerous ambivalences (e.g., biological, biographical, social, creative), comes to be dominated by so-called biological and 'life' sciences. The resulting 'life strategies' aim at systematically implementing biomedical concepts into questions regarding life and the meaning of life. Rose suggested that medicine provides answers to a public generally preoccupied with risk by counterposing risks to an "ethos of hope, anticipation, and expectation" (Rose 2007, 27). He moreover criticized the common practice of subjective self-reflection and self-management as a form of "ethopolitics" (Rose 2007, 27). Ageing, thus, turns into a task, something that has to be prevented, structured, and treated. Contingency, fate, and acknowledging weaknesses, as well as accepting helplessness and dependency, seem to have no place in the new vision of life as a (bio-)scientific and (bio-)medical 'project.'

The concept of the book

The aim of this edited volume is to examine the relevance of modern medicine and healthcare in shaping the future lives and situations of elderly people and ageing societies – and vice versa. By focusing on the field of medicine and healthcare, we want to engage authors and readers in a dialogue on the individual and social implications of recent trends in geriatric medicine, dementia research and care, advance healthcare planning, the rise of prevention and anti-ageing medicine, and the transformation of healthcare systems in ageing societies.

The volume's overall conception is international and interdisciplinary. It combines European, US, and Asian perspectives from the fields of philosophy, bioethics, sociology, cultural studies, gerontology, nursing sciences, and public health. Thus, the theoretical scope ranges from the rather individually oriented perspective of bioethics to public-health ethics to medical sociology and cultural studies. Centered around the idea of 'planning later life,' the contributions deliberately consider different types and aspects of envisioning, evaluating, and controlling individual and societal futures as well as their entanglements. In doing so, they open a synoptic perspective providing an overview of the conceptual implications and concrete practices of 'planning.' This approach unfolds the range of planning later life in its philosophical, ethical, epistemological, anthropological, and sociocultural dimensions. This comprises imagining and forecasting in the sense of different visions and conceptions of ageing and old age, hoping and fearing in the sense of emotional views and moral evaluations of individual and societal futures, and preventing and planning in the sense of individual provisions and public policies regarding later life.

As a start, the volume's first part provides general philosophical and sociological considerations regarding changing conceptions of ageing, old age, and the life course. They shed light on the normative relevance of the temporal extension and structure of human existence, the development of an ethical interpretation of ageing, and the emerging differentiation of a third and fourth age. Against this background, the second part focuses on specific perspectives and problems of old age in the context of medicine and healthcare. The contributions include critical reflections on the changing face of old age in modern societies, its developmental potentials and limits, the ethical aspects of dementia and cognitive decline, end-of-life decision-making, the prospects and problems of prolongevity and biotechnological life extension, and the appropriate ethical perspective on age-group justice. The third part turns to perspectives and procedures of dealing with the future's contingency, the idea of controlling long-term developments such as ageing and demographic change, and the risks and problems of planning later life. Here, current topics such as the expectations associated with advance directives, public images of late-onset dementia, and considerations of the ethical and social implications of medical prevention and provision methods, as well as discussions of public-health strategies and healthcare policies regarding sustainability of the welfare state and intergenerational relations, are addressed.

The contributions

In the beginning of the volume's first part on general conceptions of ageing and old age, Mark Schweda considers the life-course perspective as a starting point for a broader understanding of the role of ageing in bioethics and public health. His contribution, '"A Season to Everything"? Considering Life-Course Perspectives in Bioethical and Public-Health Discussions of Ageing,' thus proposes a new conceptual framework for discussing ethical issues of ageing in the context of biomedicine and public health. In the following chapter, philosopher Thomas Rentsch traces the fundamental ethical meaning of ageing and old age. Starting from the ancient tradition of ethics of the good life, his contribution, 'Becoming Oneself: Toward a New Philosophy of Ageing,' argues that ageing has to be interpreted as a radicalization of the basic human condition relevant to all ethical and political reasoning. Introducing a sociological perspective, François Höpflinger then turns to the implications of the influential distinction between a 'third age' and a 'fourth age.' His contribution, 'Third Age and Fourth Age in Ageing Societies,' critically discusses to which extent the emergence of two divergent cultures of ageing and two specific policies toward a third and a fourth age can be justified: an achievement-oriented culture for the 'young old' and a care-oriented culture for the 'old old.' Continuing this sociological line of thought, Paul Higgs and Chris Gilleard subsequently focus on very old age. In 'The Nature of the Fourth Age as a Challenge to Ageing Societies,' the authors claim that the fourth age acts as a 'social imaginary' of a feared old age marked by dependency and decline and that people included in this category become excluded from everyday life.

The volume's second part focuses on specific perspectives and problems of old age, such as physical and psychological potentials and limitations, dementia, end-of-life decision-making, and life extension. In the first chapter, gerontologist Andreas Kruse takes an in-depth look at the specific conditions and situations of very old age. His contribution, 'Old Age, Potentials, and Vulnerability,' argues that aspects of vulnerability and developmental potentials should both find consideration in ethical and social-science approaches to old age and pertinent issues such as dementia and care. Perla Werner and Silke Schicktanz then address ethical questions associated with the increase of the number of people with dementia and the scientific study of their competence. Their contribution, 'Competence and Cognitive Deterioration,' examines the existing empirical literature in the field of competence and cognitive deterioration and identifies ethical issues to be considered in the future. In the following chapter, the public-health scholar Hsiu-I Yang reviews the common practice of medical end-of-life decision-making for the oldest old. Her contribution, 'Opt In or Opt Out? Rethinking the Provision of Life-Sustaining Medical Technology to the "Old Old,"' argues that, for the oldest old, the paradigm of presumption for life should be replaced by the presumption for peaceful death. Changing the focus, the next chapter then explores the ethical implications of biomedical life-extension technologies. In his contribution, 'Not Growing Old – Gracefully,' bioethicist Søren Holm argues that although there is a duty to discharge one's moral duties in each particular segment of life, the precise contents of that duty cannot be fixed a priori but must be discovered by the first generations who do not grow old. Finally, Nancy Jecker reflects on the twin challenges of rising healthcare costs and the shifting nature of healthcare needs in ageing societies. Her contribution, 'How to Think about Age-Group Justice,' offers a capabilities approach to justice as an ethical framework and shows that this account has advantages over autonomy-based accounts because it places emphasis on the respect and recognition we owe to the elderly.

The volume's third part is dedicated to individual provisions and public policies in ageing societies. In the first chapter, sociologist Kai Brauer discusses the practices surrounding advance directives in Germany. His contribution, 'Final Decisions for the Final Crisis,' focuses on the paradoxes of deciding in advance for never-experienced future situations. Ralf J. Jox subsequently introduces advance healthcare planning as a further development going beyond advance directives. In 'Preparing Existential Decisions in Later Life,' he explains the rationale and practice of advance healthcare planning, discusses its ethical and social ramifications, and sketches how to further develop this model in the future. The following two contributions shift the focus to medical and public-health strategies of prevention and longevity. In 'Articulating the Case for the Longevity Dividend,' S. Jay Olshansky introduces therapeutic interventions that slow ageing in people as a plausible target for scientific research and public-health measures. He argues that delayed ageing is an efficient and promising approach for combating disease, extending healthy life, compressing morbidity, and reducing healthcare costs. Based on qualitative social research, Larissa Pfaller and Frank Adloff then discuss the practice of anti-ageing and prevention in Germany. Their chapter 'Paradoxes of Planning Later Life' argues that the attraction of contemporary anti-ageing practices can be traced to symbolic power creating a positive bodily experience and emotional security. In the following contribution, Silke Schicktanz examines 'The Visionary Shaping of Dementia Research.' The chapter discusses scenarios as social imaginations that not only influence the cultural view on very old age but also are used as arguments for justifying current research activities to diagnose, prevent, and care for people with dementia. Ruud ter Meulen then turns to the shifting public-health perspectives on care for the elderly. In his contribution, 'Solidarity and Family Care for an Ageing Population,' he criticizes neoliberal reductions of solidarity and introduces the 'communicating vessels' model, in which family caregivers are supported by professional caregivers. In the final chapter, Stephen Katz and Peter J. Whitehouse explore contemporary and emerging intergenerational ethics as a framework for anti-ageist practices and the future planning of ageing societies. Their 'Legacies, Generations, and Ageing Futures: The Ethics of Intergenerativity' also promotes The Intergenerational School (TIS) as a learning community and an ethical model of intergenerativity.

The authors would like to thank their co-editors Frank Adloff and Kai Brauer for their advice and support. All editors would like to thank the reviewers who provided valuable expertise and recommendations: Hans-Jörg Ehni (Tübingen), Joel Kramer (San Francisco), Ralf J. Jox (Munich/Lausanne), Martin Sand (Karlsruhe), Jens Schlieter (Bern), Aagje Swinnen (Maastricht), and Markus Zimmermann (Fribourg). Finally, we are very grateful for the assistance of Pia Christensen (Göttingen), Verena Klar (Göttingen), Moritz Kuhles (Erlangen), Angelika Wunder (Erlangen), and Julia Perry (Göttingen) in the process of copyediting and proofreading. The work in this volume was funded by the German Ministry of Education and Research (grant no. 01GP1004) and the Deutsche Forschungsgemeinschaft (DFG) (grant no. SCHI 631/5–1).

References

Bauman, Z. 2001. *The Individualized Society*. Cambridge: Polity.

Beck, U. 1992. *Risk Society: Towards a New Modernity*. New Delhi: Sage.

Beck, U., and E. Beck-Gernsheim. 2002. *Individualization: Institutionalized Individualism and Its Social and Political Consequences*. London: Sage.

Estes, C. L., and E. A. Binney. 1989. "The Biomedicalization of Aging: Dangers and Dilemmas." *The Gerontologist* 29 (5):587–596. doi: 10.1093/geront/29.5.587.

Giddens, A. 1991a. *Modernity and Self-Identity: Self and Society in the Late Modern Age*. Stanford: Stanford University Press.

Giddens, A. 1991b. *The Consequences of Modernity*. Stanford: Stanford University Press.
Hazan, H. 2015. *Against Hybridity: Social Impasses in a Globalizing World*. Cambridge: Polity.
Higgs, P., and C. Gilleard. 2015. *Rethinking Old Age: Theorising the Fourth Age*. Basingstoke: Palgrave Macmillan.
Imhof, A. E. 1987. "Planning Full-Size Life Careers. Consequences of the Increase in the Length and Certainty of Our Life Spans over the Last Three Hundred Years." *Ethnologia Europea* 17:5–23.
Inglehart, R., and C. Welzel. 2005. *Modernization, Cultural Change and Democracy: The Human Development Sequence*. New York: Cambridge University Press.
Kaufman, S. R., J. K. Shim, and A. J. Russ. 2004. "Revisiting the Biomedicalization of Aging: Clinical Trends and Ethical Challenges." *The Gerontologist* 44 (6):731–738. doi: 10.1093/geront/44.6.731.
Larkin, M. 2011. "The 'Medicalization' of Aging: What It Is, How It Harms, and What to Do about It." *The Journal on Active Aging* 10 (1):2836.
Laslett, P. 1987. "The Emergence of the Third Age." *Ageing and Society* 7 (2):133–160. doi: 10.1017/S0144686X00012538.
Laslett, P. 1991. *A Fresh Map of Life: The Emergence of the Third Age*. London: George Wiedenfield and Nicholson.
Leedham, C. A., and J. Hendricks. 2006. "Foucault and Successful Aging as Discourse: Explorations in Biopower and the Practice of Freedom." In *Foucault and Aging*, edited by J. L. Powell and A. Wahidin, 31–45. New York: Nova Science.
Moody, H. R. 1988. *Abundance of Life: Human Development Policies for an Aging Society*. New York: Columbia University Press.
National Center for Health Statistics. 2016. *Health, United States, 2015: With Special Feature on Racial and Ethnic Health Disparities*. Hyattsville, MD: National Center for Health Statistics.
Powell, J. L., and S. Biggs. 2000. "Managing Old Age: The Disciplinary Web of Power, Surveillance and Normalization." *Journal of Aging and Identity* 5 (1):3–13. doi: 10.1023/A:1009541314124.
Powell, J. L., and S. Biggs. 2003. "Foucauldian Gerontology: A Methodology for Understanding Aging." *Electronic Journal of Sociology* 17 (2):1–10.
Pruchno, R. 2015. "Successful Aging: Contentious Past, Productive Future." *The Gerontologist* 55 (1):1–4. doi: 10.1093/geront/gnv002.
Rose, N. 2007. *Politics of Life Itself: Biomedicine, Power and Subjectivity in the Twenty-First Century*. Princeton: Princeton University Press.
Schweda, M., and S. Schicktanz. 2012. "Das Unbehagen an der Medikalisierung. Theoretische und ethische Aspekte der biomedizinischen Lebensplanung." In *Pro-Age oder Anti-Aging. Altern im Fokus der modernen Medizin*, edited by S. Schicktanz and M. Schweda, 23–40. Frankfurt am Main/New York: Campus.
Statistisches Bundesamt. 2016. *Sterbetafel 2013/2015 – Methoden- und Ergebnisbericht zur laufenden Berechnung von Periodensterbetafeln für Deutschland und die Bundesländer*. Wiesbaden: Statistisches Bundesamt.
Taylor, C. 1989. *Sources of the Self: The Making of Modern Identity*. Cambridge, MA: Harvard University Press.
Zola, I. K. 1991. "The Medicalization of Aging and Disability." *Advances in Medical Sociology* 2:299–315.

Part 1

Conceptions of ageing and old age

1 "A season to everything"? Considering life-course perspectives in bioethical and public-health discussions on ageing

Mark Schweda[1]

About 15 years ago, the newly elected chairman of the German conservative party's youth organization declared in a newspaper interview that he did not think it right that 85-year-olds should receive hip replacements paid for by the welfare state. The German media as well as the public were scandalized. Colleagues accused the junior politician of advocating an ideology that destroys the solidary structures of our community. And the minister of family affairs even warned that a society that allowed such discussions was on its way to "a Brave New World in which 60- or 65-year-olds were expected to take the death pill." (Schweda 2013, 149).

In retrospect, what appears striking in this debate is the disparity between moral outrage and argumentative elaboration. Neither the young politician nor his opponents actually made great efforts to substantiate their respective stances on age-based limitations of medical care. What specifics of old age make it seem acceptable (or not) to withhold medical treatment from the elderly that other citizens are usually granted without any reservation? What exactly is it in senior citizens' conditions and situations that lets specifically hip replacement appear dispensable (or not)? And why does an 85th birthday mark such a significant threshold in a person's life that their whole standing within the 'welfare state' is fundamentally altered (or not)?

The controversy illustrates increasing socio-economic anxieties in ageing societies. On a more general level, it can also be regarded as a twofold example of many contemporary public, political, and academic debates on ethical and public-health questions in the context of ageing. On one hand, such questions gain relevance and immediacy as demographic ageing and its consequences move to the focus of political attention, media coverage, and public awareness. At the same time, however, the corresponding debates often express a rather limited perspective on ageing and old age. Ageing is usually only considered and discussed inasmuch as it poses a *practical problem* – that is, to the extent that it interferes with the standardized, predefined, and desired course of things within the existing framework of clinical or health-policy practices and institutions. Thus, the issues raised include the problem of meeting the special needs and requirements of elderly, frail, and demented patients; the problem of making medical decisions regarding the prolongation of life; or the problem of distributing limited health-care resources in ageing societies (Fenech 2003).

This contribution is based on the conviction that this problem-centered perspective is itself problematic. First, it considers only those aspects in ageing that seem to pose the problems, and thus it hampers a more comprehensive understanding of the phenomenon as such in its interplay of biological, psychological, and socio-cultural dimensions. At the same time, however, the problem-centered perspective itself usually tacitly relies on certain implicit, often rather traditional preconceptions and prejudices regarding ageing and the life course, thus slipping questionable assumptions into the debate without further reflection or justification. For example, the proposition to withhold hip replacements from the elderly draws upon a forceful traditional image of old age that has prevailed and has been taken for granted for such a long time that we have come to accept it as natural: the frail, decrepit elderly. In fact, the aforementioned junior politician explicitly acknowledged this traditional image in his interview when he added offhand that, after all, elderly people, in the past, also used to walk on crutches. This finally highlights a further serious issue of the problem-oriented perspective: it has a tendency to frame ageing or the elderly themselves as the problem, thus reinforcing negative stereotypes of old age and fostering ageism – that is, discrimination against individuals due to their (advanced) age (Butler 2005).

In the following, I therefore argue for broadening the theoretical perspective. The problem-oriented perspective has to be embedded in a more fundamental and comprehensive approach to ageing. Solving specific problems in bioethics and public health in the context of ageing requires an explicit discussion about what it actually means to age and to be old. I will argue that the so-called life course paradigm developed in the fields of developmental psychology and social sciences provides a suitable starting point for such a discussion. It allows for conceptualization of human life as a socio-culturally standardized sequence of phases, stages, or steps, each linked to a particular status as well as to specific roles, moral expectations, and life prospects. To substantiate my claim, I first discuss a few more examples for the relevance of implicit conceptions of ageing and the life course in contemporary bioethical debates on medical care and futility, on anti-ageing medicine and life extension, and on age-based rationing of healthcare resources. I then introduce the life-course perspective as a theoretical framework for the ethical analysis, reflection, and discussion of such conceptions. Two pertinent categories appear particularly useful and productive from an ethical point of view: 'age norms' as normative standards of age-appropriate behavior and ideals of 'ageing well' as evaluative standards of personal self-fulfillment and flourishing at different stages of life. Finally, I discuss benefits and challenges of a life-course approach to bioethics and public health, concluding that ethical reasoning needs to appreciate and theoretically accommodate the normative implications of the temporal structure of human existence.

Implicit conceptions of ageing and the life course in contemporary bioethical debates

As demographic ageing and its consequences move to the focus of public attention and to the center of public and media discourses, bioethical and public-health questions regarding old age are gaining in relevance and urgency. After all, the general changes in most Western industrialized nations' overall age structure have a particularly pronounced impact on the field of medicine and healthcare. Those belonging to the fastest-growing age groups of 65 years and older display an especially high demand for medical services and products (Congressional Budget Office 2014). They change the prevalent disease panorama and thus the focus of medical research and practice (World Health Organization 2011). This consequently also directs the attention of medical ethics and health policy toward problems that become relevant in the context of providing care to the old and the very old (Jecker 1992; Moody 1992; Wicclair 1993). In the respective debates, at least three major thematic strands can be identified: The first revolves around the adequate consideration of autonomy and care in physicians' and caregivers' interactions with elderly people (Agich 2003); the second, around the prospects of well-being and a good, fulfilled life at old age in light of new medical possibilities (Post and Binstock 2004); and the third, around the just distribution of healthcare resources among different generations (Binstock and Post 1991). As the following examples show, normative conceptions of ageing and the life course pervade and inform many of these discourses.

Conceptions of ageing and the life course in the debate on appropriate medical care

Social research clearly indicates that a person's chronological age makes a significant difference in medical practice and healthcare. Thus, there is evidence that, in the UK, doctors have a tendency to not resuscitate older people (Ebrahim 2000). Studies in the US found that the proportion of recommended healthcare patients received declined with age (Asch et al. 2006). And an analysis of hospital-discharge data from Germany's largest public health-insurance company shows that older individuals receive less costly treatment than younger ones with the same diseases (Brockmann 2002). One explanation is that physicians simply withhold certain kinds of medical measures from the elderly (Kapp 2002). This suspicion is supported by qualitative studies that indicate that age-related value judgments play an important role in treatment decisions for the elderly – for example, the notion that physical decline and, ultimately, death are somehow more natural and thus also more acceptable at an older age (Ubachs-Moust et al. 2008). Indeed, it is a common intuition that physical impairment and dying carry a different moral weight at different points in life – for example, that it makes a difference whether someone still has their whole life to live ahead of them or whether they have almost completed it (Jecker and Schneiderman 1994). We would probably be perplexed to read an obituary for a 97-year-old containing phrases like 'died unexpectedly,' 'untimely passing,' and 'torn from the midst of life.' However, it is important to acknowledge that the corresponding expectations and value judgments imply some normative conception of ageing and the human life course.

Such implicit normative conceptions also play an important role in many academic bioethical debates on medical decision-making. Take, for example, the central issue of determining the appropriate type and amount of care, usually discussed in terms of medical benefit and utility (or futility). Notwithstanding widely recognized claims to patient autonomy, most bioethicists agree that medical treatment should be beneficial to the patient and that it is therefore legitimate to withhold or withdraw treatment that promises minimal or no benefit (Schneiderman and Jecker 1990). Of course, the methods and criteria for determining the benefit or futility of a given treatment option are notoriously unclear and controversial. Statistical data indicating the probability of certain outcomes is often inconclusive, leading to widely diverging prognoses (Gabbay 2010). Moreover, judging treatment outcomes in terms of benefit or utility necessarily involves some sort of normative standard. Thus, one of the most prominent measures of utility, the concept of quality-adjusted life years (QALY), is based on the assumption that what matters in healthcare is maximizing healthy life years. This rationale has been criticized as inherently ageist since, statistically speaking, treatment of older individuals per se yields lower gains in both life years and well-being (Harris 1987). The idea that there is a connection between age and medical futility may mirror immemorial patterns of the normal course of human life and corresponding traditional notions of natural decline and inevitable death at old age (Tsuchiya 2000). Against this background, the death of an elderly person may even be seen as the "paradigm case" (Callahan 1977, 36) of a natural death. However, the mere empirical fact of a certain statistically average life expectancy alone cannot justify the normative decision to terminate a patient's treatment. Indeed, a closer look reveals that the 'natural death' at old age only appears more acceptable due to a "biographical standard" – that is, a normative conception of the life course suggesting that most of a person's history has "been achieved by that stage of life" and death now takes its "proper place as a necessary link in the transition of generations" (Callahan 1987, 24f.). The underlying traditional image of human life as an ascending and then descending curve that frames ageing as a natural process of decline, self-containment, and acceptance of finitude may have seemed inevitable in the past. In light of new technological possibilities and changing life plans, however, it is increasingly contested.

Conceptions of ageing and the life course in the debate on anti-ageing and life extension

Like under a magnifying glass, the sustained influence of such normative assumptions on ageing and the life course becomes particularly clear as soon as old age itself shifts to the focus of biomedical interventions and, consequently, bioethical discussions. This is the case in the highly controversial debates on so-called anti-ageing medicine. Starting in the 1990s, the anti-ageing movement has advocated biomedical methods to prevent or fight the effects of ageing – to decelerate, stop, or even reverse the underlying processes of biological senescence – and radically prolong human life (Mykytyn 2006). Indeed, some of the more ambitious anti-ageing protagonists explicitly announced that modern medicine is about to "forever alter our very notion of age, life, disease, and death," promising the "elimination of the disability, deformity, pain, disease, suffering and sorrow of old age" (Klatz and Goldman 2003, 13). According to them, "the traditional enfeebled, ailing elderly person" will soon be "a grotesque memory of a barbaric past" (Klatz and Goldman 2003, 13). The self-proclaimed British biogerontologist Aubrey de Grey even speculated that "the first person to live to 1,000 might be 60 already" (2004).

Declaring a biomedical 'war on old age' apparently presumes that ageing is some sort of disease that calls for medical treatment. In fact, this assumption is spelled out in the statements of the American Academy of Anti-Ageing Medicine, which explicitly addresses ageing as "a treatable medical condition" (Klatz and Goldman 2003, 12). While the diagnosis and treatment of diseases have usually been based on age-relative standards for health and functionality, implying a notion of age-associated decline as a natural physiological process, anti-ageing protagonists demand the same standards be applied to the young and the elderly. Under these premises, a process such as a decrease in hormone levels is no longer considered as a normal sign of physiological ageing but as a kind of deficiency syndrome calling for "hormone replacement therapy" (Klatz and Goldman 2003, 119). The ultimate consequence of this perspective is to view ageing itself and even "death as an unnatural process" (Caplan 2005). In contrast to such positions, opponents of anti-ageing usually insist that ageing is not a disease but a natural process we have to accept, integrate, and shape in a meaningful way. Occasionally, the experience of vulnerability, transitoriness, and mortality associated with old age is regarded as an essential aspect of the human condition or even as something positive – for example, a constitutive condition of a meaningful life (Kass 2001). Anti-ageing advocates discredit the general view underlying such apologist ideas as a gerontological "death cult" (A4M 2002, 6) that glorifies decreasing functionality, deteriorating quality of life, and ultimately death itself. They argue that it is not acceptable to reject the benefits of scientific and technological progress based on subjective 'yuck-factors' and the traditional 'pro-ageing trance' (de Grey 2005). According to them, this not only denies the elderly an equal right to life, well-being, and self-fulfillment, but also epitomizes an ageist culture that offers senior citizens no positive social roles and opportunities for personal development, only "graceful accommodation" (Bostrom 2005), with decline, impairment, and perishing. After all, an extension of the healthy lifespan would not only provide people with opportunities to fulfill a greater number of desires, attain more goods, and experience more pleasure, but also widen the scope for developing, experimenting, and realizing a whole series of different life plans and goals (Gems 2003). Thus, traditional images of ageing and the life course are explicitly challenged in the context of anti-ageing medicine (Vincent 2003).

Conceptions of ageing and the life course in the debate on resource allocation

The influence of normative conceptions on ageing and the life course also is becoming evident on the level of public-health and social policy. Against the backdrop of medical progress, ageing populations, and shrinking budgets of public healthcare systems, extensive public and policy debates have evolved around the issue of just and economically reasonable allocation of healthcare resources in ageing societies (Binstock and Post 1991). With principles such as solidarity, social justice, and Christian charity, these debates touch upon central forces of social cohesion and the moral basis of modern social and welfare states. This may be the reason why they are often led in such a fierce and controversial manner. Especially the provocative idea of age-based rationing – that is, the restriction of access to healthcare on the basis of (old) age, frequently arouses heated public discussion. Empirical research indicates that many of these debates are informed by implicit conceptions of ageing and the life course. Indeed, the aforementioned differences between the treatment of older and younger persons might be interpreted as a symptom of informal age-rationing 'at the bedside' based on widespread defeatist notions of ageing and old age (Schweda, Wöhlke, and Inthorn 2015; Ubachs-Moust et al. 2010).

As a matter of fact, some of the most important positions in the academic bioethical debate on just allocation and age-based rationing also seem to draw on normative conceptions of ageing and the life course (Agich 2001). One particularly prominent example is Daniel Callahan's so-called natural lifespan account. In his controversial book *Setting Limits: Medical Goals in an Ageing Society* (1995 [1987]), Callahan denounced modern medical hubris and argued for rationing medical interventions in old age. According to him, we have to learn once again to accept that ageing and death are meaningful phases of the life cycle instead of medically fighting them. Consequently, he argues that after a fulfilled life beyond the "natural lifespan" (1995 [1987], 65) of about 80 years, costly medical treatment to resist death and extend life should not be supported. Instead, patients should receive good nursing and palliative care (1995 [1987], 137f.). Although this plea to recognize mortality and the limits of medical feasibility might seem intuitively sensible, the argument is problematic. First of all, it remains unclear why Callahan sets the limit at around 80 years. The number seems somewhat arbitrary. But even if there were actually some objective natural limit to the human lifespan, the mere fact alone would not support any normative directives regarding resource allocation in healthcare. That something *is* the case does not imply that it also *should be* the case. An additional, normative standard is needed to draw any normative conclusions. Indeed, on closer inspection, it turns out that Callahan's natural lifespan account is based on a particular conception of the good life: The 'natural lifespan' is acceptable since it leaves us with sufficient time to accomplish the possibilities and discharge the responsibilities that are deemed essential to a decent and fulfilled human life comprising "work, love, the procreating and raising of a family, [. . .] the experience of beauty, travel, and knowledge" (1995 [1987], 66). Apparently the argument presumes a conception of the ideal life course concordant with the traditional image of the "three boxes of life" (Bolles 1978): childhood and adolescence dedicated to socialization and education, adulthood dedicated to reproduction and professional advancement, and old age dedicated to social disengagement and contemplation. Regardless of our personal stance toward this model, proposing general regulations based on one specific vision of the good life contradicts some of our basic moral intuitions. After all, the greater part of modern moral thought is based on the liberal and egalitarian idea that, on principle, *all* people have prima facie the same moral status and value and the same rights and duties whatever their origin or particular position. The *Declaration of the Rights of Man and of the Citizen* of 1789 stated that "men are born and *remain* free and equal in rights." With this in mind, to withdraw or curtail the rights of certain people simply because of the contingent fact of their date of birth appears just as gratuitous and unfair as discriminating on the grounds of sex, race, or faith (Butler 2005).

In order to avoid such quandaries, John Harris (1985) has described an alternative approach to age-based rationing: the so-called fair innings argument (Harris 1985, 91). The underlying image has been borrowed from sports, where an inning denotes one segment of a game in which one side is batting, trying to score, and the other is fielding or defending. And, in fact, Harris's argument basically stays within this metaphorical frame. According to him, everyone has the right to a full inning of, say, 70 years in order to get "what can be got out of life" (Harris 1985, 93). Someone who is denied such a complete course of life has to be regarded as deprived. It is "a tragedy and a misfortune to be cut off prematurely" (Harris 1985, 93). All further years lived, on the other hand, have to be considered a fortunate extra – biographical stoppage time, so to speak. It may be pleasant to live very long, but it is definitely "not a tragedy to die in old age" (Harris 1985, 93). Thus, under certain circumstances, "it would be morally defensible to prefer to save the lives of those who 'still have their lives before them' rather than those who had 'already lived full lives'" (Harris 1985, 94). Again, this argument seems to encapsulate moral common sense. But, again, it is more difficult to justify this intuition. Once more, we have to ask how the concept of a 'complete course' regarding a human lifespan can be made concrete or quantified. Harris's number of 70 years seems rather random. After all, life expectancy in the US, to date, is 76.9 years for men and 81.6 years for women, and these numbers are rising. Who would be satisfied with 70 years as a 'full round,' given that the phase of the 'third age' – with its promise of 'late freedom,' second chances, and new life prospects – has only just begun at that point? But even if we could indicate a specific number, it would not follow that there is a moral duty to give up one's own lifetime in favor of younger people. First of all, the very idea of actually being able and justified to dispose over one's lifetime is far from self-evident. It presupposes the emergence of a secure lifespan, which suggests that we have a justified expectation of and moral claim to a certain amount of time. And even then, a redistribution of lifetime budgets between elderly and young people seems plausible only against the backdrop of social norms that suggest that adolescence and middle age are dedicated to family, employment, growth, and personal fulfillment, while old age is left with retirement, sacrifice, and self-denial in favor of coming generations (Rivlin 2000).

Norman Daniels (1985) has developed a third approach to distributing medical resources. His basic liberalist conception explicitly claims validity independent of different notions of the good life. Drawing on Rawls's principle of equal opportunities, Daniels argues that in order for an individual to benefit from fair equal opportunities, certain physical preconditions, summarized in the concept of "normal species functioning" (Daniels 1985, 33) must be fulfilled. Public healthcare thus contributes to fair equal opportunities by maintaining or restoring normal human functioning (Daniels 1985, 35). Although the basic structure of Daniels's theory does not suggest any direct conclusions on age-based rationing, it is not indifferent toward age. The basic notion of 'normal species functioning' is a bio-statistical concept determined in relation to an organism's objectives (self-preservation and reproduction) and age groups (Boorse 1977). Different age groups have different levels of normal functioning, so that physical or mental impairments or malfunctions cannot be conceived as pathological conditions as long as they correspond to the average functioning within the respective group. Healthcare for the elderly thus has to be guided by different points of reference than care for the young. On one hand, this may seem plausible: Speech problems in young children should be regarded differently than those in adolescents or adults. However, the concrete definition of the age groups and the organism's essential objectives already presuppose a specific view on the development of human functioning over the life course. Ultimately, Daniels's concept assumes a natural diminishing of functioning and a resulting decrease of opportunities with increasing age. The range of opportunities and perspectives that we grant someone to enjoy thus, in a way, carries an age index and ultimately an 'expiration date.' Accordingly, in a different context, Daniels (1988) explicitly justifies age-based rationing under certain conditions. Interestingly, his "prudential lifespan account" (Daniels 1988, 149) frames the problem not in the sense of just allocation of resources between age groups but as the task of distributing them sensibly with regard to an individual's lifespan. In a thought experiment, he argues that if we had to distribute available medical resources over our own lifespan without knowing anything about our life expectancy and our position in life, it would only be reasonable to allot the majority of goods to the early and middle periods of life. On closer scrutiny, however, we can see that such a calculation can count as prudent only within the traditional image of a life course with adulthood as its climax and old age as its declining phase with nothing much to hope for. Knowing about the rise in life expectancy, the prolonged period of old age with a greater need for resources later in life, and higher demands and standards for old age, one might in fact plan very differently today.

Introducing life-course perspectives to ethical reasoning

As it turns out, many contemporary bioethical and public-health debates presuppose certain conceptions of ageing and the human life course. Traditional images of a 'natural lifespan' and the 'three boxes of life' play an especially important role. They usually describe an ascending and then descending curve that starts with upbringing and education in childhood and adolescence, progresses through employment and reproduction in adulthood, and finally fades into a short period of old age characterized by retirement and decline. However, these images are rapidly losing ground.

Social research shows that the long-known temporal shape and course of life is eroding. Due to increasing life expectancy and demographic ageing, we as individuals and as a society, so to speak, have grown out of the corset of traditional standard biographies. A "fresh map of life" (Laslett 1991) emerges on which the phase of old age is not only temporally extended but also differentiated. Today we envisage a 'third age' that basically seems to continue the life of late maturity, with its emphasis on activity and social participation, and a 'fourth age' characterized by failing health, progressive frailty, and increasing need for help (see Höpflinger as well as Higgs and Gilleard in this volume). At the same time, our traditional ideas and orientations concerning old age carry less and less force. The classical industrial society's model of ageing in light of retirement, deserved repose, and impending demise loses ground. The 'greying of the baby boomers,' with their pronounced orientation toward personal fulfillment and social engagement, is overturning traditional patterns of ageing and old age (Pruchno 2012). On the other hand, there is still a lack of established role models and generally accepted social rules for the emerging society of old age. In fact, in the wake of demographic ageing, a "structural lag" (Riley et al. 1994) has been diagnosed: a growing discrepancy between, on one hand, social roles and occupations traditionally assigned to the later phase of life and, on the other hand, rising life expectancy. Some warn that "[w]e are gaining time and space but we do not have any images and texts. Our culture has not prepared us. [. . .] Our ancestors have not planted anything in our imagination, they have not built and thought or written anything for an old age which lasts long and in which we are all old" (Schirrmacher 2004, 104 [own translation]).

As outdated patterns and images of ageing are dissolving, the temporal course of human life loses its semblance of naturalness and reveals its normative dimension as a path significantly shaped and standardized by socio-cultural parameters. Traditionally, it has been the task of ethics to reflect on questions of our moral orientations in view of their meaning and justification. Insofar, the outlined range of norms shaping the life course would definitely fall in its field of competence, especially as their significance and legitimacy seem to be increasingly called into question. However, philosophical as well as applied ethics have done remarkably little to engage with the elementary fact that human beings do age. Although there may be famous reflections on the advantages and disadvantages, virtues and vices of old age, there has been almost no fundamental and systematic reflection on what it means for ethical theorizing as such that human life is determined by a specific temporal structure and course marked by certain fundamental and far-reaching changes (Small 2007).

A first starting point to tackle this question is provided in developmental psychology and the social sciences: the *life course* perspective. Without going into the details of the different strands and schools of life-course research (Hagestad and Neugarten 1985; Levy et al. 2005; Mortimer and Shanahan 2007; O'Rand and Krecker 1990), the general approach can be characterized by two central premises: First, individual life is a sequence of phases, thresholds, and trajectories essentially structured by socio-cultural norms, each tied to a particular status and specific roles, expectations, and possibilities. Second, individuals appropriate this social segmentation and schematic course as a 'social clock,' a biographical timetable providing a subjective frame of reference for value judgments, life decisions, and choices.

This perspective has important implications. First, it means that the course of people's lives is not just naturally structured into a certain shape and different stages. Rather, the continual biological progress of life unfolds between the poles of individual predispositions, situations, and attitudes, on one hand, and the orienting, regulating, and controlling influence of a kind of socially institutionalized and individually internalized biographical norm, on the other. In other words, the course of human life must be considered a social construct standardized through socio-cultural norms and subjected to historical and cultural variations (Hareven 1996; Holstein and Gubrium 2000). Accordingly, history and ethnology study life-course patterns and age-group systems in different cultures and their frequently hierarchical generational structures and rites of passage (Hareven 1996; Holmes and Holmes 1995). Developmental psychology investigates the (self-)ascription and subjective experience of different age roles and phases of transition in connection with personal well-being and health, appearance, behavior and lifestyle, or place within familial and societal generations (Pulkkinen and Caspi 2002). Sociology examines modern biographies structured by the demands of industrial society, its working world, and welfare-state administration (Giele and Holst 2004). And humanities and cultural studies analyze the symbolic representations of life, ranging from ancient notions of a cyclical process embedded in cosmological cycles, to the medieval linearization of the individual 'journey of life' modeled on Christian ideas of pilgrimage and salvation, to modernity's stages of life shaped by humanistic 'Bildung' and the early-bourgeois career ladder (Bedford, Davis, and Kelly 2007; Gilchrist 2012).

From an ethical point of view, another implication of the life-course perspective is of particular interest: The life course not only represents certain social *regularities*, objective patterns which can be traced in statistical socio-demographic research on individual lives, but also embodies a set of *rules*, subjective measures and norms according to which the individual will order his or her actions and life choices and which can be explored through opinion surveys and qualitative studies. Although the interrelation and relative weight of these two perspectives in sociological life-course research is controversial (Dannefer 1996), it seems plausible to assume that they influence each other. On one hand, statistically normal, widespread behavioral patterns can take on normative, orienting significance for individuals. On the other, normative conceptions of an appropriate or ideal life course can certainly spread to the extent that they exert an influence on the dominant behavioral and life-course patterns within society so that they become statistically significant. From an ethical perspective considering the classical distinction between prescriptive and eudaimonistic ethics (Anscombe 1958), two concepts from life-course research appear particularly pertinent and productive: first, *age norms* as normative standards of age-appropriate behavior and, second, *ideals of ageing well* as evaluative touchstones for shaping later stages of life. In the following, I outline each of these two life-course concepts and point out their ethical significance.

Prescriptive ethics and the normative standards of age-appropriate behavior

Prescriptive ethics underpins the larger part of modern moral philosophy. It is concerned with formulating, justifying, and applying moral norms – that is, universally binding rules for morally acceptable behavior. In short, the prescriptive perspective comprises the whole field of actions that we may expect from or owe to each other – that is, which are morally prohibited, allowed, or required in our relationships and interactions with each other.

In the field of sociological life-course research, this perspective corresponds to the so-called age norms (Neugarten et al. 1965; Maines, Neugarten, and Passuth 1987). These are standards of age-appropriate behavior and thus determine which actions have to be regarded as appropriate or inappropriate, imperative, permissible or prohibited, commendable or reprehensible at a specific age or life stage. Such age norms are exemplarily expressed vis-à-vis a young child, a teenager, a middle-aged adult, or an elderly person when they are told to 'act their age' (Laz 1998). Thus, while we would tolerate a 3-year-old girl making a scene in public when she cannot have her way, we would hardly accept this in a 15-year-old teenager or a 20-year-old apprentice, but, under certain circumstances, we would respect a 54-year-old chief executive or a 78-year-old patriarch doing the same.

For the most part, social age norms are rather informal. They are implicit and subtle expectations toward groups that are not exactly and chronologically defined, such as 'the young child' or 'older woman.' They include general conventions of politeness, decency, and propriety – for example, referring to style of clothing or partner choice, which, if disregarded, would only be sniffed at or met with a shake of the head. Thus, the survey used by Neugarten (1965) in her large-scale study on age norms in US society contained questions on the appropriate age for a woman to wear a bikini at the beach or to consider having another child and the appropriate age for a man to prefer living with his parents rather than in his own apartment (Neugarten 1965, 731). But age norms also range to strict moral norms whose violation is severely condemned and can bring on serious social sanctions. Sometimes a system of interlocking age norms organizes the interaction of members of different age groups – for example, who should offer a seat to whom on public transport, or how financial resources and the obligations of care and maintenance should be distributed between members of different generations. Meanwhile, the age of consent and marriage as well as the intergenerational contracts presumed in many social policies already belong to the field of formalized age norms. These are explicit, sometimes juridically codified, rules that refer to chronologically determined age limits and that are reinforced by sanctions (Ruppert 2010). Examples are the right to vote, reaching legal age, and driving a motor vehicle, but such rules also include the obligation to vacate one's position at retirement age, as well as the accompanying legal claim to public retirement benefits. In the bioethical debate, fixed chronological age limits that regulate children's legal competence to give informed consent to medical treatment are increasingly being criticized (Kuther 2003).

That age norms show considerable historical and cultural variability seems to be obvious and has been pointed out in research time and again. Thus, it is striking that many traditional cultures segment and ascribe stages of life not from the point of view of chronological time but rather according to an individual's position in the reproductive cycle or the succession of generations (Holmes and Holmes 1995, 50f.). According to this calculation, for example, a relatively young person may be seen as 'old' if she already has children or grandchildren. Moreover, rights and obligations ascribed to age vary. For some tribal communities, a progressive deprivation of rights of old people, right up to a consensual ritual senicide, is reported (Holmes and Holmes 1995, 107). In contrast, people in gerontocratic communities acquire more rights and privileges with age, sometimes by transforming real power into social prestige in the form of honors, eulogies, and distinctions (Holmes and Holmes 1995, 107). Furthermore, the degree and extent according to which societies regulate the age-appropriate behavior of their members may vary. With view to late modern postindustrial societies, a progressive relaxation and increasing loss of significance of traditional age standards is frequently witnessed. Age deviations in marriage and professional careers are deemed less offensive (Maines, Passuth, and Neugarten 1987). Against this background, the development of an "age-irrelevant society" (Neugarten 1996) leveling any moral or political significance of age has been predicted. This outlook corresponds to the vision of a "post-modern life course" (Featherstone 1991) constructed without regard to traditional age norms and models of life. However, as fierce controversies on medical innovations such as reproductive technologies for postponing motherhood show, the sustained influence of (frequently gendered) age norms should not be underestimated (Bühler 2015).

From the perspective of the egalitarian universalism of modern moral philosophy, there seem to exist only two possibilities to consider age norms and the unequal age-related treatment they imply (Cole 1983). Either this difference in treatment can be morally justified with reference to egalitarian principles or it is to be criticized and rejected as a form of arbitrary discrimination. An example for the first possibility are certain egalitarian arguments in the aforementioned debate concerning a just distribution of resources in healthcare. Thus, according to the 'fair innings' argument, it can be morally acceptable to grant scarce medical resources to younger rather than older people in order to provide them a fair chance to complete a full lifespan (Harris 1985, 93f.). Consequently, this argument justifies a difference in treatment according to chronological age if it contributes to establishing equal treatment in a morally more important respect – in this case, the lifetime to be lived (Harris 1994). If such morally decisive respects of equal treatment cannot be identified, unequal treatment on the basis of age seems baseless from an egalitarian point of view and thus just as arbitrary and unjust as discrimination on account of gender, class, or race.

However, this narrow view is overhauled as soon as one leaves the pertaining theoretical perspective behind. In the course of more recent critical discussion of egalitarianism, a number of non-egalitarian approaches developed that deny that the normative core of moral justice indeed lies in the comparativist idea of equal treatment of individuals in relationship to one another. Instead they campaign for a somewhat absolutist notion of appropriateness for the particular case in question – for example, based on aspects of need, sufficiency, or merit (Steinhoff 2015). If we do not discard existing social age norms as unjust a priori but seek to ponder their content in an open and unbiased discussion, the specificities of different life stages could be considered in a similar way. Of course, such reasoning would have to refer to the findings of the relevant empirical sciences for example, developmental biology or developmental psychology – in order to avoid simply repeating popular myths, conventional prejudices, or ideological stereotypes concerning certain age groups. On the other hand, it must not degenerate into a biological or psychological positivism or reductionism, since the moral relevance of factual age characteristics, respectively differences, could never be made plausible from this perspective. A way out of this dilemma could be offered by the theoretical framework of internal realism, which strives for a systematic integration of scientific information and the historical manifestations of our ongoing cultural self-reflection and self-interpretation as human beings – for example, mythology, literature, and the arts (Nussbaum 1992). At least, such an approach could help us acknowledge and clarify the significance of biographical age norms in our moral deliberations.

Eudaimonistic ethics and the evaluative ideals of ageing well

In the last decades, philosophers have increasingly criticized the almost exclusively prescriptive approach of modern moral philosophy. This has led to a revival of ancient eudaimonistic models of ethical deliberation based on categories of virtue or the good life. Their theoretical perspective can be described as *teleological-evaluative* in the sense that they are not primarily concerned with the justification of universal norms governing our interactions but rather consider the value of the aims we pursue in our practices and lives. Eudaimonistic ethics thus asks about what has to be regarded as prudent and desirable in the context of a good life comprising aspects of happiness as well as of self-fulfillment and human flourishing.

In psychological and sociological life-course research, the teleological-evaluative perspective seems to correspond to ideals of ageing well. One prominent example is the idea of successful ageing, which marks a central field of research in contemporary gerontology (Pruchno 2015). In the respective debates, however, the actual goal or decisive standard against which the 'success' of ageing is measured is often taken for granted (usually involving certain uncritically adopted medical, psychological, or sociological notions of physical functioning, psychological well-being, or social adaptation). Similar to analogical conceptions of childhood in pedagogy, gerontological concepts of successful ageing hence frequently turned out to mirror the society and the value systems of their time, whether they recommended social disengagement in the early 1960s or continuing activity in the 1970s (Bearon 1996). In comparison, a philosophical reflection has to dig deeper: It has to address the goals and standards of ageing well as such and in general, and it has to discuss why and to what extent they can *actually* be considered desirable or definitive (see Rentsch in this volume). Of course, such a perspective must incorporate the entire range of empirical results of gerontology, albeit without already drawing any evaluative or normative conclusions from them.

It seems surprising that the teleological-evaluative perspective on the good life has generally given little consideration to the internal temporal structure of human life. After all, life is not a monolithic block or a permanent, stationary state but a process in time, characterized by a specific temporal duration and course. Indeed, we usually speak not so much of *the* good life as such and in general but consider different ideas of a good life (in terms of subjective happiness and objective flourishing) for different stages of life. For example, a good childhood is frequently associated with perceptions of a carefree existence and autotelic activities such as, above all, playing, where certain assumed traits of the child as embodiment of an original and unadulterated existence become manifest (Ariés 1962). By contrast, adulthood is usually characterized by instrumental activities and tasks in support of responsibilities and objectives in the context of one's professional career, family life, and public functions (Hudson 1999). For the higher age, traditional perspectives of social disengagement and separation are relevant, often going hand in hand with a life dedicated to reminiscence, theoretical contemplation, or spiritual opening (Tornstam 2005). Of course, these ideals are remnants of an epoch already vanishing. As mentioned above, the course and segmentation of human life, as well as the meaning given to its different stages, are changing. Currently, this is becoming particularly clear with regard to the phase of old age, whose expansion and inner differentiation involves higher expectations and an increasing need of significant roles and fulfilling life perspectives (Riley et al. 1994).

Regardless of specific ideals for different life stages, the fundamental temporal structuredness of human life entails certain general and formal conditions for any ethical analysis of the good life. This includes the seemingly trivial fact that the different phases of life follow each other and therefore stand in a certain consecutive relationship and order. In this sense, human life constitutes a temporally structured whole, comparable to a literary narrative or a musical composition. Its individual components cannot be moved, rearranged, shortened, extended, or exchanged without changing the identity and meaning of the whole, much like, for example, the beginning of a novel or the final chord of a symphony. Accordingly, the temporality of human existence appears to be decisive for the question of the good life, since life's success or failure not only depends on the summary realization of certain general goals but is bound to a specific coherent sequence of their achievement. The different phases of life build on each other, thus successively forming a structured and meaningful biographical texture (Kauppinen 2012). This includes, for example, the idea of a prime of life – common to classical ethics – a zenith or peak, where all of a person's capabilities and possibilities are developed to the fullest extent, or the consoling thought that life moves toward a final meaningful closure in the end, thus becoming a complete, well-rounded whole. The moral significance of such meaningful biographical structures is often neglected in bioethics – for example, in the debates on anti-ageing medicine and life extension, which typically dwell on the purely additive question of whether more life is better. In any case, it is important to note that biographical meaning is not simply a given fact. Rather, it has to be produced by the individual herself in the face of variable biographical discontinuities, transitions, changes, and disruptions that question the unity of the person and the wholeness of her life. In this context, special relevance must be attributed to the *narrative* construction of connections through which single events and phases can be incorporated into an overarching biographical storyline (Baars 2012).

Finally, the temporal succession of life phases results in a certain fundamental directionality and irreversibility of human life as a whole. There is simply no way back into past phases of life such as childhood or youth. What happened then is irrevocable and cannot be reversed. It forms the inevitable starting point from which everything proceeds. Life – as Kierkegaard says – must be lived forward. Different conclusions can be drawn from this temporal directionality. On one hand, psychoanalytical models and empirical research suggest that especially in early life phases people experience fundamental and far-reaching imprints that in some circumstances can be determining for one's entire future life. On the other hand, the temporal directionality of life accounts for a certain path dependency and an increasing determinacy of its course. Initially, there seems to be an unlimited number of possibilities available to the individual, but with each decision and each turn, a course is set that increasingly narrows the range of future choices and leads to an ever-increasing degree of determinacy. In any case, the common equalization of children and old persons – for example, in bioethical debates on mental capacity and proxy decision-making, becomes problematic as soon as we take the essentially temporal structure of human life seriously. And finally, the irreversibility of life once lived establishes the gravity of human existence, which as such does not provide for a tolerable hypothetical or tentative state. There is no grace period, learning phase, or dress rehearsal. With each lived moment, life time has already irretrievably passed and thus definitely counts. Only against this backdrop do the biographical drama of fundamental existential crises and individuals' desperate efforts to make the most of their lives become comprehensible. Strangely enough, this uniqueness and irreversibility of the individual process of life is often ignored in bioethical reasoning – for example, when it comes to utilitarian calculations of abstract time budgets in the debate on the cost-efficiency of medical treatment (Harris 1987).

Conclusion: toward an ethics of the life course

The public controversy about hip replacements for the elderly, as well as the examples from academic debates on medical futility, life extension, and age rationing, illustrate the importance of normative conceptions of ageing and the life course in bioethical discourse. Traditional images of the natural curve and the 'three boxes' of life play an especially important role. At the same time, current developments draw attention to the problematic lack of reflection and justification of such conceptions. As traditional images of ageing and the life course begin to lose their common acceptability and become subject to doubt, controversy, and renegotiation, they forfeit their semblance of self-evident naturalness and reveal their genuinely normative character.

Under these circumstances, ethics can no longer simply presuppose certain existing life-course patterns as though they were manifestations of some objective order of things. Instead, we have to acknowledge their normative origin and implications and raise them to the level of explicit ethical appreciation and discussion. After all, far from making ethical reflection obsolete, the fact that traditional binding models of life give way to a multitude of possible biographical orientations only makes it more necessary. The first task of such systematic ethical reflection would be a *critical* one by uncovering biases and stereotypes of old age in order to challenge them and expose them to scrutiny. Yet, in doing so, it would not be sufficient to simply counter negative stereotypes of old age with more positive ones – for example, to replace ageist images of decrepit dodderers with today's active and attractive 'young old' seniors. Rather than replacing one biased stereotype of old age with another, thus merely reversing the value system that informs ethical discourse, we need to achieve a profound understanding of what it actually means from an ethical perspective to age and to be old. In this sense, the necessary reflection entails the *constructive task* of developing a conceptual framework that allows for discussing the central significance of ageing in the context of bioethical and health-policy issues. As I have argued in this chapter, the life-course perspective constitutes a promising starting point for both tasks. On one hand, it provides suitable theoretical categories for the critical analysis of normative conceptions of human life and its stages and passages. On the other, it offers constructive theoretical perspectives for conceptualizing the normative implications of the temporal extension and structure of human existence in a fine-grained and comprehensive manner.

In two respects, these considerations point beyond the context of the specific questions discussed in this chapter. First, it seems plausible that normative life-course concepts not only impinge on bioethical debates about old age but play an important role regarding other phases of life. This particularly concerns considerations of the other end of life – childhood and adolescence – which is also often shaped by certain normative conceptions (Wiesemann 2016). But ultimately, it affects the bioethical discourse as such and in general. Whenever human life is presumed to be structured into specific segments or certain images of life phases – with their associated needs, priorities, rights, and responsibilities at stake – the significance and justification of such a presumption deserve closer examination. In this regard, bioethics is still confronted with numerous unresolved theoretical issues. Indeed, many bioethical considerations seem to be implicitly based on a certain image of adulthood and its specific demands, capabilities, and perspectives defining the normal moral subject and framing both childhood and old age as mere special cases or, normatively speaking, as deficient and deviant modes of human existence (Holm 2013).

Secondly, considering the significance of normative conceptions of the life course transcends the problems discussed here in the field of applied area-specific ethics and directs us toward key questions within philosophical ethics as such. Keeping in mind that ethics is traditionally conceived as a reflection on the normative and evaluative principles of morally acceptable actions and desirable ways of life, it seems surprising that philosophers have hardly engaged in a systematic manner with the norms and values pertaining to the temporality, structure, and segmentation of human life. Of course, there are famous works discussing the advantages and disadvantages, vices and virtues of certain life stages – for example, Enlightenment and neo-humanist writings on childhood and education such as Rousseau's *Emile*, or Cicero's and Seneca's ancient virtue ethical tracts on old age. However, these reflections usually still take the life course as a given, indispensable fact. There is almost no general reflection on the temporal structure of human life as a central *subject* of ethical discussion. What does it mean for ethical thought that human actions and lives are essentially determined by certain inevitable and irreversible changes over the life course? How far is it justified to have different moral expectations of people at different stages of life and thus apply different standards of need, sufficiency, acceptability, appropriateness, deservingness, or fulfillment over the life course? What is the role of specific images, conceptions, expectations, and norms regarding childhood, adolescence, adulthood, and old age? And how can we appropriately reflect these aspects and systematically integrate them into ethical theory? If ethics is still concerned with the reflection of our moral orientations and practices, it has to address these questions and thus engage with the attendant age norms and biographical ideals in order to foster an open debate on their significance and justification. In this sense, what we need is not a specific ethics of ageing – an ethics for old people, so to speak – but an appropriate ethical appreciation of the temporal dimension and structure of human existence as such and in general.

Note

1 I would like to thank Larissa Pfaller (Erlangen/Hamburg), Silke Schicktanz (Göttingen), and Nitzan Rimon-Zarfaty (Beer-Sheba) for helpful comments and suggestions.

References

Agich, G. J. 2001. "Implications of Aging Paradigms for Bioethics." In *Aging: Culture, Health, and Social Change*, edited by D. N. Weisstub, D. C. Thomasma, S. Gauthier, and G. F. Tomossy, 15–28. Dordrecht: Springer Netherlands.

Agich, G. J. 2003. *Dependence and Autonomy in Old Age: An Ethical Framework for Long-Term Care*. Cambridge: Cambridge University Press.

American Academy of Anti-Aging Medicine. 2002. *Official Position Statement on the Truth about Human Aging*. A4M (www.worldhealth.net/pdf/OfficialStatement_Truth-Aging-Intervention.pdf).

Anscombe, G. E. M. 1958. "Modern Moral Philosophy." *Philosophy* 33 (124):1–19.

Ariés, P. 1962. *Centuries of Childhood: A Social History of Family Life*. Translated by Robert Baldick. New York: Knopf.

Asch, S. M., E. A. Kerr, J. Keesey, J. L. Adams, C. M. Setodji, S. Malik, and E. A. McGlynn. 2006. "Who Is at Greatest Risk for Receiving Poor-Quality Health Care?" *New England Journal of Medicine* 354:1147–1156. doi: 10.1056/NEJMsa044464.

Baars, J. 2012. *Aging and the Art of Living*. Baltimore: Johns Hopkins University Press.

Bearon, L. B. 1996. "Successful Aging: What Does the 'Good Life' Look Like?" *The Forum* 1 (3) (online).

Bedford, R., L. Davis, and P. Kelly. 2007. *Early Modern English Lives: Autobiography and Self-Representation, 1500–1660*. Farnham: Ashgate.

Binstock, R. H., and S. G. Post, eds. 1991. *Too Old for Health Care: Controversies in Medicine, Law, Economics, and Ethics*. Baltimore: Johns Hopkins University Press.

Bolles, R. N. 1978. *The Three Boxes of Life and How to Get out of Them: An Introduction to Life/Work Planning*. Berkeley, CA: Ten Speed Press.
Boorse, C. 1977. "Health as a Theoretical Concept." *Philosophy of Science* 44 (4):542–573.
Bostrom, N. 2005. "The Fable of the Dragon Tyrant." *Journal of Medical Ethics* 31:273–277.
Brockmann, H. 2002. "Why Is Less Money Spent on Health Care for the Elderly than for the Rest of the Population? Health Care Rationing in German Hospitals." *Social Science and Medicine* 55:593–608. doi: 10.1016/S0277-9536(01)00190-3.
Bühler, N. 2015. "Imagining the Future of Motherhood: The Medically Assisted Extension of Fertility and the Production of Genealogical Continuity." *Sociologus* 65 (1):79–100.
Butler, R. 2005. "Ageism: Looking Back over My Shoulder." *Generations* 29 (3):84–86.
Callahan, D. 1977. "On Defining a 'Natural Death'." *Hastings Center Report* 7 (3):32–37.
Callahan, D. 1987. "Terminating Treatment: Age as a Standard." *Hastings Center Report* 17 (5):21–25.
Callahan, D. 1995 [1987]. *Setting Limits: Medical Goals in an Aging Society with "A Response to my Critics"*. Washington, DC: Georgetown University Press.
Caplan, A. L. 2005. "Death as an Unnatural Process." *EMBO Reports* 6 (1):72–75.
Cole, T. 1983. "The 'Enlightened' View of Aging. Victorian Morality in a New Key." *Hastings Center Report* 13 (3):34–40.
Congress of the United States/Congressional Budget Office. 2014. *The 2014 Long-Term Budget Outlook*. Washington, DC: Congressional Budget Office (www.cbo.gov/publication/45471).
Daniels, N. 1985. *Just Health Care*. Cambridge: Cambridge University Press.
Daniels, N. 1988. *Am I My Parents' Keeper? An Essay on Justice between the Young and the Old*. New York: Oxford University Press.
Dannefer, D. 1996. "The Social Organization of Diversity, and the Normative Organization of Age." *The Gerontologist* 36:174–177.
Ebrahim, S. 2000. "Do Not Resuscitate Decisions: Flogging Dead Horses or a Dignified Death?" *British Medical Journal* 320:1155–1156. doi: http://dx.doi.org/10.1136/bmj.320.7243.1155.
Featherstone, M., and M. Hepworth. 1991. "The Mask of Aging and the Postmodern Life Course." In *The Body: Social Process and Cultural Theory*, edited by M. Featherstone, M. Hepworth, and B. Turner, 371–390. London: Sage.
Fenech, F. F. 2003. "Ethical Issues in Ageing." *Clinical Medicine* 3 (3):232–234.
Gabbay, E., J. Calvo-Broce, K. B. Meyer, T. A. Trikalinos, J. Cohen, and D. M. Kent. 2010. "The Empirical Basis for Determinations of Medical Futility." *Journal of General Internal Medicine* 25 (10):1083–1089.
Gems, D. 2003. "Is More Life Always Better?: The New Biology of Aging and the Meaning of Life." *Hastings Center Report* 33 (4):31–39.
Giele, J. Z., and F. Holst, eds. 2004. *Changing Life Patterns in Western Industrial Societies*. Oxford: Elsevier.
Gilchrist, R. 2012. *Medieval Life: Archaeology and the Life Course*. Woolbridge: Boydell Press.
Grey, A. de. 2004. "We Will Be Able to Live to 1000." *BBC News* (3 December). http://news.bbc.co.uk/2/hi/uk/4003063.stm.
Grey, A. de. 2005. "Life Extension, Human Rights, and the Rational Refinement of Repugnance." *Journal of Medical Ethics* 31:659–663.
Hagestad, G. O., and B. L. Neugarten. 1985. "Age and the Life Course." In *Handbook of Aging and the Social Sciences*, edited by R. H. Binstock and E. Shanas, 35–61. New York: Van Nostrand Reinhold.

Hareven, T. K., ed. 1996. *Aging and Generational Relations over the Life Course: A Historical and Cross-Cultural Perspective*. Berlin: De Gruyter.

Harris, J. 1985. *The Value of Life*. London: Routledge.

Harris, J. 1987. "QALYfying the Value of Life." *Journal of Medical Ethics* 13 (3):117–123.

Harris, J. 1994. "Does Justice Require That We Be Ageist?" *Bioethics* 8 (1):74–83.

Holm, S. 2013. "The Implicit Anthropology of Bioethics and the Problem of the Aging Person." In *Ethics, Health Policy and (Anti-)Aging: Mixed Blessings*, edited by M. Schermer and W. Pinxten, 59–71. Dordrecht: Springer Netherlands.

Holmes, E. R., and L. D. Holmes. 1995. *Other Cultures, Elder Years*. Thousand Oaks: Sage.

Holstein, J. A., and J. F. Gubrium. 2000. *Constructing the Life Course*. Dix Hills, NY: General Hall.

Hudson, F. M. 1999. *The Adult Years: Mastering the Art of Self-Renewal*. San Francisco: Jossey-Bass.

Jecker, N. S. 1992. *Aging and Ethics: Philosophical Problems in Gerontology*. Totowa, NJ: Humana.

Jecker, N. S., and L. J. Schneiderman. 1994. "Is Dying Young Worse Than Dying Old?" *The Gerontologist* 34 (1):66–72.

Kapp, M. B. 2002. "Health Care Rationing Affecting Older Persons: Rejected in Principle but Implemented in Fact." *Journal of Aging and Social Policy* 14:27–42. doi: 10.1300/J031v14n02_02.

Kass, L. 2001. "L'Chaim and Its Limits. Why Not Immortality?" *First Things* 113:17–24.

Kauppinen, A. 2012. "Meaningfulness and Time." *Philosophy and Phenomenological Research* 84 (2):345–377.

Klatz, R., and R. Goldman. 2003. *The New Anti-Ageing-Revolution: Stopping the Clock for a Younger, Sexier, Happier You*. North Bergen, NJ: Basic Health Publications.

Kohli, M. 2007. "The Institutionalization of the Life Course: Looking Back to Look Ahead." *Research in Human Development* 4 (3–4):253–271.

Kuther, T. L. 2003. "Medical Decision-Making and Minors: Issues of Consent and Assent." *Adolescence* 38 (150):343–358.

Laslett, P. 1991. *A Fresh Map of Life: The Emergence of the Third Age*. Cambridge, MA: Harvard University Press.

Laz, C. 1998. "Act Your Age." *Sociological Forum* 13 (1):85–113.

Levy, R., P. Ghisletta, J.-M. Le Goff, D. Spini, and E. Widmer, eds. 2005. *Towards an Interdisciplinary Perspective on the Life Course*. Oxford: Elsevier.

Maines, D. R., P. M. Passuth, and B. L. Neugarten. 1987. "Age Norms and Age Constraints Twenty Years Later." *Psychology Today* 176:29–33.

Moody, H. R. 1992. *Ethics in an Aging Society*. Baltimore/London: Johns Hopkins University Press.

Mortimer, J. T., and M. J. Shanahan, eds. 2007. *Handbook of the Life Course*. New York/Boston/Dordrecht/London/Moscow: Kluwer.

Mykytyn, C. E. 2006. "Anti-Aging Medicine: A Patient/Practitioner Movement to Redefine Aging." *Social Science and Medicine* 62 (3):643–653.

Neugarten, B. L. 1996. "The Young-Old and the Age-Irrelevant Society." In *The Meanings of Age: Selected Papers*, edited by B. L. Neugarten, 34–46. Chicago: University of Chicago Press.

Neugarten, B. L., J. W. Moore, and J. C. Lowe. 1965. "Age Norms, Age Constraints, and Adult Socialization." *American Journal of Sociology* 70 (6):710–717.

Nussbaum, M. C. 1992. "Human Functioning and Social Justice: In Defense of Aristotelian Essentialism." *Political Theory* 20 (2):202–246.

O'Rand, A. M., and M. L. Krecker. 1990. "Concepts of the Life Cycle: Their History, Meanings, and Uses in the Social Sciences." *Annual Review of Sociology* 16:241–262.

Post, S. G., and R. H. Binstock, eds. 2004. *The Fountain of Youth: Cultural, Scientific and Ethical Perspectives on a Biomedical Goal*. New York: Oxford University Press.

Pruchno, R. 2012. "Not Your Mother's Old Age: Baby Boomers at Age 65." *The Gerontologist* 52 (2):149–152.

Pruchno, R. 2015. "Successful Aging: Contentious Past, Productive Future." *The Gerontologist* 55 (1):1–4.

Pulkkinen, L., and A. Caspi. 2002. *Paths to Successful Development: Personality in the Life Course*. Cambridge: Cambridge University Press.

Riley, M. W. E., R. L. E. Kahn, A. E. Foner, and K. A. Mack. 1994. *Age and Structural Lag: Society's Failure to Provide Meaningful Opportunities in Work, Family, and Leisure*. Oxford: John Wiley & Sons.

Rivlin, M. M. 2000. "Why the Fair Innings Argument Is Not Persuasive." *BMC Medical Ethics* 1 (1) (online).

Ruppert, S., ed. 2010. *Lebensalter und Recht: Zur Segmentierung des menschlichen Lebenslaufes durch rechtliche Regelungen seit 1750*. Frankfurt a. M.: Klostermann.

Schirrmacher, F. 2004. *Das Methusalem-Komplott*. München: Karl Blessing Verlag.

Schneiderman, L. J., N. S. Jecker, and A. R. Jonsen. 1990. "Medical Futility: Its Meaning and Ethical Implications." *Annals of Internal Medicine* 112 (12):949–954.

Schweda, M. 2013. "Zu alt für die Hüftprothese, zu jung zum Sterben? Die Rolle von Altersbildern in der ethisch-politischen Debatte um eine altersabhängige Begrenzung medizinischer Leistungen." In *Gerecht sorgen: Verständigungsprozesse über den Einsatz knapper Ressourcen bei Patienten am Lebensende*, edited by G. Duttge and M. Zimmermann-Acklin, 149–167. Göttingen: Göttingen University Press.

Schweda, M., S. Wöhlke, and J. Inthorn. 2015. "'Not the Years in Themselves Count': The Role of Age for European Citizens' Moral Attitudes Towards Resource Allocation in Modern Biomedicine." *Journal of Public Health* 23 (3):117–126.

Small, H. 2007. *The Long Life*. London: Oxford University Press.

Steinhoff, U., ed. 2015. *Do All Persons Have Equal Moral Worth?: On 'Basic Equality' and Equal Respect and Concern*. Oxford: Oxford University Press.

Tornstam, L. 2005. *Gerotranscendence: A Developmental Theory of Positive Aging*. New York: Springer.

Tsuchiya, A. 2000. "QALYs and Ageism: Philosophical Theories and Age Weighting." *Health Economics* 9 (1):57–68.

Ubachs-Moust, J., R. Houtepen, W. Dondorp, R. ter Meulen, and R. Vos. 2010. "Age and Age-Based Rationing in the Medical Decision-Making Process for Older People: A Qualitative Study of Experts' Views and Perspectives." In *From Setting Limits to Shaping Practices: Trust and Accountability in Healthcare for Older People*, edited by J. Ubachs-Moust, 23–39. Maastricht: Ridderprint.

Ubachs-Moust, J., R. Houtepen, R. Vos, and R. ter Meulen. 2008. "Value Judgements in the Decision-Making Process for the Elderly Patient." *Journal of Medical Ethics* 34 (12):863–868.

Vincent, J. A. 2003. "What Is at Stake in the 'War on Anti-Ageing Medicine'?" *Ageing and Society* 23 (5):675–684.

Wicclair, M. R. 1993. *Ethics and the Elderly*. Oxford, NY: Oxford University Press.

Wiesemann, C. 2016. *Moral Equality, Bioethics, and the Child*. Cham: Springer International.

World Health Organization (WHO). 2011. *Global Health and Aging*. Geneva: World Health Organization.

2 Becoming oneself

Toward a new philosophy of ageing

Thomas Rentsch

Our life is a process of finitization – a process that we can grasp only within the perspective of a unique, finite constitution of meaning. Ageing is *the process of the human being becoming him- or herself* within a finite, unique life situation. We feel that the phases of our life have their specific meaning because of their finitude and limitation. Internally, they form a highly complex arrangement. On one hand, they develop highly specific modes of uniqueness – in the mother's womb, as a baby, as a toddler, during childhood and adolescence, during the phase of maturity, in the many forms of becoming a person or of ageing and growing old. On the other hand, the different phases of our life flow into each other, for I am still the same physical entity that I was in my mother's womb, as the baby that was born, and I will remain so until the end of my life.

It is therefore misleading and incorrect to separate and schematize the phases of one's life. In the worst case, 'old age' then becomes a nightmare scenario along with all of its associations with disability – associations that have an almost ideological content. From the perspective of a critique of ideology, it is remarkable that we do not have similar negative ideological associations with regard to babies. It is self-evident that babies are helpless in many ways. In the case of the very old (Fishkin and Laslett 1992), this helplessness is often considered burdensome. From an ethical perspective, however, this asymmetry in our intuitive evaluation of life phases is not justified and is indeed worthy of criticism, for the gestures of sympathy and support that a small child enjoys are just as important and meaningful for our older fellow human beings (Callahan 1995; Daniels 1988; Lesser 2012).

The tendency to repress and to devalue age (and hence the finitude that informs all the phases of our life) becomes especially obvious in our all-encompassing consumerist, fitness or wellness 'culture.' Indeed, in many areas it has become dominant. Mythical and suggestive catchphrases such as 'the avalanche of ageing,' the 'flood of retirees,' and the 'Methuselah conspiracy' are widespread. Especially in the United States, an anti-ageing ideology has developed in which hostility toward the old, dreams of eternal youth, and pharmacological and economic interests are fused. Who will discover the key to extending life by 100, 200, or even 300 years (and, naturally, remaining fit throughout this time)? Or, as some research projects (without joking) specify their goal: 'the elimination of death'?

(For debate on the anti-ageing movement, see Callahan 1995; de Grey 2007; Fukuyama 2002; Harris 2007; Sell, Lorenzini, and Brown-Borg 2009; Vincent 2006, 2009). Of course, wanting to live a healthier life for longer is completely rational and understandable, and in the Western industrialized nations, we have indeed come very far in this respect. Yet, these developments have nothing to do with the aforementioned demonization of ageing, of finitude, or, indeed, of death. The project of anti-ageing is a medical project, whose social, ethical, and moral foundations are still controversial and hence the subject of discussion. Thus, the current debate has centered on images of ageing as a negative process and age discrimination rather than on the age-based rationing of medical resources we have witnessed until now.

What is more important is – and this is the key ethical and philosophical thesis of my reflections – to make the connection between finitude and meaning much clearer in our child-rearing and our education, in politics, and in the media, as well as to differentiate between the limits of our life and the meaning of our life. I have, for some time now, in my training sessions for ethics teachers and also in the volume *Gutes Leben im Alter: Die philosophischen Grundlagen* (*Good Life in Old Age: The Philosophical Foundations*) (Rentsch and Vollmann 2012), been pursuing the project of a *clarification about life as a whole*. Although 'clarification' in this context is, importantly, almost synonymous with the concept of 'sexual clarification,' my aim, from an ethical perspective, has been to clarify to people what life *as a whole* – that is, life that includes the experience of sickness, disability, susceptibility to injury, finitude, mortality, and death – is.

In the following, my aim will be to show the means by which ageing, finitude, vulnerability, and mortality can be reintroduced into public consciousness and the understanding of society and how these aspects can be integrated in a new way. I will also explicate the medical and healthcare consequences of this urgently needed project of enlightenment. Philosophically, the anthropological and ethical foundations, as well as the normative implications, of the process of becoming a human being, of growing old, and of the finitude of all life, will be brought to the reader's attention, and the associated practical, social, and political tasks of creating a new human culture will be presented.

Toward a new philosophy of ageing

The late modern society of the West faces the great task of bringing ageing, advanced age, and mortality back into life and back into its common life. This also holds for the values we attach to the nursing profession and to our relationship with dementia and Alzheimer's disease; indeed, it also holds for end-of-life care, for palliative medicine, and for the time and money that we are willing to spend for these basic human needs (Piven 2004). The challenges of an ageing society have great significance for medical practice and healthcare. Assistance, care, and monitoring need to be valued as forms of a humane praxis rather than as issues of mere supply and demand. This also has economic and social consequences. I will return to this problem in the conclusion.

Furthermore, we could point to the asymmetry in our relationship with very young people as compared with our relationship with very old, invalid individuals. It is considered self-evident that we support babies in all their needs and emergencies. When it comes to advanced age, however, we very quickly raise the question of whether such support is worth it, especially in regard to its costs. We here risk relativizing or quantifying human dignity and hence infringing upon it and violating it. The many reports from old-age homes about overextended and underpaid nursing professionals and about the limited time available for caring for individual residents' needs also attest to a worrying and problematic development.

Thus, our goal must now be – as it is in my overarching project about finitude, susceptibility to injury, mortality, and death – to initiate and further develop a similar project at universities, for the training of ethics teachers, and to raise awareness through education and public information. Here, too, in what may be the greatest social task over the next decades, we shall see that the classic modern achievements of the Enlightenment – such as those of Kant, but also those of Marx and Freud – are by no means fully exhausted. Rather, they confront us ever anew in different forms. Freud placed at the center of his analysis two primordial anthropological phenomena: sexual desire and the fear of death (Meyer 2008; Piven 2004). Whereas the project of sexual clarification appears to be finished (here I also have my doubts, at any rate with respect to other cultures), the repression and taboo associated with finitude, ageing, susceptibility to injury, and death is still dominant. The reference to psychoanalysis is intended only to make clear that, in this project about clarification of the limits and the meaning of our life, about age and age-related restrictions, we are faced with something that, to put it casually, we have bottled up, and this is something that has to do with our existential self-understanding. This is precisely why the project must be planned in such a way that it has a strong interdisciplinary component and foundation. Almost every subject that deals with the human being in one way or another can contribute.

It is essential to reintroduce the topic of human ageing into philosophy. The modern age and the Enlightenment addressed their normative claims to all rational beings. However, their universal ethics ignored the conditions and the relative nature of human life – for example, the phases of life. Consequently, Immanuel Kant (1956) directed his unconditional categorical imperative not to older or younger people, but rather formally and universally, as well as abstractly, to all free, potentially moral individuals. In his abstract ethics of reason, he made no mention at all of the embodiment, finitude, and vulnerability of beings. In contrast, the ancient tradition of ethics focused on happiness and asked, as did Aristotle (1984), 'How can human beings lead a good life (Greek: *eu zen*)?' Ancient ethics was not concerned with a categorical imperative or a universal 'you ought' for all human beings; it focused on questions related to the success and the happiness of the individual: his or her 'eudaimonia.' The ancient ethics of the good life thus had to take into consideration and to respect the particular circumstances of a human life to be able to help people achieve an appropriate understanding. The ethics of the good life cannot refer to humans in general but must instead refer to concrete individuals in order to provide valuable insight into the possibility of happiness. An ethics of the stages of life was therefore developed in the tradition of ancient philosophy. If we want to deal with the problem of ageing in modern society thoughtfully, we must have the courage to overcome the practical inadequacy of the modern ethics of reason: We must look back at ancient ethics and at the tradition of practical wisdom with a view to developing a culture that treats ageing in a humane way.

Happiness and communicative praxis

The first fundamental insight of ancient ethics was its principle that all human beings pursue happiness. All human beings want to be happy (Meyer 2008). Human actions can be understood as an attempt to lead a meaningful life. The result of the extensive discussion about happiness – let me put this simply – is that happiness is nothing special. Happiness is nothing extraordinary, separated from our normal actions. Basically, happiness comes about if we conduct ourselves satisfactorily in our ordinary activities. Connected with this view is a critique of the idea that happiness is the highest or the ultimate goal, to be placed at the tip of a pyramid of aims that one chases after in vain. In contrast, we have to begin with the intrinsic value of the supposedly lower and inferior projects and fulfillments – which are actually elementary and fundamental; for example, eating, drinking, sleeping, listening and seeing, talking with others, and doing something meaningful.

In addition to their basic functions with regard to more complex and meaningful projects, such elementary aims also have an intrinsic value and modest core. To see all human action as a mere means directed at, and as a function of, a final end – namely happiness – is a misunderstanding, because in this view, all the different meaningful forms of successful life are not acknowledged as such. We must therefore go beyond this view and grasp the diverse forms of the good – that is, of happiness. That all human beings pursue happiness does not necessarily mean that there is only one form of happiness. On this basis, we can now ask about the specific forms of fulfillment for different stages of life.

In the tradition of the ethics of the good life, something else is clear. We become ourselves in a medium of communicative praxis through a common life with others. In this sense, ancient practical philosophy defined the human being as a linguistic and political creature whose natural environment was the city. The process of becoming human is made possible by the communicative, social forms of fulfillment in a common life. This is clearly the case for childhood, early adulthood, education, and professional training. The question is 'In what sense is this relevant to the phase of life in which we grow old?'

Despite the emphasis placed on the social essence of human beings, the existential sense of loneliness is a presupposition of the human condition. In fact, only by being with other people is it possible to experience loneliness, subjectivity, and awareness of individuality. The life of the individual is not completely absorbed into the communicative essence of humans. On the contrary, every life is a unique whole, a singular totality that appears definite in the limited bodily form of humans. Plato called the human body "the principle of individuation" (Charlton 1972). Also, the totality of life, which develops in time, should not be regarded as anything special or superior to ordinary life. Instead, it appears only in practical situations.

Becoming human

How can the developing human being be understood in its temporal finitude? Life forces us to give it a specific form – that is, an existential configuration of ourselves. We must continuously produce this form, in youth and old age, on a daily basis. The extensive activity of this process can be called 'leading one's own life.' From the beginning of our lives, we are distinct, physically constituted beings with the feature of uniqueness – that is, a factual irreplaceability and distinctiveness. In our lives, we are always working on shaping this unique totality that we already are. Whether we like it or not, our life is first and foremost the process of forming the singular totality we ourselves are.

The unique totality of every life appears to genuinely split into a dialectical process of forming. On one hand, individual actions are always movements in the context of life as a whole, albeit situated in particular life situations, and they gain or lose their meaning in relation to the whole. On the other hand, the framework of this totality is modified by individual actions and meaningful projects in the local situations. Given this dialectic of uniqueness and totality, a conceptually irretrievable form of the world – individuality – constitutes itself as a concrete life form.

The totality of life can never be experienced outside of the particular situation and outside of the concrete stages of life. Moreover, singular situations can be grasped more closely only in the perspective of the totality. This statement preserves the complete rigor we find in the viewpoint of a morally conceived unique totality of life. In this context, we can speak of the ethical time of responsibility as the absolute time of a finite human life, the time that is really at stake.

In modern ethics, the ancient theme of the good and successful life has re-entered through the back door, namely with the concept of identity or personal identity. Developmental psychologists such as Piaget (1978) and Kohlberg (1981), who, on the basis of their empirical investigations, showed the step-by-step formation of children's ability to make moral judgments, brought the fully enlightened philosophers of reason closer to the facts. 'Pure' reason develops in fragile and vulnerable little bodies in difficult and continuously jeopardized processes and nowhere else. The formation of personal identity is linked to the process of moral development precisely because of humans' natural dependency. Furthermore, the past 30 years have seen a comprehensive renaissance of an ethics of the good life in practical philosophy (Nussbaum 2001; Raz 1994; Taylor 2003).

What is true of the genesis of the development of personal identity for childhood, youth, and young adulthood seems just as true for later life, which is, so to speak, the reverse of early development and thus requires an extension of the theory of moral development.

Life as a task of interpretation

How is becoming oneself constituted in time? It is not completed upon reaching adulthood. On the contrary, this is when the complex processes of protecting and testing identity begin. We experience ourselves as essentially identical during and after decisive and impressionable experiences of change. The form of our life preserves its unmistakable quality because we experience profound changes in ourselves and must react to these transformations.

One look at the natural structure of our life in childhood and youth, adolescence and adulthood, ageing, and the end of life makes this clear. These changes within a meaningful and enduring life are connected to adjustments in our way of seeing the world. The point is that the unique totality of life represents a continuous task of interpretation; on one hand, it develops in accordance with the existential dialectic of the concrete individual situation and the concrete action. On the other hand, it progresses in accordance with the perspective of the totality of our existence, through the changes of life.

In growing up and maturing, one's perspective within a life that is perceived as meaningful changes. Human beings are to be understood not just as significant projects in themselves, but rather as beings who are capable of fundamental changes in perspective. They have to be capable of this, too, for the unique totality of life entails that everything fundamental happens only once: Every one of us is a child, a young person, and an adult only once; only once is there an entry into later life. All these stages occur without a chance to rehearse: Life is a constant premiere. Every new opportunity in life is simultaneously a loss; every loss, a gain. Therefore, Kierkegaard (2000) says life can only be understood backward but must be lived forward (Strawser 1997).

On the social level, the unique totality of life is obvious in the very objective irreplaceability of any individual in the lives of others: My life experiences show that I can be no other person. This irreplaceability is, in practical terms, an inexchangeability. In this aspect of life, we can see the reason for its seriousness: The common expression 'seriousness of life' ('life is serious business') refers to the absolute necessity of leading one's own life. In my existential particularity, in the singularity of my individual life, and according to my genuine abilities, I am a practical fulfillment of perspectives for others. We become acquainted with certain natural forms of life – daughter or son, mother or father, sister or brother, grandparents. We are irreplaceable in these forms. We must therefore grasp the internal complexity and nuances of the unique totality of life in the course of life.

This irreplaceability in the lives of others varies according to the stages of life and changes during the development of identity. There is always the chance of fulfillment or of failure in which we have a stake – as a child, as a daughter, as a teacher, as a grandfather, as a sick person, as a healthy person, as a fragile person, as a youthful or vigorous person, as an experienced or inexperienced person. In every instance, this depends on what we do or can be. The isolation of generations, which is characteristic of modern society, can be analyzed as a communicative impoverishment of the forms of fulfillment in life that we owe to the differentiated irreplaceability of others. A moral understanding of life is measured most unmistakably by the ability to see the other as the other in his difference; it is measured by the strength and sensitivity to put oneself in someone else's position, to have the existential imagination to make clear to oneself as a young person that I am potentially this older person.

The fundamental ethical meaning of finitude

The unique totality of life has its concrete form in the bodily existence of humans. This bodily existence does not end at the surface of our skin; rather, we reach out to the world by acting, speaking, planning, and reflecting. The body is not a shell in which we are 'hidden.' It is not the outside of an inside. We do not sit 'inside' ourselves like drivers of the machine that is our body. Nor are we ethereal spiritual beings standing above our bodies. More precisely, the human body is the center of our dynamic reality, where its natural basis and its communicative being are made possible and are mutually related. The question is 'What do the demonstrated characteristics of the unique totality of life actually mean for the process of becoming oneself in old age?'

In order to answer this question, we have to philosophically consider the fundamental ethical meaning of human finitude, because the temporality of human life becomes more radical in old age, as we will see in a moment. We always exist as a temporally finite being, but the process of ageing intensifies the experience of finitude. Finitude shows itself in the inability to repeat and the inability to retrieve the common and solitary life; it manifests itself in the irreversibility of the movement of life, in the inevitability of the entry into and the exit from the stages of life, in the irrevocability of the past, in recalling significant attempts at a meaningful and conscious life that we failed to attain, and in the unpredictability of the future. The finitude of life means that many aspects of our past remain hidden from us as humans, the future is evasive, and the present is a place in which we may experience such insecurity that it threatens our very autonomy.

Before I discuss the consequences of these reflections for an ethics of later life, I would like to emphasize that I think it is entirely wrong, considering the fact of ageing, to develop a pessimistic or even tragic anthropology of the poverty of human existence (Améry 1999). I would like to offer the view that the normality, universality, and continuity of being human occur in all the phases of life. It is wrong to think that the elderly and the very old are, as it were, an exotic foreign tribe in the midst of otherwise young, carefree, healthy human beings in love, happy and consuming rapturously. This distorted picture is superficial and mistaken insofar as vulnerability, the threat of suffering and defenselessness, and existential fragility shape all phases of a human life. We need not speak of the helpless baby. Instead, let us think of the problems of adolescence, professional training in a frequently harsh and mercilessly competitive society, the large and complex problems of love, relationships, marriage, and education, to mention but a few. It then becomes clear that the constitutive orientation of meaning for human beings should be seen in the context of this fragility.

We should not forget the normality, universality, and continuity of the fragility of being human in our reflection on the peculiarity of ageing: Problems, crises, conflicts, fear, and dangers are just as characteristic of the life phases as is the chance for happiness. With this in mind, we can see ageing as an opportunity. In ageing, one can continue to speak of the very specific elements of becoming oneself. I will now discuss these elements as a radicalization of the human condition in order to shed light on its ethical implications.

Ageing as the radicalization of the human condition

The process of ageing is the radicalization of the basic human condition, since ageing can be grasped philosophically and anthropologically as an insistent manifestation of the human constitution of meaning. The abstract ethics of reason are of no assistance in explaining this point; the same can be said about metaphysics insofar as it concerns a-temporal spiritual beings.

Therefore, we must seek a conceptual understanding of the reality of life if we want to describe the radicalization of the human situation and the appearance of the human constitution of meaning. First, the following aspects can be distinguished: physical ageing, psychological ageing, social ageing, and cultural ageing. The physical changes during the ageing process can be described as the radicalization of the bodily constituted basic condition of human existence. Parts of the body that once functioned normally, such as the joints and the heart, all begin to deteriorate, reminding us of the basis of a finite life: its dependence upon nature. The human being has been defined as 'a deficient being' (*Mängelwesen*) because of an extremely long phase of helplessness as an infant, as well as because of his constitutive defenselessness: He is without a coat of hair – at the mercy of the climate – without special protection or an organ that involves the instinct for preserving himself, and without reliable instincts for security (Gehlen 1988). This deficiency once again increases with age. This is when the physical, social, and cultural components of the ageing process appear. It is in accordance with the unique totality of the human being that ageing concerns the singular totality of our entire situation in life.

Oscar Wilde (2005) addressed the issue of ageing in his novel *The Picture of Dorian Gray.* He made the paradoxical statement: "The tragedy of ageing is not based on the fact that one is old but rather that one is young" (Wilde 2005, 182). What does Wilde imply here? One takes a personal identity developed in one's youth into old age. The individual trusts this identity and creates it in his or her active years. Developed and regularly affirmed, this identity comes into conflict with the beginning of the physical fragility that becomes increasingly dominant. This fragility is opposed to the self-chosen and developed form of one's own existence, an identity created through youth and adulthood, appearing clearly as it becomes threatened by the bodily process of ageing.

The radicalization of the physically constituted basic condition of humans is accompanied by psychological ageing. It is connected to the finite temporality of life and the basic modifications of the life experience. The period of time during which life is experienced becomes ever longer, and yet the time left to live becomes ever shorter. Thus, the experience of becoming a body in the physical sense has an analogue in the process of becoming conscious of time in relation to the experience of consciousness. This increased awareness of time comes about through the disappearance of expected life and the increase of experienced life. Schopenhauer wrote:

> From the standpoint of youth, life seems to stretch away into an endless future; from the standpoint of old age, to go back but a little way into the past; so that, at the beginning, life presents us with a picture in which the objects appear a great way off, as though we had reversed our telescope; while in the end everything seems so close. To see how short life is, a man must have grown old, that is to say, he must have lived long.
>
> (Schopenhauer 1924, 137)

In addition to becoming a body and becoming conscious of time, there is social and cultural ageing. The ruptures in becoming oneself and the radicalized experience of time are reinforced by the loss of partners, relatives, family members, and friends of one's own generation. Because of human beings' communicative nature, this aspect of ageing is one of the most difficult ones – that is, accepting the loss of someone close is one of the most difficult existential tasks for human beings to come to grips with. The very old complain they can no longer converse with anyone because the familiar context of life and everyday things – the horizon of common experience and acquaintances – has disintegrated, insofar becoming oneself appears as an isolation and is accompanied by being estranged from the world.

The ethical implications

What are the ethical implications of all this? Let us keep the basic question in mind. Our postmodern society is characterized by a phenomenal and abhorrent pace that is without historic precedent. Further, the process of technological development is ever accelerating. This high-speed civilization fosters social and cultural alienation. Paul Virilio analyzes the 'polar inertia' generated in our late modern society by the digitalization of information networks (which now control all aspects of life) and the processes of technical acceleration (Lotringer and Virilio 1998; Rosa 2003, 2004a, 2004b; Virilio 2005). One result is the tendency to misunderstand one's own life-world. Personal identities and normative systems together with impressionable experiences have been developed in a social and cultural sphere that no longer exists. It has become 'remembered time.' The rate of social change and historical transformation has increased to such an extent that it is quite commonplace to find that old people can no longer cope. Having grown up as a young child in the 1950s, it seems to me that some aspects of present-day life make intuitively unreasonable demands. Even if there were an easy and cheerful conformity and lively willingness to pick up new things on the part of the 'young old'; even if a steady decline in curiosity about interesting developments in society and culture were not observable: The legitimate and far-reaching experience of finitude can be smoothed over but ultimately cannot be overcome.

It is through the radicalization of the physical and temporal human condition, through the appearance of physical, temporal, social, and cultural conditions of the meaning of human life, that becoming a human being takes place in ageing. From an ethical point of view, the question is 'What possible forms of fulfillment, of broken and endangered processes of becoming oneself, are specific to the elderly?' Traditionally, this perspective was developed with the concept of wisdom or the wisdom of old age, which is unfortunately no longer common today. In the tradition of wisdom, to learn from ageing can mean to set concrete, practical forms of life, such as slowing down and taking it easy, against the 'polar inertia' of late modern processes of technical acceleration, to gain a new sense of the definitive, temporal reality of our lives, the reality that is so precious. Normative and practical research into ageing that focuses on regaining the tradition of wisdom shows that the ageing process is capable of uncovering important sources for the constitution of the meaning of life and of happiness in life, changes that can help us gain a more life-supporting insight into our lives (Baltes and Smith 1990; Baltes and Staudinger 1993). This perspective was developed in close connection with life experience: It is in no sense 'idealistic,' nor does it gloss over or romanticize anything. Here, old age essentially appears as a chance to gain primary insight into the limited possibilities of human beings. There is no doubt about the continuous orientation toward fulfillment and happiness in old age. I would like to say, however, that it is the increasing 'immediate' experience of this limitedness that allows us to understand our own lives as the forming of a singular totality, as really becoming oneself. Growing old in many respects aids the development of ethical insights, because as one ages, one is able to intensely experience the finitude and the fragility of life. The human dependency on communication and solidarity is manifold and can be experienced through loss. The experience of transience and the ease with which some forms of happiness slip away can lead to disillusionment, but they may ultimately bring about a calm view, a view without self-deception – a state that Goethe called renunciation (*Entsagung*) (Bahr 1998). This is not a pitiful renouncement but rather the highest form of existential sovereignty and human self-assertion.

The unique totality as a temporal and finite process of becoming a self is conceived ethically if becoming oneself is understood as becoming final. Becoming final means that life has attained its final form in old age and becomes its whole time – the whole time of life. This whole time of the singular totality of life is the ethical time, since it is the time in which guilt and responsibility, autonomy and solidarity, transgressions against the self, and fulfillment have become real. To consciously grasp finality means that the brevity of life and its entirety can be seen, experienced, and understood, and there is a chance to distinguish between the important and the numerous unimportant things in life.

Old age is grasped from a theological point of view as grace, and the becoming-final of the person is called 'eternal life.' Since I am a philosopher, I cannot adopt this theological way of speaking. However, I think we might be able to preserve its meaning if we understand old age as a time in life in which the entanglement of finitude and meaning, fulfillment and limitedness can be recognized and understood.

Consequences for a culture of human ageing

We can now formulate some consequences for a culture of human ageing. We have described ageing as a communicative, self-reflective process of forming a unique totality, a formation that is essentially highlighted by a change of view toward a meaningful and enduring life. Ancient ethics is preferable to the modern ethics of reason since it is closely related to life. Its focus on happiness and fulfillment appears to be unparalleled. We could ask where reason should go if not there.

Furthermore, we have seen that the ancient form of enquiry has returned in modern theories through the back door – the return of the repressed – as an enquiry into the presuppositions of personal identity. Whereas modern ethical debate and moral philosophy discuss this form of questioning in connection with developmental psychology and especially in the field of child psychology and early human development, it follows that we should extend this form of questioning to life as a whole and, above all, to the later stages. It becomes clear that personal identity in this sense is absolutely inconceivable prior to or outside of morality. This can already be seen in the category of existential irreplaceability through and for others.

Like every other phase of life, old age appears to be a process that is in constant jeopardy but also rich in opportunities. In the past, we would have said it is a *way* to preserve and to test identity, making clear that this identity is not something static that is given once and for all but something linked to a dynamic process that we have characterized as becoming a body, becoming conscious of time and, ultimately, ethically, as becoming final. Given this background, the radicalization of the human condition implied in the keywords 'becoming-a-body,' 'becoming-conscious of time,' and 'becoming-final,' we can define this radicalization of the human condition with a view to the traditional category of wisdom as the time for developing a meaningful life. If we understand the process of becoming a self in its finitude and finality, this leads to a more conscious life; more conscious insofar as it follows from the insight into the entanglement of finitude and meaning. Following Aristotle (1984), we can say that true enduring happiness is based on this insight.

Conclusions: what does old age mean for human cultures?

With this in mind, I would like to finally address the question of the conditions of a culture of human ageing, in which I turn the tables and ask 'What does old age mean for human culture?' What does a highly advanced modern society learn ethically from the fact of ageing, which can neither be eliminated nor be repressed, and what does it learn from the presence of more and more older people? If we turn the tables from the point of view of ethics, we would not ask how a being that is restricted, disadvantaged, handicapped, useless, slow, and dependent on the help and conduct of others is able to cope with the end of old age in a modern, sophisticated, highly complex, rapidly changing society, but rather – and this is the ethical turn – ask: 'What can this society learn from the fact and meaning of ageing? Indeed, what is it required to learn?'

It can and has to learn a lesson in modesty. The principle of higher and higher, faster and faster, further and further, more and more complex, more and more perfect, more intense, more and more excessive, louder and louder, more and more informed, remains, ethically, existentially, and in terms of meaning, nothing more than a system designed to quantify. However, trees do not grow to heaven. We need an awareness of the human significance of finitude, limitation, and vulnerability, a consciousness of the worth of slowing down, of pausing, of calmly looking backward, of oral communication, of genuine conversation between real people, and of being able to admit one was wrong. Slowing down, pausing, and concrete oral communication are, paradoxically, the essential tools for defeating the process of perishing through the attainment of the profound. Only a calm look backward can help us achieve an emancipated clarification of life.

A meaning of life that is both ethically and morally demanding and truly sustainable has to do with not just the positive satisfaction of desire but also the way we deal, both as individuals and as a group, with the many negative aspects that shape our existence, whether we want them to or not. Against this background, ageing, illness, suffering, and death can be understood as opportunities to open up specific dimensions of meaning that are often overlooked: the dependence of each and every human on meaningful communication, on mutual assistance and sympathy, on solidarity, and, decisively, on the conscious awareness of his or her own limitation. These dimensions belong to a stage of maturity and of reflected self-knowledge – and hence, in essence, to a truly meaningful, self-reflexive and aware existence. Formulated in an emphatic way: These dimensions belong, from a philosophical perspective, to a knowledge of what is really real. We need to understand not only from a medical or ethical perspective but also from an existential perspective that health is not simply the absence of pain, disorders, and infirmity, of finitude and mortality, but rather, seen in a holistic perspective, the strength to live with these. As humans, we are psychosomatically irreducible wholes; we cannot be divided into the body and the mind, into objectivity and subjectivity. Self-knowledge and the clarification and deepening of life are also and especially enabled and developed by the experience of suffering, pain, and finitude.

This insight can be applied to the entire problem of the purpose of suffering and dying. We can change this perspective of a transformed understanding of human life using key approaches from the philosophical tradition. For instance, using the classic 'golden rule' or a form of Kant's categorical imperative, we can say: 'We should treat the sick, the suffering, and the dying as we ourselves would like to be treated in similar situations.' On a social and ethical level, this existential, individual principle, which concerns our moral self-understanding, has to be given a *constitutional* status: as justice between generations. Respect for the irreducible dignity of humans, as the German constitution states in a preamble to our entire legal order, cannot be reduced or quantified. This respect is owed to the sick, the suffering, the dying, and the needy just as it is to the healthy and the young. An earnest, honest burial ceremony makes it poignantly clear that a human remains a person and thus deserves the irreducible dignity due to him in the human world even after his death. This is true as unrestrictedly for the senile, the comatose, or the dying. What argument might convince us to restrict or, indeed, to deny them their dignity? No one would deny children who are helpless and constantly in need of assistance their personal dignity (Rentsch 1999).

What consequences can we draw from the practical and philosophical analyses discussed up to this point for medicine and the provision of healthcare? What are the consequences for the provision of medical assistance and care for the old and those suffering from dementia, for the discussion surrounding assisted suicide and euthanasia, and for the question of a public healthcare system? Firstly, there must be adequate caregivers for the old, the disabled, and children; a minimum number of caregivers should be legally required. Secondly, criteria for good treatment as well as for fair treatment must be clarified and institutionalized anew at appropriate intervals; this holds from a technical as well as from a legal perspective. Thirdly, patients should be permitted to determine their own care as far as possible. Fourthly, the management staff at healthcare facilities should possess expertise in medicine and care and not just in economics. Fifthly, an elaborate communication between patients, doctors, and caregivers is utterly necessary, and more time and money should be made available for this. And, sixthly, a revision of the rules for hospital services and costs should take place on a continuous and critical basis; otherwise there will be an oversupply of lucrative services and care will be offered only where it is essential. Furthermore, we have to avoid employing untrained caregivers, as they will most likely be overstrained. All responsible staff must be given training relevant to the specific form of assistance required (for example, loss of hearing). Only once these six central aspects have been wholeheartedly taken into consideration can new, sustainable answers be provided to difficult questions urgently in need of resolution, such as those surrounding assisted suicide and euthanasia (Cohen 2005; Greve and Staudinger 2006; Jochimsen 2010; Kontos 2005; Martin and Kontos 2013; Mol 2008). The finite constitution of meaning in the life-world is structured through interpersonal relationships. The singular totality of the specific, unique, personal, individual is constituted through communication and social interaction and can only come into its own and become itself in this way.

In conclusion, I would like to emphasize that a philosophical and ethical analysis shows that we must strive for *a new culture of ageing as well as of dying*. Ageing and dying are multifaceted and are far more complex processes than a universal ideology of feasibility suggests. It is a task for society as a whole to develop this new culture centered not on availability, but on human respect and care conveying solace and assurance. In order to enable this new culture, a project of education and clarification for society as a whole is required. This project of education and clarification has to begin with child-rearing and in school – much earlier than previously assumed. For when the reflection on finitude, mourning, and the reflexive look back at one's life – the process of finding meaning in the face of finitude – begins in an acute stage of dying, it has begun, by any measure, too late. Ageing and dying must be brought back into life.

References

Améry, J. 1968. *Über das Altern. Revolte und Resignation.* Stuttgart: Klett-Cotta.

Améry, J. 1999. *On Suicide: A Discourse on Voluntary Death*, translated by J. D. Barlow. Bloomington: Indiana University Press.

Aristotle. 1984. "Nicomachean Ethics." In *The Complete Works of Aristotle: The Revised Oxford Translation*, Vol. 2, edited by J. Barnes, 1729–1867. Princeton: Princeton University Press.

Bahr, E. 1998. *The Novel as Archive: The Genesis, Reception, and Criticism of Goethe's Wilhelm Meisters Wanderjahre*. Suffolk: Camden House.

Baltes, P. B., and J. Smith. 1990. "Towards a Psychology of Wisdom and Its Ontogenesis." In *Wisdom: Its Nature, Origins, and Developments*, edited by R. J. Sternberg, 87–120. Cambridge: Cambridge University Press.

Baltes, P. B., and U. M. Staudinger. 1993. "The Search for a Psychology of Wisdom." *Current Directions in Psychological Science* 2 (3):75–80. doi: 10.1111/1467-8721.ep10770914.

Callahan, D. 1995. *Setting Limits: Medical Goals in an Aging Society*. Washington, DC: Georgetown University Press.

Charlton, W. 1972. "Aristotle and the Principle of Individuation." *Phronesis* 17 (3):239–249. doi: 10.1163/156852872X00051.

Cohen, G. D. 2005. *The Mature of Mind: The Positive Power of the Aging Brain*. New York: Basic Books.

Daniels, N. 1988. *Am I My Parent's Keeper? An Essay on Justice between the Young and the Old*. Oxford: Oxford University Press.

Fishkin, J., and P. Laslett. 1992. *Philosophy, Politics, and Society, Sixth Series: Justice between Age Groups and Generations*. New Haven: Yale University Press.

Fukuyama, F. 2002. *Our Posthuman Future: Consequences of the Biotechnology Revolution*. New York: Farrar, Straus and Giroux.

Gehlen, A. 1988. *Man: His Nature and Place in the World*, translated by C. McMillan and K. Pillemer. New York: Columbia University Press.

Greve, W., and U. M. Staudinger. 2006. "Resilience in Later Adulthood and Old Age: Resources and Potentials for Successful Aging." In *Developmental Psychopathology*, 2nd ed., edited by D. Cicchetti and A. Cohen, 796–840. Hoboken: John Wiley & Sons.

Grey, A. de, and M. Rae. 2007. *Ending Aging: The Rejuvenation Breakthroughs That Could Reverse Human Aging in Our Lifetime*. New York: St. Martin's Press.

Harris, J. 2007. *Enhancing Evolution: The Ethical Case for Making Better People*. Princeton: Princeton University Press.

Jochimsen, M. 2010. *Careful Economics: Integrating Caring Activities and Economic Science*. Boston/Dordrecht/London: Springer Science and Business Media.

Kant, I. 1956. *Critique of Practical Reason*. Indianapolis: Library of the Liberal Arts.

Kierkegaard, S. 2000. *The Essential Kierkegaard*, edited by H. V. Hong and E. H. Hong. Princeton: Princeton University Press.

Kohlberg, L. 1981. *Essays on Moral Development*. San Francisco: Harper & Row.

Kontos, P. C. 2005. "Embodied Selfhood in Alzheimer's Disease: Rethinking Person-Centred Care." *Dementia* 4 (4):553–570. doi: 10.1177/1471301205058311.

Lesser, H. 2012. *Justice for Older People*. Amsterdam: Rodopi.

Lotringer, S., and P. Virilio. 1998. *Pure War*. Dunfermline: Better World Books.

Martin, W., and P. C. Kontos. 2013. "Embodiment and Dementia: Exploring Critical Narratives of Selfhood, Surveillance, and Dementia Care." *Dementia* 12 (3):288–302. doi: 10.1177/1471301213479787.

Meyer, S. S. 2008. *Ancient Ethics*. Abingdon/New York City: Routledge.

Mol, A. 2008. *The Logic of Care: Health and the Problem of Patient Choice*. London/New York: Routledge.

Nussbaum, M. C. 2001. *The Fragility of Goodness: Luck and Ethics in Greek Tragedy and Philosophy* (Revised edition). Cambridge: Cambridge University Press.

Piaget, J. 1978. *The Development of Thought*. Oxford: Blackwell.

Piven, J. S. 2004. *Death and Delusion: A Freudian Analysis of Mortal Terror*. Greenwich: Information Age Publishing.

Raz, J. 1994. *Ethics in the Public Domain: Essays in the Morality of Law and Politics*. Oxford: Clarendon Press.

Rentsch, T. 21999. *Die Konstitution der Moralität. Transzendentale Anthropologie und praktische Philosophie*. Frankfurt am Main: Suhrkamp.

Rentsch, T., and M. Vollmann, eds. 2012. *Gutes Leben im Alter. Die philosophischen Grundlagen*. Stuttgart: Reclam.

Rosa, H. 2003. "Social Acceleration. Ethical and Political Consequences of a Desynchronized High-Speed Society." *Constellations: An International Journal of Critical and Democratic Theory* 10 (1):3–33. doi: 10.1111/1467-8675.00309.

Rosa, H., ed. 2004a. *Fast Forward: Essays zu Zeit und Beschleunigung*. Hamburg: Edition Körber-Stiftung.

Rosa, H. 2004b. "Four Levels of Self-Interpretation: A Paradigm for Interpretive Social Philosophy and Political Criticism." *Philosophy & Social Criticism* 30 (5–6):691–720. doi: 10.1177/0191453704045761.

Schopenhauer, A. 1924. *Counsels and Maxims, Being the Second Part of Arthur Schopenhauer's Aphorismen zur Lebensweisheit*, translated by T. B. Sanders. London: George Allen & Unwin Ltd.

Sell, C., A. Lorenzini, and H. Brown-Borg. 2009. *Life-Span Extension*. New York: Humana Press.

Strawser, M. 1997. *Both/And: Reading Kierkegaard: From Irony to Edification*. New York: Fordham University Press.

Taylor, C. 2003. *The Ethics of Authenticity*. Cambridge/London: Harvard University Press.

Vincent, J. A. 2006. "Anti-Ageing Science and the Future of Old Age." In *The Future of Old Age*, edited by J. Vincent, C. Philipson, and M. Downs, 203–210. London: Sage.

Vincent, J. A. 2009. "Ageing, Anti-Ageing, and Anti-Anti-Ageing: Who Are the Progressives in the Debate on the Future of Human Biological Ageing?" *Medicine Studies* 1 (3):197–208. doi: 10.1007/s12376-009-0016-6.

Virilio, P. 2005. *City of Panic*. Oxford: Berg Publishers.

Wilde, O. 2005. *The Picture of Dorian Gray*, edited by L. M. Miller and J. Langham. Clayton: Prestwick House.

3 Third age and fourth age in ageing societies – divergent social and ethical discourses

François Höpflinger

Introduction

Quantitative changes in the age distribution of the population (demographic ageing) intervene with qualitative changes of attitudes, behaviors, and lifestyles among older men and women. The combination of new generations of elderly (baby boomers) and concepts of active ageing results in new dynamics in later life. Gerontological theories try to conceptualize these new developments by distinguishing between the 'young old' and the 'old old' or by differentiating between a third and fourth phase of life after retirement. The ambivalence of concepts such as 'young old' versus 'old old' illustrates the difficulties of dealing with historically new developments within ageing societies.

In this contribution, life situations, attitudes, and images emerging among the 'young old' and the 'old old' in central Europe are analyzed and discussed. The main research question is how far the increasingly popular concepts of 'young old' versus 'old old' are associated with significant divergence in social and ethical discourses for different phases of later life. Many of the trends mentioned are rapidly evolving, and some behavioral trends are observed only among a selective minority of elderly men and women. Therefore, some points of discussion indicate possible future developments and ethical challenges rather than empirically validated facts.

Societal changes within ageing societies

Ageing European societies are confronted with three major societal changes: First of all, low fertility and high life expectancy among the elderly population result in a strong demographic ageing – a development reinforced in many European countries by the ageing of the large birth cohorts of men and women born after World War II (baby boomers) who themselves had fewer children. While the demographic and social effects of low fertility on the age distribution have been extensively analyzed, the second dimension of demographic ageing – increasing life expectancy of older men and women – has been less discussed, to some extent because trends toward longevity have been underestimated (Höpflinger 2012). Not only do European societies have more retired citizens, but the retired men and women live much longer (resulting in recent discussions on the longevity risks of pension systems).

Second, as new birth cohorts (or generations) of men and women enter later phases of life, we observe significant changes in ageing processes. New birth cohorts of elderly are in many dimensions ageing differently from earlier birth cohorts. As a result of better education, new forms of family formation (and dissolution), and changing socio-economic conditions since the 1980s, the new generations of elderly have a different attitude regarding life after retirement. At least in some European countries, improved social security has reduced poverty rates among the elderly, and an increasing proportion of retired people remain healthy longer than in earlier generations (Unger 2016). Life perspectives regarding retirement and ageing are evolving in the direction of more active lifestyles, at least among healthy and affluent European retirees.

Third, new concepts of ageing have been developed, resulting in more positive and dynamic views on the chances of remaining healthy longer, of learning new things even at old age, and of being able to participate in new engagements after retirement. Individual ageing is no longer seen as a process one has to passively endure; it is seen as a process that can be actively shaped. Deficit-oriented concepts of ageing have been replaced by concepts of active or even successful ageing (Klott 2014). A radical consequence of these new developments is the emergence of anti-ageing medicine to prevent or to at least slow down biological ageing (Stuckelberger 2012).

Quantitative changes in the age distribution of the population are therefore linked with qualitative changes in lifestyles among older men and women (Karl 2012). Observations made for earlier cohorts of elderly are no longer valid for the elderly of today and tomorrow. At the moment, new forms of lifestyles after retirement are observed primarily among affluent groups of retired men and women, particularly in wealthy urban regions (Simpson 2015).

The trend toward a more active and 'youthful' life after retirement is an important countervailing factor to traditional concepts of demographic ageing. When men and women at age 70 have lifestyles that correspond to the lifestyles of much younger generations, demographic ageing does not lead to a socially or culturally ageing society. New socio-demographic approaches are therefore discussing how far traditional measurements of demographic ageing (defining people aged over 64 as belonging to the elderly population) are still valid. Measurements of demographic ageing based on prospective age and not chronological age result in much lower old-age dependency ratios, putting into perspective political discourses on the social problems of demographic ageing (Sanderson and Scherbov 2007, 2010).

In general, chronological age is a poor indicator for ageing processes, as people age differently depending on gender, economic status, biographical experiences, and health behavior. At the same time, men and women at age 65 are confronted with different life challenges and health problems than men and women at age 90 (even after controlling for cohort effects). Since the 1970s, this has resulted in distinguishing between at least two different types of older individuals. In this (heuristic) schema, the traditional notion of old age bifurcates between a new and rapidly expanding population of healthy and independent 'young old' (third age) and a frail or dependent population of 'old old' (fourth age).

The term 'young old' was first used by American gerontologist Bernice Neugarten (1974) and developed into an elaborate theory of a third age by Peter Laslett

(1989).[1] While the beginning of the third age is characterized by an important social transition (retirement), the more recent term 'fourth age' remains conceptually more ambivalent, as the start of the fourth age is not structurally defined (Kohli 2013). The concept of fourth age refers either to very old people aged over 80 or to frail or dependent old individuals (Baltes and Smith 2003; Lalive d'Epinay 1994). In recent discussions of the fourth age, the concept of frailty has been emphasized, and the transition from third to fourth age is characterized by decreasing functional health and increasing frailty (Lalive d'Epinay et al. 2008). The main advantage of such a conceptualization is the possibility of a clear empirical classification of people (Dapp et al. 2012). The disadvantage is a primarily deficit-oriented perspective of the fourth age (see Higgs and Gilleard in this volume).

The third age – the 'young old'

Life expectancy at age 65 has increased, and life after retirement has extended. In some countries, such as Germany and Switzerland, the gender gap in life expectancy at old age has decreased. More important for the emergence of a new third age is the fact that many men and women not only live longer but remain healthy longer, or at least without severe functional impairments. This reinforces the development of active lifestyles after retirement. More men and women remain able (and willing) to live a fulfilled and active life after retirement due to good functional health. The Austrian gerontologist Leopold Rosenmayr (1983) introduced the image of 'late freedom': being able to remain active without having to work within fixed employment structures.

National differences in socio-economic affluence, social welfare, and health systems result in significant inequalities in health expectancies at older age between European countries (Table 3.1) (see also Jagger et al. 2011).

Table 3.1 Life expectancy and healthy life expectancy at age 65 in selected European countries, 2013

	Women			*Men*		
	A	*B*	*B in % of A*	*A*	*B*	*B in % of A*
Austria	21.5	8.8	41%	18.2	8.9	49%
France	23.6	10.7	45%	19.3	9.8	51%
Germany	21.1	7.0	33%	18.2	7.0	38%
Great Britain	20.9	10.7	51%	18.6	10.6	57%
Italy	22.6	7.1	31%	18.9	7.7	41%
Spain	23.4	9.0	38%	19.2	9.7	51%
Sweden	21.3	13.8	65%	18.8	12.9	69%
Switzerland	22.4	14.2	63%	19.4	13.6	70%

A: Average life expectancy at age 65 in years.

B: Average healthy life expectancy at age 65: good health defined as absence of health-related functional limitations on everyday life.

Source: Eurostat (health statistics), for Switzerland: Federal office of statistics.

In Sweden and Switzerland, women and men aged 65 not only live for a relatively long time, but also in many cases remain healthy longer than, for example, in Italy, Spain, or Germany. In Germany, one can expect that the proportion of healthy retirees will increase, particularly as ageing white-collar workers with lower occupational hazards outnumber ageing blue-collar workers. Furthermore, the proportion of highly educated men and women in younger cohorts of the elderly is increasing, and with increasing educational attainment people generally stay healthy longer (Lampert, Kroll, and Dunkelberg 2007; Richter and Hurrelmann 2006; Valkonen 2006).

The data in Table 3.2 confirm that – with the exception of Poland and the Czech Republic – a majority of 55-to-74-year-olds define their subjective health as good. Most men and women aged 55 to 74 experience no functional impairments in their daily activities. Particularly good health values are observed in Sweden and Switzerland, two continuously affluent countries (not involved in the Second World War). However, in the Netherlands, Belgium, and Austria, about two-thirds of the 'young old' also define themselves as healthy.

An important factor underpinning active and healthy ageing is a good socio-economic situation. Looking at the socio-economic situation, large differences between and within countries exist. In Denmark, Sweden, and Switzerland, a majority of the 'young old' profit from a 'golden retirement.' In Germany and France, the picture is less positive. Less than 40 percent define themselves as affluent. In Southern and Eastern European countries, widespread poverty among the elderly is observed – a situation reinforced in some European regions by the recent economic crisis (Cavasso and Weber 2013). Economic conditions and health at old age are strongly interrelated. Comparing 28 European countries for the year 2012, a high positive correlation (r = 0.83) between the proportion of

Table 3.2 Health indicators and financial situation of people 55 to 74 years of age in selected European countries, 2014

	Subjective health good/very good	*Functional health intact**	*Living comfortably***
Austria	65%	69%	33% (N: 550)
Belgium	67%	68%	32% (N: 493)
Czech Republic	49%	58%	11% (N: 613)
Denmark	68%	69%	70% (N: 456)
France	56%	73%	36% (N: 436)
Germany	52%	63%	42% (N: 970)
Netherlands	68%	65%	52% (N: 611)
Poland	37%	52%	5% (N: 482)
Sweden	72%	64%	66% (N: 552)
Switzerland	77%	74%	60% (N: 431)

*Hampered in daily activities by illness/disability/infirmary/mental problem: no.

**Feelings about household income nowadays: living comfortably on present income.

Source: European Social Survey 2014 (weight data) European Social Survey Round 7 Data (2014). Norwegian Social Science Data Services, Norway – Data Archive and distributor of ESS data.

respondents with good subjective health and the proportion of respondents living comfortably is evident. Looking at individual data for Europe for 2012, we find a positive correlation (r = 0.39, N: 6914) between subjective health and feelings of living comfortably among elderly respondents aged 65 to 74. In many European countries, the concepts of active and healthy ageing are ideals primarily observed within an elite of affluent elderly, and only in few long-term affluent countries (such as Sweden, Switzerland, and the Netherlands) is active and healthy ageing experienced by a majority of new generations of older men and women.

In the context of new ideals of life after retirement, many of the 65-to-74-year-olds do not define themselves as being 'old' in the classical sense of deficit-oriented images of old age. A new trend is the fact that surprisingly many of the elderly respondents identify themselves with post-modern values such as creativity, spontaneity, and flexibility. Looking at the value of new ideas among younger and older respondents in some countries (such as France, Germany, Netherlands, and Switzerland), no age difference can be observed. To remain innovative and adaptive to new ideas is – at least on the level of attitudes – important for many European respondents, even at old age. New generations of the 'young old' emphasize a pattern of 'old and innovative' as a new frame of reference. The lower proportion of elderly people who find it important to try new and different things in life indicates that – at least for some men and women – new ideas do not necessarily mean new activities. As expected, there is a strong association between post-modern values and socio-economic situation, indicating that post-modern life values among the 'young old' are primarily concentrated among more affluent elderly men and women.

In recent debates, the orientation of new generations of elderly toward an active lifestyle has been linked to a new ethics on ageing: Healthy ageing is possible

Table 3.3 Post-modern values at higher ages in selected European countries, 2014

	*New ideas**		*New activities***	
Age:	*15–34*	*55–74*	*15–34*	*55–74*
Austria	64%	50%	53%	30%
Belgium	51%	50%	57%	39%
Czech Republic	59%	45%	53%	30%
Denmark	59%	67%	55%	37%
France	55%	59%	46%	42%
Germany	61%	61%	50%	41%
Netherlands	56%	52%	50%	36%
Poland	56%	42%	55%	40%
Sweden	59%	53%	46%	32%
Switzerland	66%	67%	61%	46%

*Important to think new ideas and being creative: % like me, very much like me.

**Important to try new and different things in life: % like me, very much like me.

Source: European Social Survey 2014 (weight data) European Social Survey Round 7 Data (2014). Norwegian Social Science Data Services, Norway – Data Archive and distributor of ESS data.

and should be promoted and perhaps even enforced. If people can learn to remain healthy and active even at old age, then they have an individual and social responsibility to remain healthy and active. The moral change from 'can' to 'must' is not yet final, but the new ethics of active, healthy, and successful ageing, particularly among the 'young old,' become more forceful as the perceived challenges of demographic ageing – for example, for health costs – become more salient (van Dyk and Lessenich 2009). In the same sense, processes of healthy ageing underscore socio-economic arguments to increase retirement age.

Fourth age – the 'frail old'

The construction of a fourth age, as well as the differentiation between 'young old' and 'old old,' is an attempt to transcend traditional demographic classifications based on chronological age. Chronological age definitions have been replaced by functional concepts of age. In some debates, the fourth age has been explicitly defined as a phase of increasing frailty, as well as higher risk of functional dependency in basic and instrumental daily activities (Lalive d'Epinay et al. 2008). Other definitions of the fourth age include concepts of increasing vulnerability, high risk of cognitive impairment, and the limits of individuals' and medicine's ability to combat ageing processes (Motel-Klingebiel, Ziegelmann, and Wiest 2013).

Within an intergenerational perspective, the fourth age has been associated with the loss of peers and the perception of living within a society dominated by much younger generations (Höpflinger 2011). Old age is inevitably associated with the loss of friends and confidants within the same generation and with the death of a spouse. Widowhood is perceived as a critical life event in old age (Perrig-Chiello et al. 2016). The combination of higher life expectancy and younger age at marriage has the effect that at old age, more women experience widowhood than men. In Germany for example, in 2011, 64 percent of all women aged 80 or over were widows, compared to 30 percent of men (Nowossadeck and Engstler 2013). On the other hand, the birth of grandchildren or even great-grandchildren can result in a widening of family relationships. However, even for highly socially integrated old men and women, one fact of life becomes more and more salient: They live in a society clearly dominated by much younger generations, and they lose more and more of their peers in their age cohort – a process that can result in a feeling of intergenerational isolation.

The risks of negative health developments resulting in functional dependency and cognitive impairments (such as dementia) increase at old age. Frail and vulnerable old men and women are dependent on a barrier-free environment, an elaborate care system, or sheltered housing (Albrecht 2011; Höpflinger and van Wezemael 2014). Adapted housing conditions and care systems are even more important for old people afflicted by functional impairment or dementia. The fourth age also remains determined by socio-economic differences. End-of-life analysis illustrates that better educated old men and women are less affected by functional limitations during their last year of life than less educated individuals (who at the same time do not live as long) (Andersen-Ranberg et al. 2008).

Table 3.4 Dependence on care and prevalence of dementia by age group

Proportion in need of care for basic daily activities					
Age	*70–74*	*75–79*	*80–84*	*85–89*	*90+*
Germany (2013)	5%	10%	21%	38%	64%
Switzerland (2014)	4%	6%	13%	26%	54%
Prevalence of dementia					
European countries (2009)	4%	7%	16%	26%	43%

Source: Prevalence of dementia: EuroCoDe 2009, In need of care: Switzerland: Höpflinger, Bayer-Oglesby, and Zumbrunn 2011, adapted to 2014 Germany: Pflegestatistik 2013.

Table 3.4 shows the proportion of people in Germany and Switzerland in different age groups who are dependent on care in basic activities of daily life and the prevalence of dementia. Whereas in Germany, only a tenth of people aged 75 to 79 need care, these proportions increase to a fifth of those aged 80 to 84 and nearly two-fifths of those aged 85 to 89. Today, most men and women aged 90 or over depend on the care of younger generations. In Switzerland – due to higher healthy life expectancy – the proportions are lower, but at age 90 and over, most people are in need of care.

At very old age, most people are affected by health problems, but not all become functionally dependent. Karen Andersen-Ranberg (2001) entitled her contribution on centenarians 'Healthy centenarians do not exist, but autonomous centenarians do.' Nonetheless, in actual social discussions and professional debates, the fourth age is generally perceived as characterized by social losses, vulnerability, frailty, and dependency (while the third age is increasingly seen as a phase of new competences and activities). The 'old old' are thought to be affected by functional and cognitive deficits. The greatest social fear of old age is dementia, and the loss of cognitive functions is perceived as a major risk of the fourth age.

Divergent social and ethical discourses for different phases of later life?

Whether two divergent cultures of ageing and two specific social policies toward a third and a fourth age in life are emerging is open to discussion, particularly as many new socio-cultural developments are at an early stage or are observed only among selected, affluent groups of older men and women. Regarding social policies, there is in fact a certain tendency toward a differentiation between two main policies for the elderly. One policy aims at activating the healthy elderly toward a positive contribution to society – for example, as experienced professionals or senior experts, to compensate for a demographically shrinking workforce, but also as participants in voluntary work and intergenerational projects (Kubisch and Störkle 2016). Some of the social policies toward an active and productive ageing intend to engage healthy elderly people in helping frail or dependent old ones – a strategy seen as part of a new solidarity pact of the 'young old' for the 'old old.' A second policy concentrates on improving the care system for the very old, on strengthening the independence of frail old persons, or on securing the dignity of people affected by dementia. Within a policy for the 'old old,' the immigration of care professionals is seen as one possible strategy to compensate for demographically induced gaps in family or professional care systems. In the same sense, a lot of energy is spent on inventing technologies that compensate for functional impairments. When ethics of participation and empowerment are considered, the social policy toward the fourth age deals primarily with functional deficits, while new social policies toward healthy retirees emphasize the potentials and experience of the elderly.

As the boundaries between the 'third age' and the 'fourth age' vary individually and are constantly changing, there is a lot overlapping of concepts and definitions, giving room to social and ethical discussions on ageing that have no final solutions. Thus, rather than clear-cut social and ethical conflicts within an ageing society, we have a permanent ambivalence between an achievement-oriented culture of ageing (for the 'young old') and a culture of dealing with the limits of human life for the 'old old.'

In this context, two general trends are noticeable: First, the emphasis on competence-oriented concepts of ageing has resulted not in less deficit-oriented perspectives on age, but simply in changing the time segment of 'old age.' Traditional cultural images of old age are deferred in time, as retirement is no longer the start of old age. 'Real old age' begins later, when functional impairments affect daily life. Many retired persons consider themselves to not be 'really old' as long as they live at home without extensive help (Graefe, van Dyk, and Lessenich 2011, 304). Second, the emergence of a healthy phase of retirement, oriented toward new activities or at least continuing previous activities, is to some extent reinforcing fears about old age. Individualistic independence after retirement constitutes a social and cultural contrast to (assumed and real) dependency at old age. Adapting to functional and cognitive impairments seems to be more difficult after a long period of healthy ageing; becoming dependent on the care of others is more difficult to accept after a long history of independent living. The positive developments among the 'young old' highlight the contrast to the challenges of old age. In any case, it is conspicuous that the positive re-evaluation of the 'young old' – who are increasingly perceived as socially and politically forceful and active men and women – contrasts with more negative attributes associated with the 'old old.' German gerontologist Ludwig Amrhein (2013) poses the thesis that the social upgrading of the third age is complementary to a social devaluation of the fourth age. While the 'young old' are perceived as active subjects, the 'old old' are still primarily seen as passive objects in need of help and care.

From a social and ethical point of view, there are valid reasons to criticize this simple but increasingly popular taxonomy of later stages of life. Recent studies demonstrate valid possibilities for successful ageing even for very old individuals, questioning the purely negative concepts of the fourth age (Gondo, Nakagawa, and Masui 2013). A comparison of two cohorts of German centenarians indicates positive cohort changes even at old age (Jopp et al. 2013). Personally, I am not convinced that it will be possible to redefine the fourth age in a more positive frame of reference – at least not in the next decade. The main social trend is to delay the onset of frail and dependent age as long as possible. The – in a first phase heuristic – taxonomy of different phases of age has become a metaphor of the ongoing social and medical reconstruction of ageing processes. The ever more powerful pro-ageing industry promoting healthy and productive ageing among affluent baby boomers is partly legitimated by emphasizing deficit-oriented reference groups. Or, to put it more bluntly: The promised 'heaven' of a third age is not marketable without referring to the dark sides of the fourth age.

Note

1 The concept of third age was first practically applied in 1975 in Lyon (France) when the first university of the third age (université du troisième âge) was founded.

References

Albrecht, P.-A., ed. 2011. *ServiceWohnen als Zukunftsaufgabe einer alternden Gesellschaft.* Berlin: Berliner Wissenschafts-Verlag.

Amrhein, L. 2013. "Die soziale Konstruktion von 'Hochaltrigkeit' in einer jungen Altersgesellschaft." *Zeitschrift für Gerontologie und Geriatrie* 46 (1):10–15. doi: 10.1007/s00391-012-0459-3.

Andersen-Ranberg, K., J. M. Robine, M. Thinggaard, and K. Christensen. 2008. "What Has Happened to the Oldest Old SHARE Participants after Two Years?" In *First Results from the Survey of Health, Ageing and Retirement in Europe (2004–2007)*, edited by A. Börsch-Supan, A. Brugiavini, H. Jürges, A. Kapteyn, J. Mackenbach, J. Siegrist, and G. Weber, 66–73. Mannheim: Mannheim Research Institute for the Economics of Aging.

Andersen-Ranberg, K., M. Schroll, and B. Jeune. 2001. "Healthy Centenarians Do Not Exist, but Autonomous Centenarians Do: A Population-Based Study of Morbidity among Danish Centenarians." *Journal of the American Geriatrics Society* 49 (7):900–908. doi: 10.1046/j.1532-5415.2001.49180.x.

Baltes, P. B., and J. Smith. 2003. "New Frontiers in the Future of Aging: From Successful Aging of the Young Old to the Dilemmas of the Fourth Age." *Gerontology* 49 (2):123–135. doi: 10.1159/000067946.

Cavasso, B., and G. Weber. 2013. "The Effect of the Great Recession on the Wealth and Financial Distress of 65+ Europeans." In *ASGREC: Active Ageing and Solidarity Between Generations in Europe*, edited by A. Börsch-Supan, M. Brandt, H. Litwin, and G. Weber, 28–36. Berlin: De Gruyter.

Dapp, U., J. Anders, S. Golgert, W. von Renteln-Kurse, and C. E. Minder. 2012. "Ressourcen und Risiken im Alter. Die LUCAS-I-Marker zur Klassifizierung älterer Menschen als Fit, pre-FRAIL und FRAIL. Validierung und erste Ergebnisse aus der Longitudinalen Urbanen Cohorten-Altersstudie (LUCAS)." *Zeitschrift für Gerontologie und Geriatrie* 45 (4):262–270. doi: 10.5167/uzh-63972.

Dyk, S. van, and S. Lessenich, eds. 2009. *Die jungen Alten. Analysen zu einer neuen Sozialfigur*. Frankfurt am Main: Campus.

EuroCoDe, European Collaboration on Dementia. 2009. *Prevalence of Dementia in Europe. Workpackage 7/06. Final Report, 7. Aug. 2009* (mimeo.).

Gondo, Y., T. Nakagawa, and Y. Masui. 2013. "A New Concept of Successful Aging in the Oldest Old: Development of Gerotranscendence and Its Influence on the Psychological Well-Being." *Annual Review of Gerontology and Geriatrics* 33 (1):109–132. doi: http://dx.doi.org/10.1891/0198-8794.33.109.

Graefe, S., S. van Dyk, and S. Lessenich. 2011. "Altsein ist später. Alter(n)snormen und Selbstkonzepte in der zweiten Lebenshälfte." *Zeitschrift für Gerontologie und Geriatrie* 44 (5):299–305. doi: 10.1007/s00113-012-2224-x.

Höpflinger, F. 2011. "Die Hochaltrigen – eine neue Grösse im Gefüge der Intergenerationalität." In *Hochaltrigkeit, Herausforderung für persönliche Lebensführung und biopsychosoziale Arbeit*, edited by H. G. Petzold, E. Horn, and L. Müller, 37–53. Wiesbaden: VS Verlag für Sozialwissenschaften.

Höpflinger, F. 2012. *Bevölkerungssoziologie. Eine Einführung in demographische Prozesse und bevölkerungssoziologische Ansätze*. Weinheim: Beltz Juventa.

Höpflinger, F., L. Bayer-Oglesby, and A. Zumbrunn. 2011. *Pflegebedürftigkeit und Langzeitpflege im Alter. Aktualisierte Szenarien für die Schweiz*. Bern: Huber.

Höpflinger, F., and J. van Wezemael, eds. 2014. *Wohnen im höheren Lebensalter. Grundlagen und Trends. Age Report III*. Zürich: Seismo.

Jagger, C., C. Weston, E. Cambois, H. V. Oyen, W. Nusselder, G. Doblhammer, J. Rychtarikavo, J.-M. Robine, and the EHLAIS team. 2011. "Inequalities in Health Expectancies at Older Ages in the European Union: Findings from the Survey of Health and Retirement in Europe (SHARE)." *Journal of Epidemiology and Community Health* 65 (11):1030–1035. doi: 10.1136/jech.2010.117705.

Jopp, D. S., C. Rott, K. Boerner, K. Boch, and A. Kruse. 2013. *Zweite Heidelberger Hundertjährigen-Studie: Herausforderungen und Stärken des Lebens mit 100 Jahren*. Stuttgart: Robert Bosch Stiftung.

Karl, F., ed. 2012. *Das Altern der "neuen" Alten. Eine Generation im Strukturwandel des Alters*. Münster: Lit-Verlag.

Klott, S. 2014. "Theorien des Alters und des Alterns." In *Lehrbuch Gerontologie. Gerontologisches Fachwissen für Pflege- und Sozialberufe – eine interdisziplinäre Aufgabe*, edited by S. Becker and H. Brandenburg, 37–74. Bern: Hans-Huber.

Kohli, M. 2013. "Alter und Altern der Gesellschaft." In *Handwörterbuch zur Gesellschaft Deutschlands*, edited by S. Mau and N. Schöneck, 11–23. Wiesbaden: Springer VS.

Kubisch, S., and M. Störkle. 2016. *Erfahrungswissen in der Zivilgesellschaft. Eine rekonstruktive Studie zum nachberuflichen Engagement*. Wiesbaden: Springer VS.

Lalive d'Epinay, C. 1994. "La construction sociale des parcours de vie et de la vieillesse an Suisse au cours du XXe siècle." In *Le poids des ans. Une histoire de la vieillesse en Suisse romande*, edited by G. Heller, 127–150. Lausanne: Editions d'en bas.

Lalive d'Epinay, C., and D. Spini (eds.). 2008. *Les années fragiles. La vie au-delà de quatre-vingts ans*. Quebec: Presse de l'université Laval.

Lampert, T., L. E. Kroll, and A. Dunkelberg. 2007. "Soziale Ungleichheit der Lebenserwartung in Deutschland." *Aus Politik und Zeitgeschichte* 42:11–18.

Laslett, P. 1989. *A Fresh Map of Life: The Emergence of the Third Age*. London: Weidenfeld and Nicolson.

Motel-Klingebiel, A., J. P. Ziegelmann, and M. Wiest. 2013. "Hochaltrigkeit in der Gesellschaft des langen Lebens. Theoretische Herausforderung, empirisches Problem und sozialpolitische Aufgabe." *Zeitschrift für Gerontologie und Geriatrie* 46 (1):5–9. doi: 10.1007/s00391-012-0458-4.

Neugarten, B. L. 1974. "Age Groups in American Society and the Rise of the Young-Old." *Annals of the American Academy of Political and Social Science* 415 (1):187–198.

Nowossadeck, S., and H. Engstler. 2013. *Familie und Partnerschaft im Alter: Report Altersdaten* 3. Berlin: Deutsches Zentrum für Altersfragen.

Perrig-Chiello, P., S. Spahni, F. Höpflinger, and D. Carr. 2016. "Cohort and Gender Differences in Psychosocial Adjustment to Later-Life Widowhood." *Journals of Gerontology, Series B: Psychological and Social Sciences* 71 (4):765–774. doi: 10.1093/geronb/gbv004.

Richter, M., and K. Hurrelmann, eds. 2006. *Gesundheitliche Ungleichheit. Grundlagen, Probleme, Perspektiven.* Wiesbaden: VS Verlag für Sozialwissenschaften.

Rosenmayr, L. 1983. *Die späte Freiheit. Das Alter – ein Stück bewusst gelebten Lebens.* Berlin: Severin und Siedler.

Sanderson, W. C., and S. Scherbov. 2007. "A New Perspective on Population Aging." *Demographic Research* 16 (2):27–58. doi: 10.4054/DemRes.2007.16.2.

Sanderson, W. C., and S. Scherbov. 2010. "Remeasuring Aging." *Science* 329 (5997):1287–1288. doi: 10.1126/science.1193647.

Simpson, D. 2015. *Young-Old: Urban Utopias of an Aging Society.* Zürich: Lars Müller.

Stuckelberger, A. 2012. *Le guide des médecines anti-âge. De la prévention aux traitements.* Lausanne: Editions Favre.

Unger, R. 2016. "Lebenserwartung in Gesundheit. Konzepte und Befunde." In *Handbuch Bevölkerungssoziologie*, edited by Y. Niephaus, M. Kreyenfeld, and R. Sackmann, 565–594. Wiesbaden: Springer VS.

Valkonen, T. 2006. "Social Inequalities in Mortality." In *Demography: Analysis and Synthesis*. Vol. 2, edited by G. Caselli, J. Vallin, and G. Wunsch, 195–206. Amsterdam: Elsevier.

4 The nature of the fourth age as a challenge to ageing societies

Paul Higgs and Chris Gilleard

Introduction

Conventionally, the sociology of old age has treated the final stage of the life course as a 'residual category' of social and health policy, a category that affords little autonomy from the structuring processes of modernist institutions and individual biographies (Macnicol 2015, 20). As such, it has received relatively little sociological theorizing. In recent decades this *lacuna* has been challenged both by the 'de-standardization' of the life course and the emergence of the third age (Brückner and Mayer 2005; Gilleard and Higgs 2008). This latter development has been the subject of a number of theoretical formulations, which have established it as a way of understanding some of the coordinates of contemporary later life (Carr and Komp 2011; Weiss and Bass 2002). Relatively less attention, however, has been paid to the other constituent part of the re-articulation of old age, namely the 'fourth age.' Although this phenomenon has its roots in traditional discourses surrounding the dependency and decline of old age, in contemporary circumstances it has become much more than a final stage of life. In the context of the agentic cultures of the third age, giving rise to longer, healthier, and more productive later lives as well as their associated lifestyles, the fourth age acts as a 'social imaginary' for a feared old age of decline, dependency, and social death. The impact of this social imaginary of the fourth age is not confined to any section of society but can be observed on people of all ages, from the young who seek to minimize any signs of potential ageing to the retired who wish to show that they are still capable of the agency that marks out their active participation in the third age. In part, this is recognition of the fact that those who come to be ascribed as being in this category have passed into a position of 'ageing without agency' and are deemed through social and health policies to be sequestered from everyday life (Gilleard and Higgs 2010).

The argument of this chapter is that whereas old age was once a relatively uncomplicated residual category that could be used to embrace all old people, in contemporary society, the unity of later life has been fragmented. Old age does not disappear, however, but re-emerges in a more concentrated form as a fourth age of dependency and infirmity. In this chapter, we will point out that the fourth age is not a social institution or structure but exists as a social imaginary. We will be drawing on the work of the theorist Cornelius Castoriadis (1997), using his ideas regarding the nature of social imaginaries to position the fourth age as an example of one such imaginary. By utilizing this framework, we distinguish between the kind of 'apocalyptic demography' based on chronological age (Robertson 1997) and approaches that focus on social attributions and cultural interpretations of the 'challenge' that is widely assumed to confront ageing societies.

The changing nature of later life

Most societies are ageing as a consequence of rising life expectancy and falling fertility. The number of people reaching retirement age is growing. This has led governments in many countries to implement a variety of social policies to address these changes; these include reforming pension systems as well as changing the eligibility criteria for state retirement pensions. The specifics vary from country to country, and there is a continuing debate about what are the most appropriate policies to follow (Hyde and Higgs 2016). More significant for the purposes of this chapter, however, is not the policy responses of governments but the profound transformation of old age into what can be better described as 'later life,' often represented as the 'new' ageing (Gergen and Gergen 2000; Torres-Gil 1992). Central to this transformation have been the changes to the institutionalized life course, with its once stable divisions between education, work, and retirement. The emergence of a differentiated consumer society allowing for individual distinction and the construction and re-construction of lifestyle has since the 1960s resulted in a very different terrain on which new forms of post-working life have been established. This has been noted by a number of social theorists, who have put different slants on what has changed or why (Bauman 2000; Beck 1992; Schulze 1997).

Within the sociology of old age, a gradual awareness of these changes has slowly emerged. Social gerontology has shifted from being oriented in large part toward social administration to becoming much more conversant with, and engaged by, the 'cultural turn' in the social sciences (Twigg and Martin 2015). This has manifested in the growth of cultural gerontology and the development of approaches focusing around the emergence of a third age (see Höpflinger in this volume). The third age is typically represented as a more expansive experience of later life than that previously outlined by accounts centered upon the 'structured dependency' of older people or the political economy of ageing (Phillipson 1982; Townsend 1981; Walker 1981). The concept of the third age is now extensively debated, and while there has been considerable resistance to accepting that the incomes, lives, and health of older people have improved substantially, there is now more general recognition that on the whole, the majority of the retired population in the West are not the most 'residualized' individuals in society (Phillipson 2015). In fact, older people have generally weathered the recessions of the early 21st century better than the young (Grech 2015; Higgs and Gilleard 2015a; Jenkins et al. 2012). This transformation in the material circumstances of the older population has fueled talk of generational conflict, at least among some political commentators (Higgs and Gilleard 2010). Whatever the interpretations made of the phenomenon, there is a general awareness that the majority of the older population have in current circumstances escaped their status as a residual category of social policy.

This has meant that the idea of old age as a unitary category defined by lack and dependency is no longer sustainable. Old age/later life has been fragmented into a multiplicity of lifestyles and locations, leading to a divergence of concerns, interests, and needs. The category of retirement, which was earlier fashioned as a mainly male exit from the labor market (on the grounds of potential ill health and declining productivity), has been transformed into a complex and more potentially fulfilling period of life, largely disconnected from the previously overshadowing notions of economic dependency and fragile health. This has underpinned the culture of the third age and the related concepts of active, productive, and successful ageing (Gilleard and Higgs 2011a). As health and relative affluence have become aspirations increasingly realized by successive cohorts of retirees in the developed economies of the world, some have begun warning that such aspirations serve only as a denial of the difficulties still experienced by many older people and the profound challenges to health facing societies growing ever older (Grenier 2012; Komp 2011; Lloyd et al. 2014).

If the third age suggests the possibility of a later life removed from the limitations of ill health, how does the connection between ageing, illness, and impairment re-enter the equation? That there is a profound link between these phenomena has been at the heart of most social policies focusing on old age (Gilleard and Higgs 2011a). In contemporary Western society, the emergence of the third age has removed many older people from a social position defined by their health status. The fading of the once modern idea that one medical specialty – geriatric medicine – could be responsible for all the health issues faced by older people is one particular consequence of this change. This has led to some positing that if there is a third age for some, is there a 'fourth age' for others? If this is the case, what defines this fourth age, and how might such a concept help us understand the changing nature of later life? Some have argued, for example, that concepts such as the fourth age are used primarily to divide up the older population in ways that are inimical particularly to the more vulnerable members of the older population 'excluded' from the cultures of the third age (Bury 1995). We would argue that in much the same way that the third age has a number of different formulations, we need to be aware that the fourth age, too, can be understood in a variety of ways. The implications of these differing approaches throw light on important features of ageing societies, such as the creation of new as well as the maintenance of older divisions in later life.

Modeling the fourth age

Discussing the nature of the fourth age is a complex issue because, although the term is of recent origin, it has very old roots. There are three broad approaches that can be discerned in the literature on the topic. The first sees the fourth age principally in population terms and focuses on the increase of those who have been termed 'the oldest old' as a proportion of the population aged over 60. Drawing on a well-established tradition of dividing the life course into different stages (Burrow 1986; Sears 1986), this 'stages of life' framework is built on an older distinction between a 'vital,' 'green,' or 'mature' old age, which is contrasted with a subsequent 'decrepit' or 'senile' old age, prefiguring mortality. Although pre-modern use of this 'two stages of old age' approach varied widely in the choice of a particular chronological age used to distinguish between the stages, contemporary accounts have located the point between them as being around age 75, with more recent writers taking it to be 80 or even 85. This division echoes a distinction first made by American sociologist Bernice Neugarten (1974) when she divided the older population into 'the young old' (those aged 55 to 74) and 'the old old' (those aged 75 and older). In this formulation, the fourth age is assumed to be a stage of life associated with the 'old' old, whose oldness is marked by the distinctions of chronology.

The second approach is organized more by reference to disability and frailty than by chronology. This articulation emphasizes the distinction between infirmity and able-bodiedness in later life. Again, such views can be traced back into history, particularly the early modern tradition of distinguishing between the 'deserving' and the 'undeserving poor.' The former were those whose poverty reflected their inability to fend for themselves in the light of unchosen circumstances, while the latter those whose situation was seen to be of their own doing (or lack of action). Along with orphans and widows, the old and infirm constituted the bulk of the deserving poor, those who were entitled to be provided with alms and charity, while other groups such as the 'idle beggars' had less of a claim. In later centuries, these groups would become recipients of more formal systems of poor relief that were organized under the rubric of the 'poor laws' (Higgs and Gilleard 2015b). Within the newly emerging welfare states of the 20th century, this distinction became more carefully delineated. Documented chronological age formed the basis for retirement pensions, while 'chronic sickness/infirmity' served as the criterion for determining access to healthcare and social services (Gilleard and Higgs 2011b). This latter distinction elevated infirmity – or 'frailty,' as it is now designated – to serve as the point of distinction around which the idea of a fourth age would eventually congeal. In this model, frailty and infirmity define the fourth age. This position has been combined with the earlier 'demographic' delineation to define the fourth age as "very old age, or the fourth age, [. . .] usually seen as the age of vulnerability and frailty" (Kruse and Schmitt 2015, 133).

A third model focuses less upon the individual's length of life and more on their proximity to death. It treats the fourth age as a period of 'terminal decline.' Terminal decline theories assume that during the last years of life a process of general mental and physical decline that is distinct from the general trajectory of ageing is initiated (Kleemeier 1962; Riegel and Riegel 1972). Palmore and Cleveland have outlined it in the following way:

> The essence of this theory is that many human functions are not primarily related to chronological age as such but tend to show marked decline prior to

> death during a period ranging from a few weeks to a few years. A corollary is that normal aged persons are able to maintain most of their functions on a fairly stable level until they enter the terminal decline phase shortly before death. The theory assumes that whatever combination of genetic and environmental factors causes death also causes the marked decline in functions prior to death.
>
> (Palmore and Cleveland 1976, 76)

The 'theory' of terminal decline was initially concerned with decline in cognitive functioning. In more recent years, it has grown to include a more extensive list of functions, including subjective health and well-being (Gerstorf et al. 2013). Given the expansiveness of such functional decline, some researchers have chosen to put forward a 'two stage' model of human ageing, differentiating between a longer 'pre-terminal' phase of relative stability and a shorter, more acute period of 'terminal' decline, lasting from a few years to as long as a decade (Bäckman and MacDonald 2006; Gerstorf and Ram 2015). Within this framework, the 'pre-terminal' phase is viewed as being capable of modification, while the terminal phase is considered relatively fixed and directed more clearly toward death (Gerstorf et al. 2013).

Theorizing the fourth age as a distinct life stage

Although the term 'the fourth age' is not present in the works of key writers such as Bernice Neugarten and Robert Kleemeier, their views on old age nevertheless depend on the premise that there is a binary opposition operating within later life: that there is a 'good' against a 'bad' old age, that there is a 'successful' against an 'unsuccessful' form of ageing. This latter distinction – successful versus unsuccessful ageing – was first outlined by Rowe and Kahn (1987) in their seminal paper on 'usual' versus 'successful' ageing. In their paper, they sought to take issue with "a gerontology of the usual" (Rowe and Kahn 1987, 143) by highlighting the differences between 'normal' ageing as disease-free and healthy and 'ageing as usual' with its accompanying 'natural' decline. It has been pointed out that there is a tendency to merge 'usual' with 'successful' in subsequent discussion, which has had the effect of representing ageing as usually successful, with pathological or unsuccessful ageing being treated as the exception to this general rule (Strawbridge, Wallhagen, and Cohen 2002). As a result, research examining the prevalence of 'successful' ageing has produced varying estimates of its 'normality' among community samples of older adults from as low as 0.4 percent to as high as 95.0 percent (Depp and Jeste 2006).

In addition, a further issue needs to be addressed when thinking of the fourth age primarily as a life stage. If there is indeed a divide in the nature of old age, is it possible to state what exactly constitutes the alternative outcome to 'successful ageing'? For Rowe and Kahn, it was not failure but 'normal' or 'usual' ageing. Gradually, however, a different and more pessimistic image has come into focus, that of failed age and frail old people. While Kahn acknowledged that there was a risk that those seen as not ageing successfully could be seen as "unsuccessful and therefore as failing," he also thought that such categorization reflected much more the American cultural values of "succeed-or-fail" (Kahn 2002, 726) than it did the inevitable outcome of proposing a concept such as successful ageing. This has not convinced more critical writers, who have contended that models of successful ageing "have been and continue to be criticized for being most applicable to the relatively healthy 'third age' of life or 'young old' populations and not to the 'fourth age' or the 'oldest old' which comes with significant constraints in functional capacity, frailty, and psychological losses, and limited effectiveness of interventions" (Flatt et al. 2013, 947).

Although this precise terminology may not have existed previously, the division between the third and fourth ages can be discerned to be widespread in an immanent form. The term itself – 'the fourth age' – was brought into the wider gerontological community by the English historian Peter Laslett, in his book *A New Map of Life* (Laslett 1989, 1996). Significantly, and in line with the work of Rowe and Kahn, Laslett's book was not really about 'deep' old age. His concern instead was to put forward an argument for the existence of a more positive 'third age,' which could function as the 'crown of life' rather than life's decline (Laslett 1989, 1996). His introduction of a 'terminal' fourth age was meant to serve as a sharp contrast with the third age. Laslett's fourth age follows the third as a transition, one that he sees as "greater than either of the previous life course transitions"; from childhood to adulthood or from adulthood to the third age. Framing it as a period "of dependence and decrepitude" (Laslett 1996, 192–194), he delineates the fourth age as "the onset of final decline," when individuals become "passengers or encumbrances" within society (Laslett 1996, 194). By exalting the opportunities of a successful third age, Laslett, like Rowe and Kahn, ended up inadvertently drawing out the failures of the fourth. As if to sum up this view, the only positive suggestion he could make was that future generations develop the wisdom better to manage the transition or, preferably, learn how to defer it as long as possible.

A somewhat different approach to the fourth age has been followed by German psychologist Paul Baltes, whose research was concerned particularly with intellectual change over the life course. Much of his earlier work argued against the notion that there was a universal necessary decline in mental and behavioral competence over the adult life course (Baltes 1987; Baltes and Baltes 1990; Baltes and Schaie 1976). In his later work, he became more convinced that there were limits to the plasticity of mental and behavioral competence. Adopting a more explicit 'stages of life' approach, he wrote:

> For the younger-old, those in the Third Age, the prospects seem bright [. . .] modern societies have the potential to create a better future for the younger of the older ages and [. . .] empower individuals to become 'successful agers' [but] for most of the older-old however the prospects are not so bright. From my point of view 'hope with a mourning band' may be the motto best suited to this situation. [. . .] As demographers celebrate each month gained in the

lives of the oldest-old, researchers focused on improving quality of life worry about the associated increase in the gap between longevity and vitality.

(Baltes 2006, 38)

Baltes and Smith (1999, 2003) argued that there were important differences in the capacities and adaptability of people before and after the age of 80. This difference manifested as an increased dependency on culture and society, as well as a reduced capacity to benefit from them. Risk of adverse outcomes increased significantly after this age, while the potential to deal with disease, dysfunction, and external stress was greatly diminished.

Following on from this, Baltes therefore ended up utilizing a chronologically bound 'stages of life' model that contended that there are qualitative as well as quantitative differences between the periods of later life. At the same time, he introduced a variant of the terminal-decline model to define these differences. In a similar fashion to the position developed by Laslett, he used the trope of a final decline as a predictable life-course trajectory that is unlikely to be halted or overcome and that involves decline across multiple domains as his general model. This differs from those who put forward a simple model of the deleterious consequences of chronic or degenerative diseases such as arthritis, dementia, or heart disease. These diseases of later life may constrain ill health to particular areas or organ systems, but by implication each degenerative disease remains open to effective intervention and 'recovery,' whereas for Baltes this is unlikely. In this sense, the Baltes approach could be said to be similar to that of Linda Fried's model of frailty, namely an age-related syndrome of multi-system failure that is distinct from disease and disability itself and that in turn leads toward 'an end stage' that is "irreversible and presage[s] death" (Fried et al. 2001, 154).

The fourth age as a social imaginary

Although Laslett (and to some extent Baltes) have sought to frame the fourth age as a stage of 'late' late life defined by its chronology, others have pursued the idea that a qualitative change takes place in later life that is linked not with years lived but rather with closeness to death; it is this latter association that brings about 'frailty' and 'failure.' In an approach located in sociology rather than psychology or biomedicine, Gilleard and Higgs (2010; Higgs and Gilleard 2015b) have proposed viewing the fourth age in a very different light, seeing it as a cultural or social imaginary framed by the experience of decline and the deterioration present in later life. This term, the 'social imaginary,' is borrowed from French theorist Cornelius Castoriadis (1997). Castoriadis argued that all social structures possess a central imaginary, situated "on the level of elementary symbols or of global meaning," that link their functional role with their symbolic form. "[E]very society," he writes, "posits a 'view of itself' which is at the same time a 'view of the world' [. . .] [which] is part of its truth or its reflected reality [. . .] without being reducible to it" (1997, 39). Social structures therefore can only be understood through the organization or network of signifiers and signified that is held within the social imaginary. Just as the life course as a whole can be conceived as a social structure, in the sense of the 'institutionalized' life course (Kohli 2007), so can its stages and segmentations (Gilleard and Higgs 2013).

Rather than assuming anything directly about the fourth age as either an interior condition or as a social fact, Gilleard and Higgs argue that the fourth age is fashioned by the meanings attributed to old age rather than by any particular set of biological, demographical, or psychological indicators. These meanings have their historical roots in pre-modern distinctions between seniority and senility; between the sturdy and the infirm, and between a ripe and a rotten old age. In modern times, they have taken on a distinctly new resonance as contemporary influences have reshaped this imaginary, leading to the emergence and success of third-age cultures. These cultures, as we have noted, reflect a concern with lifestyle as well as the embedding of a consumerist habitus across the life course (Gilleard and Higgs 2011a, 2011c). Through the promotion and consumption of various products and practices, mid-life individuals are offered the chance of remaining participants in third-age lifestyles as long as they want to, and these engagements continue well after retirement (Higgs 2012). Accompanying the imperatives of choice, autonomy, self-expression, and pleasure that are associated with third-age culture, Gilleard and Higgs (2010; Higgs and Gilleard 2015b) have argued, lies a fear or distaste of unacceptable ageing – of ageing without agency – that itself serves as one of the drivers toward such consumerism. This habitus of active consumption is promoted by the market and the state, often as a recipe for avoiding real, costly old age (Jones and Higgs 2010).

The cultures of the third age, Gilleard and Higgs argue, help sustain the belief in two types of ageing – one that permits a lifestyle unhampered by the unwanted, undesirable aspects of age associated illness and impairment, the other a fourth age in which irremediable frailty and irreversible disease is realized. This distinction, of a 'real' old age that lies beneath the surface of 'normal' or 'usual' old age, is one acknowledged by many old people themselves. Degnen's (2007) anthropological research into ageing in a Northern English community notes the "distinctions made by older people themselves about the boundaries and distinctions between 'real' and 'normal' old age. While a great deal of physical change and a certain amount of shifts in mental states are accommodated in older people's notions of normal ageing, the most important gauge of the onset of real old age is a decline in mental acuity and related shifts in comportment" (Degnen 2007, 79).

Gilleard and Higgs have consequently argued that the fourth age can be most usefully understood as an imagined boundary within later life, a social divide internalized by older people themselves, as well as by health and welfare professionals, the state and the market (Higgs and Gilleard 2015b). It represents a line of fracture that embodies more than simple chronology, disease, and disability, drawing upon a long cultural history of distinguishing between the good and the bad sides of ageing (Minois 1989). However, as a result of the cultures of 'successful' ageing becoming much more influential in setting the aspirations of later life in contemporary society, these darker aspects of 'real' old age have become a new social and cultural terrain on which the future of old age is contested and its identity marginalized once more (Kruse and Schmitt 2015, 133). But what exactly constitutes this fourth-age imaginary, and how might it be socially realized?

Dimensions of the social imaginary of the fourth age

Four components constitute the axes for a social imaginary of the fourth age in Gilleard and Higgs' work. These are frailty, abjection, the loss of agency, and care (Higgs and Gilleard 2015b). Frailty can be seen as the equivalent of infirmity and is used in a similar fashion to the historical category of the 'aged and infirm.' Frailty includes both mental and physical infirmity as well as the idea of a material and moral vulnerability. The second aspect of the fourth-age imaginary is that of abjection. Abjection is embodied within those aspects of infirmity that society finds most distasteful; it constitutes what could be said to be the fourth age's material and moral repugnancy. Still, abjection carries a number of different connotations. It reflects, in part, membership of a social location (a category of person), but it is considerably more than that. It also reflects the inability of a person to look after himself or herself and is compounded by its capacity to elicit further disgust through the evident incapacity of the aged infirm person to recognize his or her inabilities. This, in turn, leads to an inability for the individual to assert himself or herself as a potential agent; to be the agent and representative of his or her own inabilities, a position of subjectivity that has been achieved in the disability-rights movement.

Frailty and abjection imply not just social distancing – social exclusion – but also and equally elicit a moral responsibility for the care of those so categorized. Such a moral responsibility is not unique to the fourth age; it has long existed alongside the need to provide aid to other equally deserving groups whose vulnerabilities have also been acknowledged, *inter alia* widows and orphans, the deaf and the blind, and, to use the terminology of the time, 'the halt and the lame.' These are all categories of the 'impotent poor.' The 'moral imperative of care' underlying care in the fourth age, however, creates a paradox. Care both shapes and is shaped by the fourth-age imaginary. Whether provided informally by family and friends or formally by public or private institutions, care is both a response to, and a definer of, need. It involves narratives and practices that can work together or creates ones that can lead to conflict and contradiction. In the circumstances of advanced old age, care is therefore carried out within the shadow of the fourth age and often continued through into its deepest shadows, at the end of an individual's life.

Agency (or rather the loss of agency) serves as the fourth vector framing the social imaginary of the fourth age. In many ways, the concepts of agency, identity, and personhood represent key elements sustaining the habitus of the third age, with its emphasis upon autonomy and choice, individual distinction, and lifestyle. Threats to the free exercise of autonomy and agency and the possibility of exclusion from the arenas of choice and distinction constitute perhaps the essential vulnerabilities associated with becoming 'abject' or 'frail' and with being assigned to the category of the fourth age. Most of the social movements of the 1960s emphasized identity and youth; but equally they emphasized choice and voice, being a voice that demanded to be heard. The loss of agency, of identity, casts those with neither voice nor choice into a position of exclusion and marginality – a kind of dark matter, whose presence is felt but never identified, what has been described as akin to the 'black holes' of deep space identified by astronomers through the effects of their gravitational pull on other celestial bodies (Gilleard and Higgs 2010). While the market and the marketized state privilege choice and voice, such 'third age' rhetoric sits uneasily with the circumstances of those enveloped by the fourth age's imaginary.

Implications of the fourth age

Out of these different ways of understanding the fourth age, there emerge different challenges for ageing societies, in terms of both policy and personal experience. For Laslett's model, the key issues were how to compress morbidity and foster the progressive rectangularization of the life course (Fries 1980, 2003). This could include support for measures to shorten the fourth age, ranging from the promotion of advance directives to the legalization of assisted dying. For Baltes' model, there is a need for instituting the revision of lifestyles based upon the optimizing of what can be optimized and the minimization of what is lost, early in old age, all the while preparing for the worst. This position (similar to that of the terminal-decline model) implicitly recognizes the importance of long-term-care insurance and the value of effective palliative care toward the end of life. It supports the development of mid-life healthcare checks that can promote interventions in mid-life, where the chances of effecting change are greatest. For Gilleard and Higgs, there is the need to confront the social realization of the fourth-age imaginary while seeking to support and sustain the possibilities of extending the cultures of the third age across the potential barriers of class, community, and cohorts (Higgs and Gilleard 2016). This might involve greater investment in long-term care in order to improve access, quality, and variety. While others have argued that the possibilities of civic engagement in the fourth age need to be promoted, such proposals confuse chronology with capacity (Kruse and Schmitt 2015). Being aged 80 or 90 does not automatically draw down the shadows of the fourth age. Likewise, others have argued that severe infirmity is no automatic barrier to the realization of a citizenship modeled on that of the disability movement (O'Connor and Nedlund 2016). However, those exemplifying such a position often need to reconstruct the basis of citizenship in order to make the principles work (Sonnicksen 2016). In such reconstructions, old connections are lost and new hierarchies are established.

Although each approach might lead to some difference in policy emphases, they share a number of themes that simultaneously recognize the impossibility of maintaining a common framework to improve the experience and opportunities of everyone in later life. It is little use to employ "a third age rhetoric for a fourth age reality" (Gilleard and Higgs 1998); equally it is unhelpful to insist upon a state determined 'active' old age shaped as a kind of antidote to the state-structured dependency of old age (Gilleard and Higgs 2000). Working life arguably is, and will continue to be, the principal arena from which third-age cultures and the opportunities they promise can be established. This is as true in terms of how the different factors maintaining post-work income and expenditure are likely shared between employers, employees, the state, and the market as it is for the material underpinning that the cultures of the third-age need in order to thrive. As pension policy continues to evolve and change, it is therefore particularly important that the failures of the state, and not just the market, are compensated for if the benefits of third-age cultures are to be as widely shared as is possible. Although this is a much debated and contested topic, it is not the object of this chapter. Rather, our focus is on the implications that flow from the discourses of the fourth age, however conceptualized. These are often quite different. Here, the emphasis is less upon personal income, benefits, and pension accrual and more on care, services, families, and households.

What then constitutes the particular challenges posed by the fourth age? We would argue that over the course of the 20th century, and particularly in its second half, much policy and professional rhetoric was aimed at removing the scandal of the alms-house, the workhouse, and the poor law infirmary. All had the intention to put an end to the exclusion of the old poor and sick from good-quality healthcare and social services. Despite much investment in medicine, nursing, and social care, the shadows of the fourth age, we would argue, have once again darkened and deepened the scene. Where once the aged poor feared entering the workhouse, now the fear is of ending up in a nursing home with Alzheimer's disease (Gilleard and Higgs 2011d). The fourth age has become considerably more widespread, although it is no less abject. Long-term care remains the Cinderella service, where the lowest paid and least resourced battle to sustain the dignity of life's ending. Although palliative care services are extending their remit from a particular concern with cancer, they have yet to engage more fully with the dilemmas posed by mental infirmity, personal incapacity, and complex multi-morbidity toward the end of life.

It needs to be recognized that although a fourth age is by no means a universal prospect, this does not mean that it is optional for society. To make its presence less inevitable means challenging what constitutes good care, investing in care at the deep end, and focusing research on remediating, not simply measuring, frailty. Most importantly, research and policy should be directed at preventing, reducing, or mitigating the impact of infirmity, preventing the abjection both of those who work in and those who receive long-term care, and finally focusing upon the subjectivities of old, infirm, and impaired people rather than concocting narratives of their potential agency (Higgs and Gilleard 2016). Although there are good reasons to believe that the financial impoverishment of later life is being progressively minimized within our ageing societies, the impoverishment brought about by the fourth-age imaginary will prove a much harder nut to crack. It is one of the biggest challenges facing our ageing societies; in the end, it may not be possible fully to realize such a goal. That requires an acknowledgment that for some people, some of the time, the fourth age will have to serve as a haven when the effort of living otherwise is simply too great.

References

Bäckman, L., and S. W. S. MacDonald. 2006. "Death and Cognition: Synthesis and Outlook." *European Psychologist* 11 (3):224–235. doi: 10.1027/1016-9040.11.3.224.

Baltes, P. B. 1987. "Theoretical Propositions of Life-Span Developmental Psychology: On the Dynamics between Growth and Decline." *Developmental Psychology* 23 (5):611–626. doi: 10.1037/0012-1649.23.5.611.

Baltes, P. B. 2006. "Facing Our Limits: Human Dignity in the Very Old." *Daedalus* 135 (1):32–39. doi: 10.1162/001152606775321086.

Baltes, P. B., and M. M. Baltes. 1990. "Psychological Perspectives on Successful Aging: The Model of Selective Optimization with Compensation." In *Successful Aging: Perspectives from the Behavioral Sciences*, edited by P. B. Baltes and M. M. Baltes, 1–34. Cambridge: Cambridge University Press.

Baltes, P. B., and J. Smith. 1999. "Multilevel and Systemic Analyses of Old Age: Theoretical and Empirical Evidence for a Fourth Age." In *Handbook of Theories of Aging*, edited by V. L. Bengston and K. W. Schaie, 153–173. New York: Springer Publishing.

Baltes, P. B., and K. W. Schaie. 1976. "On the Plasticity of Intelligence in Adulthood and Old Age: Where Horn and Donaldson Fail." *American Psychologist* 31 (10):720–725. doi: 10.1037/0003-066X.31.10.720.

Baltes, P. B., and J. Smith. 2003. "New Frontiers in the Future of Aging: From Successful Aging of the Young Old to the Dilemmas of the Fourth Age." *Gerontology* 49 (2): 123–135. doi: 10.1159/000067946.

Bauman, Z. 2000. *Liquid Modernity*. Cambridge: Polity.

Beck, U. 1992. *Risk Society: Towards a New Modernity*. London: Sage.

Brückner, H., and K. Mayer. 2005. "The De-Standardization of the Life Course: What It Might Mean? And If It Means Anything, Whether It Actually Took Place?" *Advances in Life Course Research* 9:27–54. doi: 10.1016/S1040-2608(04)09002-1.

Burrow, J. A. 1986. *Ages of Man: A Study in Medieval Writing and Thought*. Oxford: Clarendon Press.

Bury, M. 1995. "Ageing, Gender and Sociological Theory." In *Connecting Gender and Ageing: A Sociological Approach*, edited by S. Arber and J. Ginn, 15–30. Buckingham: Open University Press.

Carr, D. C., and K. Komp, eds. 2011. *Gerontology in the Era of the Third Age: Theory, Research and Critique*. New York: Springer.

Castoriadis, C. 1997. *The Imaginary Institution of Society*. Cambridge: Polity.

Degnen, C. 2007. "Minding the Gap: The Construction of Old Age and Oldness Amongst Peers." *Journal of Aging Studies* 21 (1):69–80. doi: 10.1016/j.jaging.2006.02.001.

Depp, C. A., and D. V. Jeste. 2006. "Definitions and Predictors of Successful Aging: A Comprehensive Review of Larger Quantitative Studies." *The American Journal of Geriatric Psychiatry* 14 (1):6–20. doi: 10.1097/01.JGP.0000192501.03069.bc.

Flatt, M. A., R. A. Settersten, R. Ponsaran, and J. R. Fishman. 2013. "Are 'Anti-Aging Medicine' and 'Successful Aging' Two Sides of the Same Coin? Views of Anti-Aging Practitioners." *The Journals of Gerontology, Series B: Psychological Sciences and Social Sciences* 68 (6):944–955. doi: 10.1093/geronb/gbt086.

Fried, L. P., C. M. Tangen, J. Walston, A. B. Newman, C. Hirsch, J. Gottdiener, T. Seeman, R. Tracy, W. J. Kop, G. Burke, and M. A. McBurnie. 2001. "Frailty in Older Adults: Evidence for a Phenotype." *The Journals of Gerontology, Series A: Biological Sciences and Medical Sciences* 56 (3):M146–M156. doi: 10.1093/gerona/56.3.M146.

Fries, J. F. 1980. "Aging, Natural Death, and the Compression of Morbidity." *New England Journal of Medicine* 303 (3):130–135.

Fries, J. F. 2003. "Measuring and Monitoring Success in Compressing Morbidity." *Annals of Internal Medicine* 139 (5 Part 2):455–459. doi: 10.7326/0003-4819-139-5_Part_2-200309021-00015.

Gergen, K. J., and M. M. Gergen. 2000. "The New Aging: Self Construction and Social Values." In *The Evolution of the Aging Self: The Societal Impact on the Aging Process*, edited by R. W. Schaie and J. Hendricks, 281–306. New York: Springer.

Gerstorf, D., and N. Ram. 2015. "A Framework for Studying Mechanisms Underlying Terminal Decline in Well-Being." *International Journal of Behavioral Development* 39 (3):210–220. doi: 10.1177/0165025414565408.

Gerstorf, D., N. Ram, U. Lindenberger, and J. Smith. 2013. "Age and Time-to-Death Trajectories of Change in Indicators of Cognitive, Sensory, Physical, Health, Social, and Self-Related Functions." *Developmental Psychology* 49 (10):1805–1821. doi: 10.1037/a0031340.

Gilleard, C., and P. Higgs. 1998. "Old People as Users and Consumers of Healthcare: A Third Age Rhetoric for a Fourth Age Reality?" *Ageing & Society* 18 (2):233–248. doi: 10.1017/S0144686X98006904.

Gilleard, C., and P. Higgs. 2000. *Cultures of Ageing: Self, Citizen, and the Body*. Harlow: Pearson Education.

Gilleard, C., and P. Higgs. 2008. "The Third Age and the Baby Boomers: Two Approaches to the Social Structuring of Later Life." *International Journal of Ageing and Later Life* 2 (2):13–30. doi: 10.3384/ijal.1652-8670.072213.

Gilleard, C., and P. Higgs. 2010. "Aging without Agency: Theorizing the Fourth Age." *Aging & Mental Health* 14 (2):121–128. doi: 10.1080/13607860903228762.

Gilleard, C., and P. Higgs. 2011a. "The Third Age as a Cultural Field." In *Gerontology in the Era of the Third Age*, edited by D. Carr and K. Komp, 33–49. New York: Springer.

Gilleard, C., and P. Higgs. 2011b. "Frailty, Disability and Old Age: A Re-Appraisal." *Health* 15 (5):475–490. doi: 10.1177/1363459310383595.

Gilleard, C., and P. Higgs. 2011c. "Consumption and Aging." In *Handbook of Sociology of Aging*, edited by R. A. Settersten and J. L. Angel, 361–375. New York: Springer.

Gilleard, C., and P. Higgs. 2011d. "Ageing Abjection and Embodiment in the Fourth Age." *Journal of Aging Studies* 25 (2):135–142. doi: 10.1016/j.jaging.2010.08.018.

Gilleard, C., and P. Higgs. 2013. "The Fourth Age and the Concept of a 'Social Imaginary': A Theoretical Excursus." *Journal of Aging Studies* 27 (4):368–376. doi: 10.1016/j.jaging.2013.08.004.

Grech, A. G. 2015. "Convergence or Divergence? How the Financial Crisis Affected European Pensioners." *International Social Security Review* 68 (2):43–62. doi: 10.1111/issr.12065.

Grenier, A. 2012. *Transitions and the Lifecourse: Challenging the Constructions of "Growing Old."* Bristol: Policy Press.

Higgs, P. 2012. "Consuming Bodies: Zygmunt Bauman on the Difference between Fitness and Health." In *Contemporary Theorists for Medical Sociology*, edited by G. Scambler, 20–32. London: Routledge.

Higgs, P., and C. Gilleard. 2010. "Generational Conflict, Consumption and the Ageing Welfare State in the United Kingdom." *Ageing & Society* 30 (8):1439–1451. doi: 10.1017/S0144686X10000425.

Higgs, P., and C. Gilleard. 2015a. *Key Social and Cultural Drivers of Changes Affecting Trends in Attitudes and Behaviour Throughout the Ageing Process and What They Mean for Policymaking*. London: Government Office for Science.

Higgs, P., and C. Gilleard. 2015b. *Rethinking Old Age: Theorising the Fourth Age*. London: Palgrave Macmillan.

Higgs, P., and C. Gilleard. 2016. "Interrogating Personhood and Dementia." *Aging & Mental Health* 20 (8):773–780. doi: 10.1080/13607863.2015.1118012.
Hyde, M., and P. Higgs. 2016. *Ageing in a Global Era: The Spatialities of Later Life*. Bristol: Policy Press.
Jenkins, S. P., A. Brandolini, J. Micklewright, and B. Nolan, eds. 2012. *The Great Recession and the Distribution of Household Income*. Oxford: Oxford University Press.
Jones, I. R., and P. F. Higgs. 2010. "The Natural, the Normal and the Normative: Contested Terrains in Ageing and Old Age." *Social Science & Medicine* 71 (8):1513–1519. doi: 10.1016/j.socscimed.2010.07.022.
Kahn, R. L. 2002. "Guest Editorial: On 'Successful Aging and Well-Being: Self-Rated Compared with Rowe and Kahn'." *The Gerontologist* 42 (6):725–726.
Kleemeier, R. W. 1962. "Intellectual Changes in the Senium." *Proceedings of the American Statistical Association* 1:290–295.
Kohli, M. 2007. "The Institutionalization of the Life Course: Looking Back to Look Ahead." *Research in Human Development* 4 (3–4):253–271. doi: 10.1080/15427600701663122.
Komp, K. 2011. "The Political Economy of the Third Age." In *Gerontology in the Era of the Third Age*, edited by D. Carr and K. Komp, 51–66. New York: Springer.
Kruse, A., and E. Schmitt. 2015. "Shared Responsibility and Civic Engagement in Very Old Age." *Research in Human Development* 12 (1–2):133–148. doi: 10.1080/15427609.2015.1010353.
Laslett, P. 1989. *A Fresh Map of Life*. London: Weidenfeld & Nicolson.
Laslett, P. 1996. *A Fresh Map of Modern Life*. London: Macmillan.
Lloyd, L., M. Calnan, A. Cameron, J. Seymour, and R. Smith. 2014. "Identity in the Fourth Age: Perseverance, Adaptation and Maintaining Dignity." *Ageing & Society* 34 (1):1–19. doi: 10.1017/S0144686X12000761.
Macnicol, J. 2015. *Neoliberalising Old Age*. Cambridge: Cambridge University Press.
Minois, G. 1989. *History of Old Age: From Antiquity to the Renaissance*. Cambridge: Polity.
Neugarten, B. L. 1974. "Age Groups in American Society and the Rise of the Young-Old." *The Annals of the American Academy of Political and Social Science* 415 (1):187–198. doi: 10.1177/000271627441500114.
O'Connor, D., and A. C. Nedlund. 2016. "Editorial Introduction: Special Issue on Citizenship and Dementia." *Dementia* 15 (3):285–288. doi: 10.1177/1471301216647150.
Palmore, E., and W. Cleveland. 1976. "Aging, Terminal Decline, and Terminal Drop." *Journal of Gerontology* 31 (1):76–81. doi: 10.1093/geronj/31.1.76.
Phillipson, C. 1982. *Capitalism and the Construction of Old Age*. London: Macmillan.
Phillipson, C. 2015. "The Political Economy of Longevity: Developing New Forms of Solidarity for Later Life." *The Sociological Quarterly* 56 (1):80–100. doi: 10.1111/tsq.12082.
Riegel, K. F., and R. M. Riegel. 1972. "Development, Drop, and Death." *Developmental Psychology* 6 (2):306–319. doi: http://dx.doi.org/10.1037/h0032104.
Robertson, A. 1997. "Beyond Apocalyptic Demography: Towards a Moral Economy of Interdependence." *Ageing and Society* 17 (4):425–446. doi: 10.1017/S0144686X97006521.
Rowe, J. W., and R. L. Kahn. 1987. "Human Aging: Usual and Successful." *Science* 237 (4811):143–149. doi: 10.1126/science.3299702.
Schulze, G. 1997. "From Situations to Subjects: Moral Discourse in Transition." In *Constructing the New Consumer Society*, edited by P. Sulkunen, J. Holmwood, H. Radner, and G. Schulze, 38–57. Basingstoke: Palgrave Macmillan UK.

Sears, E. 1986. *The Ages of Man: Medieval Interpretations of the Life Cycle*. Princeton: Princeton University Press.

Sonnicksen, J. 2016. "Dementia and Representative Democracy: Exploring Challenges and Implications for Democratic Citizenship." *Dementia* 15 (3):330–342. doi: 10.1177/1471301216638998.

Strawbridge, W. J., M. I. Wallhagen, and R. D. Cohen. 2002. "Successful Aging and Well-Being Self-Rated Compared with Rowe and Kahn." *The Gerontologist* 42 (6):727–733. doi: 10.1093/geront/42.6.727.

Torres-Gil, F. M. 1992. *The New Aging: Politics and Change in America*. New York: Auburn House Publishing.

Townsend, P. 1981. "The Structured Dependency of the Elderly: A Creation of Social Policy in the Twentieth Century." *Ageing & Society* 1 (1):5–28. doi: 10.1017/S0144686X81000020.

Twigg, J., and W. Martin. 2015. "The Challenge of Cultural Gerontology." *The Gerontologist* 55 (3):353–359. doi: 10.1093/geront/gnu061.

Walker, A. 1981. "Towards a Political Economy of Old Age." *Ageing & Society* 1 (1):73–94. doi: 10.1017/S0144686X81000056.

Weiss, R. S., and S. A. Bass, eds. 2002. *Challenges of the Third Age: Meaning and Purpose in Later Life*. New York: Oxford University Press.

Part 2

Perspectives and problems of old age in the context of medicine and healthcare

5 Old age, potentials, and vulnerability

Andreas Kruse

Introduction: key themes

This contribution considers a differentiated view of old age and, in so doing, addresses different perspectives. The first one is the view that still dominates today, namely the interpretation of age as a primarily physical process – this needs to be replaced by highlighting the simultaneity of physical losses and the potential mental and spiritual growth processes. Here then, another perspective is developed which understands ageing as a psycho-spiritual process. In it, the burden on the individual, brought about by physical ageing with its ensuing limitations and losses, is not denied. However, physical ageing should not be seen as the salient feature of ageing. If one were to focus solely on physical processes, the potential wealth that can unfold in the ageing process would be overlooked and lost.

In this context, it therefore seems appropriate to refer to the integration of two perspectives: the perspective of potential and the perspective of vulnerability. On one hand, this expresses the fact that we cannot simply take the mental and spiritual development in the ageing process as a 'given' fact; rather, it is the result of a successful interaction between an individual who is open to mental and spiritual processes and a socio-cultural environment that offers a sufficient level of ideas and thus has a positive effect on the development of potential and self-realization. On the other hand, it expresses that not only must we interpret physical development in old age in terms of multi-morbidity and functional impairment, but also we need to develop a more comprehensive approach, particularly due to the morphogenesis that takes place in the ninth decade of life and that increases human susceptibility to diseases. This is why the restitution and compensation capacity recognizably declines – it is a normal biological event. We do not live infinitely, because of our limited cell-division capacity, but also due to the fact that, during the course of our lives, more and more damage occurs in our cells, as well as in our DNA (our genetic material), thus ensuring our lifetime is limited. In addition, at an advanced age, we are confronted with biological limits; wanting to 'remove' these would really be rather naive.

However, we must not underestimate the fact that we can make significant contributions to *designing* physical ageing – as well as cognitive and emotional ageing – by means of health promotion, disease prevention, and rehabilitation.

The capacity for self-design needs to be considered explicitly in all the theories of ageing. This statement constitutes a *cantus firmus* in this contribution. Self-design is also reflected in the potential and the efforts of the individual to gain a growing understanding of himself or herself (self-understanding). A review of one's biography, as well as the anticipation of the future – in which limitations and finitude become ever more important – and the assumption of responsibility not just for oneself, but also for other people, are processes that repeatedly trigger the question of one's own identity.

The processes of self-understanding are of particular importance when old people find themselves in borderline situations, such as when faced with serious physical illness, dementia, or the loss of loved ones. In this contribution, an examination of borderline situations (also from a perspective of potential output and growth) is to be undertaken, as well as a more detailed analysis of the emotional, motivational, and cognitive processes of dementia. It will also be shown that dementia is not associated with the loss of *all* cognitive resources: Emotional and perception-related resources remain for a long time. In addition, particularly important processes and points in the biography have a subjective effect long into the dementia – in the sense of 'islands of the self.'

The complexity of ageing – also of ageing when ill – requires a society and culture that is aware of this complexity and is able to offer differentiated responses to it. For this reason, at the end of this contribution – after a number of statements on the anthropology of age have been made – questions are asked regarding the essential features of an age-friendly culture.

Potential and vulnerability in old age

Population ageing does not necessarily imply inevitable decreases in societies' competitiveness or decreases in intergenerational solidarity, but current demographic change does contribute to an increasing societal (and also scientific) interest in the possible contributions of older generations to the development and cohesion of society. The respective question refers to both an individual and a societal perspective: to actual and future resources and potentials of older people, as well as to societal conditions necessary for developing, expanding, and realizing the potentials of older people.

The psychological consideration of old age elucidates three potentials in this phase of life (Kruse 2014). The first is introspection or self-reflection – that is, an in-depth grappling of the person with himself or herself allowing for new insights and a more profound understanding of the self; the second is openness – that is, the susceptibility to new impressions, experiences, and insights that may result from a new view of himself or herself, as well as from the surrounding social and spatial world; and, finally, the third is generativity – that is, the conviction that the individual has a place in the succession of generations and has to assume responsibility within this succession.

More and more limitations and the finiteness of one's own existence enter the center of experience, and this requires concentrated, in-depth self-analysis

(Erikson 1998). This expresses, on one hand, one's knowledge about life and the knowledge of the individual gained from the biography; on the other hand, this knowledge about life, as well as the individual's self-knowledge, is differentiated. The individual's in-depth analysis of himself or herself is promoted by openness to new impressions, experiences, and insights (Randall 2013). This openness is paraphrased in psychological literature as the concept of 'cathectic flexibility,' which is expressed in old age, especially in the 'transcendence of the body,' and in very old age in the 'transcendence of the self' (Peck 1968). In contrast, cathectic impoverishment is associated with a significantly reduced sensitivity to emotional, mental, and social processes; the person is 'trapped in the body' and unable to experience meaning and connectedness within a chain of generations (Ardelt et al. 2013). A need for 'symbolic immortality' – that is, to invest resources and potentials into things that outlive the self – is conceptualized as a significant motivator in old age (Blumenberg 1986; Tornstam 2005).

Cultural demand for generativity can change substantially over time. Against the background of demographic change, interest in the possibilities and preconditions of development and effective use of strengths and potentials of old age has grown worldwide. However, generativity is prompted not only by society, and not only societies benefit from generative action. Inner desire, as a second motivational source of generativity, refers to two complementary basic human needs: a 'need to be needed' (that is, to have meaningful relations to others) and a need for 'symbolic immortality' (to invest resources and potentials into things that outlive the self) (McAdams and de St. Aubin 1992). The aforementioned motivational sources of generativity are reflected in two further facets of generativity: a conscious concern for the next generation and a commitment to take responsibility for the next generation. The translation of concern and commitment into generative action depends on what has been described as "belief in the species" (Erikson, Erikson, and Kivnick 1986) – that is, "to place hope in the advancement and betterment of human life in succeeding generations, even in the face of the strong evidence of human destructiveness and deprivation" (McAdams and de St. Aubin 1992). Moreover, generativity is conceived within the larger context of the life-story theory of adult identity (McAdams 2013). From this perspective, adults construct and try to live out a 'generativity script' that not only reflects past generative action, but also is important for current generative concerns and commitments, as well as an understanding of what is worth outliving the self and what can and should be transmitted to others through generative efforts.

The potential perspective expressed here – which describes not only an individual, but also a social potential – is to expand by a perspective of vulnerability that primarily affects the physical features but at the same time can affect brain functions. The organism's vulnerability increases in significance particularly at very old age, from the middle of the ninth decade of life.

Susceptibility to a growing number of diseases, a growing number of physical symptoms – polypathy – the probability of needing care, and a notably increased risk of dementia are all seen in the ninth and tenth decade of life. At a very old age, people regularly report that they no longer feel in control of their own bodies; they complain about a growing number of symptoms, as well as fluctuations in their physical condition and sometimes also in their cognitive ability.

Very old age – which we understand as beginning at about the middle of the ninth decade of life – is not genetically encoded. That is, it is not in our DNA, our genetic material. In addition, it should be considered that our DNA's ability for genetic control becomes increasingly more restricted due to an accumulation of damage. One consequence is the reduced protection of our bodies against noxa and disease: Very old people cannot fight diseases and degenerative processes as well as they could in younger years; they become bio-genetically increasingly vulnerable.

This *modus deficiens* – to borrow a term from medieval Jewish-Arabic doctor Moshe ben Maimon – demands an increasing degree of activation, stimulation, and motivation from the social, spatial, and institutional environment; it requires a growing number of supportive participatory structures, and it needs a barrier-free environment as a preventative measure.

Very old people are particularly dependent on good medical treatment, rehabilitation, and care. With the measures mentioned, we help compensate for the *modus deficiens*, the increased vulnerability at very old age, and better protect the elderly.

As we age, our increasing loss of biological protection and our decreasing genetic control demand greater social and cultural protection. The elderly, with their physical vulnerability, are a special responsibility, a challenge for society. In the middle of the ninth decade of life, significant changes occur in our physical and cognitive parameters, reminding us of a morphological change of the whole organism. This is accompanied by a growing vulnerability in terms of physical and organic brain disease – which does not mean that all elderly people will suffer severe physical and cognitive losses; this generalization must be ruled out (Bano and Benbow 2010; Huxhold, Fiori, and Windsor 2013; Shmotkin et al. 2013). However, the probability of such losses does increase detectably, and this can be deduced by the fact that, in the ninth decade of life, chronic physical diseases, as well as the various forms of dementia, are significantly more likely. What needs to be considered here is that it is precisely *this* advanced age that is showing a remarkable demographic dynamic; it is here that we are finding the steepest population growth.

In Western European countries today, 5.5 percent of the population is over 80 years. By the year 2040, this figure will be more than 12 percent. This means that we have to increasingly concern ourselves not just with vulnerability, but also with the transience and finitude of human existence. We must find cultural forms of dealing with this borderline situation in order to support people in accepting these borders and to realize their potential for self-design in these borderline situations – a big social and cultural task, and indeed a political one. Furthermore, population ageing implies a *real gain* for society from a psychological and existential perspective, and both aspects need to be considered when we think about age and society.

Self-understanding and self-design as a challenge and a developmental potential in old age

Following the lifespan developmental theory of Erikson, establishing ego integrity in the context of life review is an indispensable task at the end of human life; if people do not succeed in confronting this task, they are expected to suffer from despair and feelings of weariness toward their own lives. This last psycho-social crisis is initiated by changes in older people's situation at the end of life and is reinforced further by social demand. Ego integrity is conceptualized as a positive ending point of the lifelong development of identity. Reaching ego integrity implies being able to accept one's life as a whole, including lost opportunities and unfulfilled aspirations and expectations.

Re-configurations of the self can become subject to renegotiation in old age for several reasons. From a sociological perspective, cohort flow implies changing age structures, changes in individual ageing processes, and – more basically, as considered by German (later British) philosopher and sociologist Karl Mannheim in the late 1920s – new approaches to understanding the self, the world, and society. From the tradition of psychoanalysis, it has been argued that defense mechanisms might lose effectiveness in old age; others have argued that age-related impairments and losses can force people to give up "protective illusions" (Filipp 1999). 'Reality' is inevitably ambiguous; specific events and developments do not have a definite significance for re-configurations of the self but are selected from a multitude of possible relevant events and developments, which, moreover, can be interpreted and evaluated in very different ways. As a consequence, basic assumptions of our understanding of the self and the world can be challenged by critical life events and experiences.

The potential for self-reflection in old age is very nicely expressed in a poem by romantic writer Josef von Eichendorff, who lived from 1788 to 1857, and who, incidentally, spent one year studying law at the University of Heidelberg.

> My God, I give thanks to you that you, for me, beyond all the treetops bathed my youth in aurora and sound, and at the summit of life before the day ended unguarded by the heart turned towards the false brilliance that I did not stagger blinded by glory, because now the night darkens in grave splendor.
>
> (Eichendorff: poem "Dank" – translated by the author)

In an essay on self-recognition in old age, the philosopher Arthur Schopenhauer (1788–1860) describes the process as follows:

> Towards the end of life, much the same happens as at the end of a masked ball when the masks are removed. We now see who those really were with whom we had come in contact during the course of our life. Characters have revealed themselves, deeds have borne fruit, achievements have been justly appreciated, and all illusions have crumbled away. But for all this time was necessary. The curious thing, however, is that only towards the end of our

> lives do we really recognize and understand even ourselves, our real aim and object, especially in our relations to the world and others. Very often, but not always, we shall have to assign to ourselves a lower place than we had previously thought was our due. Sometimes, we shall give ourselves a higher, the reason for this being that we had no adequate notion of the baseness of the world, and accordingly set our aim higher than it. Incidentally, we come to know what we have in ourselves.
>
> (Schopenhauer 2000, 491)

Striving for ego integrity in processes of self-reflection and life review implies the usage of one's accumulated knowledge about oneself and the world, as well as the differentiation of respective knowledge systems. Processes of self-reflection and life review are promoted by openness to new impressions, experiences, and insights. The theory of gerotranscendence (Tornstam 2005) postulates an increasing willingness for incorporating one's own life into comprehensive (or 'full') terms of reference. Being beyond oneself – as the key element of gerotranscendence – encompasses the feeling of being absorbed into other people's lives (especially into the life of younger generations), as well as the feeling of being embedded in an extensive context or cosmic order. When characterizing gerotranscendence, it is helpful to take up the differentiation between lifetime (*Lebenszeit*) and universal time (*Weltzeit*) (Blumenberg 1986). Differentiating between individual lifetime and cosmic universal time highlights the human being's motive for *transcendence*, which can be defined as one's motive for feeling embedded in a cosmic order in which he or she can trust. Gerotranscendence is also discussed in the context of religiosity or spirituality – empirical results point to the increasing willingness of the elderly to interpret their own lives from a universal perspective in cases of a positively evaluated religious socialization. The universal perspective in this case not only refers to a cosmic transcendence, but also includes the advance toward generativity – that is, to identify with younger people's lives, to feel with them, to share their concerns, and to motivate and support them.

Limit situations

Karl Jaspers describes 'limit situations' as fundamental situations of our existence, which are part of existence itself; that is, these situations belong to our existence; constitute our existence (Jaspers 2014). Limit situations, such as those of suffering, of loss, of dying, are of a final character: They cannot be changed by us; they bring us only clarity, without the ability to explain and to derive them from another situation. Due to their finality, limit situations themselves cannot be altered; they require people themselves to change – in terms of the further differentiation of their experience, their knowledge, and their actions through which they also obtain a new attitude toward themselves and their existence.

What Jaspers describes as entering with open eyes can be considered psychologically in terms of reflected and responsible actions – that is, in terms of the orientation of a person on values of which they have become conscious – this is closely linked with the definition of self-responsibility in the next part of this contribution. When Jaspers writes that limit situations demand everything from one's existence, development in the limit situation is interpreted in the sense of a 'leap,' and this insofar as the individuals attain a deeper understanding of themselves by successfully grappling with the situation: After the leap, my life is a different one than my existence, if only I am there. I say "I myself" in a new context.

Following Jaspers, limit situations represent a downright provocation to obtain answers from people. As existences, we can avoid limit situations only by closing our eyes to them. In the world, we want to retain our existence by extending it; we refer to it without questioning, mastering it and enjoying it or, alternatively, suffering from it and succumbing to it, but, ultimately, there is no choice for us but to submit to it. We therefore react to limit situations not expediently, with plans and calculations, but rather through a completely different activity, the development of an existence possible within us; we become ourselves by walking into the limit situations with our eyes open.

The way elderly people handle limit situations such as increased physical vulnerability, the loss of people close to them, and increasing consciousness of their own finality is also to be considered as a potential influence on cultural guiding principles for a successful life: Here, the elderly can function as role models. They can provide subsequent generations with insights regarding the limits of life, the capability of people to handle these limits reflectively, and the conscious acceptance of dependence on the assistance of others.

Dementia: resources in addition to accentuated vulnerability?

The reflection of our image of humanity is significant in understanding the quality of life of people with dementia and the ways to influence them positively. Depending on how we understand the individual with dementia – how we understand his or her cognitive, emotional, feelings-related, everyday living and social communicative qualities – it becomes possible to identify his or her processes of self-actualization, even in severe dementia cases.

Self-actualization describes the tendency of the psyche to express, to communicate, to differentiate itself. Important for the understanding of self-actualization is that personality encompasses many qualities – cognitive skills, emotional skills, feelings-oriented skills, aesthetic skills, communication skills, and everyday practical skills – in which the tendency of the psyche for self-actualization can be realized.

Recent research has shown that, even in cases of severe dementia, a differentiated emotionality may still enable people to respond differently to various kinds of situations, thus expressing personal preferences and subjective quality of life, albeit in a rudimentary form (Kruse 2015). Insofar as dementia sufferers are in a position to express their emotions non-verbally at least, it is in principle possible for medical practitioners, care workers, and relatives to 'access' them and to maintain meaningful contact. Even in cases of advanced dementia, the emotional state of people with dementia can therefore, in all probability, be assessed by qualified nursing staff through trained observation.

The availability of a number of positive everyday situations, as well as the absence of emotionally stressful situations, can be considered as direct indicators of subjective well-being and as a promising starting point for individualized intervention strategies: On the basis of a predefined list of situations, and after close observation in all these situations, professional care workers can determine the situations in which positive or negative emotions are recognizable, as well as the frequency with which they occur in a defined period, for each resident. In the research project entitled "Demenzkranke Menschen in individuell bedeutsamen Alltagssituationen" (DEMIAN) ("People with Dementia in Individual Everyday Situations"), we were able to show that, in the context of individualized care planning, it is possible to systematically arrange situations in which the resident shows positive emotions. Here, appreciative communication and reminding people of important events and relationships in their biographies proved essential. It is also possible to successfully build on earlier interests and inclinations. To sum up, the results of DEMIAN show that emotions are important intervention resources; in addition, it again highlights that self-actualization is recognizable as long as mental abilities exist.

Ethics of responsibility and the need for a new understanding of old age

Proceeding from *coram-structure* as a figure of thought, three spheres of human responsibility are differentiated, which – taken together – elucidate the meaning of old age for individuals, as well as for societies. The first sphere is the person's responsibility for and toward himself or herself. The second sphere is the individual's shared responsibility, or willingness to engage with others and society. The third sphere of responsibility is the individual's obligation toward God and creation – in other words, joint responsibility for the following generations, including those not yet born.

The term 'shared responsibility' implies the individual's ability and motivation to empathize with others, to engage with others, to contribute to the fulfillment of other people's needs, and to engage with society as a whole. As a concept, shared responsibility refers to the principle of subsidiarity, which is founded in the Christian social ethics of Nell-Breuning (1977) and states that matters of social welfare should ideally be handled in their immediate place of origin – that is, by the smallest, lowest, or least centralized competent authority. Central authority should have a subsidiary function, performing only those tasks that cannot be performed effectively at a more immediate or local level. The concept of subsidiarity refers to both (a) the utilization of existing potentials (of the individual, the family, or municipalities) to manage tasks and challenges and (b) the obligation of more global social structures to offer the necessary structures and support. Accordingly, the principle of shared responsibility and solidarity accentuates both the obligations of the elderly and the obligations of society: The elderly should take responsibility for development and maintenance of old-age potentials and use them in support of themselves and of others, and society must guarantee the underlying conditions necessary for the development, maintenance, and realization of old-age potentials.

The concept of caring communities – in which neighbors, acquaintances, and friends provide the many services people need, not only in old age, but over their whole lifespan, to (re-)establish and maintain an independent and responsible life – is closely related to the idea of subsidiarity. Caring communities are defined by their members' willingness to take joint responsibility for others. Obviously, non-profit civil engagement of caring communities contributes not only to social cohesion in the respective locality, but also to a substantial relief of social security systems. In this regard, supporting the development of caring communities is a potential way to compensate for impending deficits in the sustainability and effectiveness of social services.

In terms of social policy, determining the appropriate structures for the balance of individual and societal responsibility is crystallized in the principle of *institutional subsidiarity*. Subsidiarity means that the individual and the community as it is should act first, and that the state should intervene only when there is no alternative. Firstly, the individual's resources should be strengthened so that he or she is able to lead an independent, self-determined, and socially active life. Here, it is important to assist the individual in creating or changing environmental conditions in accordance with personal needs and values. Where the individual is not able to help himself or herself, assistance should be sought first from family members, neighbors, self-help groups, and voluntary welfare organizations – the state should be called in only as a last resort. This aspect gains special importance in cases of high vulnerability – a risk that increases in the fourth age. Vulnerability is a demand not only for the individual, but also for society. To what extent does society provide support for the individual in his or her effort to sustain or regain an independent and personally responsible existence? How clearly defined is the obligation of society to make the social security system's resources (for example, health insurance) available for the support of old people? With a glance at the demographic development in many developed countries, to what extent will the decision-makers and the policy-makers in society be prepared to take the side of older people when the social security system's resources are even more severely stretched than is the case today? Will the needs of people who rely on extensive treatment, rehabilitation, and long-term care still be sufficiently represented and acknowledged in public?

An anthropological approach to old age

Elsewhere (Kruse 2013), we suggested an anthropological approach to old age as a basis for understanding the potentials and challenges of population ageing, sustainable ageing policy, and scientific policy advice. This approach is based on the following six statements:

(1) The topic of *self-design* in old age does not decrease in importance, but actually continues to be important until the end of life. This means that in old

and very old age, people can still be guided by the motivation to shape their lives according to their own needs, interests, values, and goals (*autopoiesis*). However, this also means that in the case of a (feared or actual) restriction of the self-design – be it due to disease and the associated functional decline, or due to financial hardship, or as a result of the loss of a stimulating and supportive social network – an individual may react with protest and accusation, but also self-blame, reduced commitment, loss of drive, or dejection. In many cases, deviant behavior is interpreted as 'behavioral disorder' without asking whether it is caused, or even conditioned, by a restriction of self-design.

(2) Understanding old age, like all life phases, requires the integration of two perspectives: the perspective of potential and the perspective of vulnerability. We must consider the individual's strengths, development, and positive change options, as well as physical losses, pre-frailty, or frailty. This double perspective is of particular significance in old and very old age, when vulnerability (in physical and cognitive, as well as social aspects) notably increases. However, potential strengths – the development potential – must always be considered.

(3) Like all life phases, old age implies developmental demands; there is a developmental necessity due to a changed role and activity spectrum, due to changes in social networks and due to late freedom following retirement, but also due to the heightened vulnerability and, not least, the confrontation with the increasingly urgent theme of mortality.

(4) People are not indifferent to their own mortality as has hitherto sometimes been presumed. The notion of no longer being part of this world, of no longer living, is seen as anything but a triviality. Moreover, death is seen as an end, but also as an aim (the Latin *finis* has this dual meaning); thus, individual development should be understood not just from the perspective of conception and birth, but also from that *of death*: We are not only distancing ourselves ever further from our origins (as defined by conception and birth), but also increasingly approaching the end, the aim of our lives, which can most certainly be seen as a return to our origins or even as a transition.

(5) Pivotal for the anthropology is the relatedness of the individual to other people – and this, of course, also applies in old and very old age. However, when looking at this life phase, relatedness can be taken even further, in the direction of the experienced responsibility of older people for future generations. In this context, the construct of generativity becomes even more meaningful. Erikson (1998) pointed to the inner pre-occupation with the future of subsequent generations, as well as to respective actions: Old age cannot be understood without the context of intergenerational relationships.

(6) The different dimensions of responsibility are important for anthropology; we justify our decisions and actions to ourselves, to other people, and to creation. Self-justification is what self-responsibility really means, the justification of treating other people with the concept of shared responsibility, the justification of thinking of creation and subsequent generations – those living today, as well as those who are not yet born – with the concept of sustainability and responsibility.

Age-friendly culture as a principal aim of ageing policy and respective guidance

The definition of an age-friendly culture emphasizes three aspects in particular: (1) When society is spoken of, it refers specifically to the elderly, who form a significant, increasingly important part of society. (2) In the creation of framework conditions for the realization of potential, in the addressing of older people as co-responsible active citizens, the recognition of their participation rights expresses respect for these rights. (3) The same applies to vulnerability; older people should be able to show their vulnerability without having to worry about being excluded from the heart of society or being limited in their participatory rights or participation opportunities.

A profound reservation against old age in Western societies is reflected in the world of work (Finkelstein et al. 2015), particularly in the formerly popular practice of early retirement. There is comparatively little use of the employment potential of older people, coupled with an increased risk of long-term unemployment and a lower participation in training at an older age. In addition, the aforementioned reservations toward age are clear in the current discussion about necessary reforms of the social security system, the risks of old age, and the resulting financial burdens, which are unilaterally emphasized (Kruse 2013). With a view to civic engagement (Kruse and Schmitt 2012), it can be seen not only that older people's existing engagement is not acknowledged, but also that older people are rarely approached as co-responsible citizens whose contribution is indispensable for society. The fact that people at old and very old age continue to develop and that – through their reflected experiences, their knowledge, and their strategies, but also just due to how they live – they can make a contribution to our society's human capital (Ardelt et al. 2013) is simply not sufficiently recognized.

Drawing attention to existing potentials does not mean that an optimistic forecast in respect of the course of ageing processes in future cohorts, the development of the labor market and innovation capacity, or the sustainability of existing support systems, has been made. The potentials of age refer much more to a twofold design option, which is to be understood in the sense of opportunity and challenge (for the individual and for society). From an individual perspective, on the basis of the stated potentials, and when compared to previous generations, there are now significantly better possibilities for older people to fulfill their own life plans, goals, and values, as well as to participate in social development and to engage with others and the community. From a societal perspective, the potentials of age refer firstly to the opportunity to contribute, by means of motivational, social, cultural, and institutional conditions, to the growing proportion of older people being able to lead an independent, self- and co-responsible life for as long as possible, whereby attention must be directed toward reducing social inequality – not just at old and very old age, but also in the preceding stages of life (Kruse and Schmitt 2015).

Moreover, the question arises as to what extent a society can benefit from the experiences older people gain when dealing with critical situations, especially at old and very old age. In this context, the works of Rentsch (2014) show that, at an advanced age, the increase in limitations – the 'radicalization of our physically captured basic situation' – offers the chance of a qualitatively new fulfillment option of individuation in which the individual can experience his or her own life as 'the coming into existence of the singular totality' or as a 'becoming oneself' (see also Rentsch in this volume).

A major social issue that is addressed through the potential and vulnerability at old and very old age relates to intra-generational justice, which also has consequences for the design of intergenerational relations: Potentials of age can and should be used in a socially responsible manner. Through them, society should be in a position to effectively support older people who find themselves in health-related, social, and/or financial distress.

How can age-friendly culture be defined?

(1) First of all, we understand age-friendly culture as the involvement of older people in social, political, and cultural discourse, as well as in social and cultural progress. Only too frequently is there the tendency to talk *about* the elderly in public discourse, but not *with* them; this is an expression of the neglect of older people, or even hidden discrimination. Talking *about* the elderly, but not talking *to* them, suggests that older people are not perceived as active, co-responsible parts of society – that their potentials are not being taken seriously. In an age-friendly culture, elderly women and men have as much of a voice and are treated with as much respect as younger people. An age-friendly culture does not generalize the group of older people but respects the 'uniqueness of being' of older women and men.

(2) Related to the first-mentioned feature of an age-friendly culture, but with a slightly different emphasis, is an intergenerational perspective, whereby it must be explicitly stated that – and empirical findings support this statement – there is an active exchange of ideas, knowledge, experience, of assistance and of sympathy between the generations. Being embedded in a sequence of generations is an important expression of participation, more so for the elderly than for the young. Moreover, the motivations of generativity and transcendence, which are so important in old age, can be realized. Prominent examples of this intergenerational perspective are generation tandems and mentoring opportunities in the workplace, as well as sponsorship of older people in civic matters.

(3) An age-friendly culture articulates a vital interest in the potentials of age (which can, of course, vary considerably from person to person) and creates conditions that are conducive to the realization of such potentials – such as the introduction of the flexible retirement age in the world of work (not to be construed as a relinquishment of legally defined age limits), as well as the removal of all age limits in the field of civic engagement. Worth mentioning are also the opportunity structures, such as community centers, where the generations can meet, enrich, and support each other: an important incentive to realizing potentials in old age.

(4) An age-friendly culture encounters older women and men, in whom vulnerability is clearly expressed, with respect and sensitivity. It provides socio-spatial contexts that promote independence and responsibility and secure participation – such as neighborhood meeting places; differentiated, target-group-specific service systems; and barrier-free environments, all of which have a positive impact on the maintenance or recovery of independence and mobility.

(5) In the case of severe physical and cognitive losses in an older person, an age-friendly culture respects the individual's uniqueness, expresses respect for the dignity of this individual, avoids trying to determine the quality of life of this person from an external position, and denies the individual neither the fundamental right of participation nor expert and ethically sound medical care. A 'grading' of human dignity is avoided, as is an age-determined scaling down of the extent and quality of healthcare. Decisive for healthcare provision is the diagnosis alone, made by an expert, not the age of the individual concerned.

(6) An age-friendly culture is determined to reduce social inequality among the group of older people and to ensure that every person – regardless of education, income, or social class – receives the social and medical services necessary for his or her specific life situation.

(7) An age-friendly culture does not deny the rights, claims, and needs of younger people but endeavors to identify and recognize the rights, claims, and needs of all the generations, whereby no single generation is preferred or disadvantaged.

References

Ardelt, M., S. D. Landes, K. R. Gerlach, and L. P. Fox. 2013. "Rediscovering Internal Strengths of the Aged: The Beneficial Impact of Wisdom, Mastery, Purpose in Life, and Spirituality on Aging Well." In *Positive Psychology: Advances in Understanding Adult Motivation*, edited by J. D. Sinnott, 106–143. New York: Springer.

Bano, B., and S. Benbow. 2010. "Positive Approaches to the Fourth Age." *Quality in Ageing and Older Adults* 11 (2):29–34. doi: http://dx.doi.org/10.5042/qiaoa.2010.0287.

Blumenberg, H. 1986. *Lebenszeit und Weltzeit*. Frankfurt am Main: Suhrkamp.

Erikson, E. H. 1998. *The Life Cycle Completed: Extended Version with New Chapters on the Ninth Stage by Joan M. Erikson*. New York: Norton.

Erikson, E. H., J. M. Erikson, and H. Q. Kivnick. 1986. *Vital Involvement in Old Age*. New York: Norton.

Filipp, S.-H. 1999. "A Three-Stage Model of Coping with Loss and Trauma: Lessons from Patients Suffering from Severe and Chronic Disease." In *Post-Traumatic Stress Disorder: A Lifespan Developmental Perspective*, edited by A. Maercker, M. Schuetzwohl, and Z. Solomon, 43–80. Seattle: Hogrefe.

Finkelstein, L., D. Truxillo, F. Fraccaroli, and R. Kanfer, eds. 2015. *Facing the Challenges of a Multi-Age Workforce: A Use-Inspired Approach*. New York: Routledge.

Huxhold, O., K. L. Fiori, and T. D. Windsor. 2013. "The Dynamic Interplay of Social Network Characteristics, Subjective Well-Being, and Health: The Costs and Benefits of Socio-Emotional Selectivity." *Psychology & Aging* 28 (1):3–16. doi: 10.1037/a0030170.

Jaspers, K. 2014. *Man in the Modern Age*. New York: Routledge.

Kruse, A. 2013. *Alternde Gesellschaft – eine Bedrohung? Ein Gegenentwurf*. Freiburg: Lambertus.

Kruse, A. 2014. "Entwicklungspotenziale und Verletzlichkeit im hohen und sehr hohen Alter. Eine theoretisch-konzeptionelle und empirische Annäherung." *Psychotherapie im Alter* 11 (2):177–198.

Kruse, A. 2015. "Selbst und Selbstaktualisierung." In *Demenz und Palliative Geriatrie*, edited by M. Kojer and M. Schmidl, 295–309. Heidelberg: Springer.

Kruse, A., and E. Schmitt. 2012. "Generativity as a Route to Active Ageing." *Current Gerontology and Geriatrics Research*, Epub Aug 7. doi: 10.1155/2012/647650.

Kruse, A., and E. Schmitt. 2015. "Shared Responsibility and Civic Engagement in Very Old Age." *Research in Human Development* 12 (1–2):133–148. doi: http://dx.doi.org/10.1080/15427609.2015.1010353.

McAdams, D. P. 2013. *The Redemptive Self: Stories Americans Live By* (Revised and Expanded edition). New York: Oxford University Press.

McAdams, D. P., and E. de St. Aubin. 1992. "A Theory of Generativity and Its Assessment through Self-Report, Behavioral Acts, and Narrative Themes in Autobiography." *Journal of Personality and Social Psychology* 62 (6):1003–1015. doi: 10.1037/0022-3514.62.6.1003.

Mannheim, K. 1928. "Das Problem der Generationen." *Kölner Vierteljahreshefte für Soziologie* 7 (2):157–185.

Nell-Breuning, O. v. 1977. *Soziallehre der Kirche*. Wien: Europaverlag.

Peck, R. 1968. "Psychologische Entwicklung in der zweiten Lebenshälfte." In *Altern – Probleme und Tatsachen*, edited by H. Thomae and U. Lehr, 376–384. Wiesbaden: Wissenschaftliche Buchgesellschaft.

Randall, W. L. 2013. "The Importance of Being Ironic: Narrative Openness and Personal Resilience in Later Life." *The Gerontologist* 53 (1):9–16. doi: 10.1093/geront/gns048.

Rentsch, T. 2014. "Werden zu sich selbst: Das Altern und die Zeitlichkeit des guten Lebens." *Zeitschrift für Praktische Philosophie* 1 (1):263–288.

Schopenhauer, A. 2000. *Parerga and Paralipomena: Short Philosophical Essays*. Oxford: Clarendon Press.

Shmotkin, D., A. Shrira, N. Eyal, T. Blumstein, and A. Shorek. 2013. "The Prediction of Subjective Wellness among the Old-Old: Implications for the 'Fourth-Age' Conception." *Journals of Gerontology, Series B: Psychological Sciences and Social Sciences* 69 (5):719–729. doi: 10.1093/geronb/gbt052.

Tornstam, L. 2005. *Gerotranscendence: A Developmental Theory of Positive Aging*. New York: Springer Publishing.

6 Competence and cognitive deterioration

Are we paying enough attention to ethical issues?

Perla Werner and Silke Schicktanz

Introduction

Due to advances in modern healthcare, medical technology, and improvements in social and environmental conditions, industrialized societies are now confronted with the challenges of a dramatic increase in the average lifespan of elderly persons (Bloom et al. 2014). This increase will be accompanied by a concomitant rise in the number of persons with Alzheimer's disease (AD) and other types of age-related dementia. Indeed, it has been estimated that approximately 35 million individuals lived with dementia worldwide in 2010; this number is expected to double every 20 years, reaching up to 115 million in 2050 (Prince et al. 2013).

In preparation for these striking demographic changes, researchers have discussed several issues related to how AD and dementia will impact public-welfare systems, society, families, and, of course, individuals. The ethical questions associated with these changes have until yet attracted only limited attention. Upon close examination, the main ethical issues dealt within the literature include disclosure of the diagnosis, the efficacy and cost of symptomatic drugs (especially in mild to moderate stages of dementia), and end-of-life issues (Gauthier et al. 2013). Competence issues and ethical questions associated with cognitive deterioration (Nuffield Council on Bioethics 2009) have been addressed only by a few expert reports (e.g., Nuffield Council on Bioethics 2009). However, clarifying how these ethical issues related to competence should be practically solved is a necessary requirement for future care and research in dementia, especially because the current underlying hypothesis implies a shift from disease to early prediction and detection of early cognitive deterioration.

In the following, we will examine in detail the existing debate by using five steps:

a defining the concepts of *competence* and *capacity*;
b explaining the relationship between competence, capacity, and cognitive deterioration;
c summarizing studies assessing competence and cognitive deterioration;
d reassessing main underlying assumptions of competence and cognitive deterioration;
e presenting and discussing ethical aspects complementing the current debate of competence and cognitive deterioration.

It should be noted that this chapter does not intend to present a systematic review of the topic or provide clinicians with recommendations and guidelines; rather, we will focus on the main ethical questions.

Defining the concepts of competence and capacity

Defining the terms of *capacity* and *competence* has proven an arduous task over the years. Although the two terms are obviously related, researchers, clinicians, and legal professionals have long debated whether they are synonymous (Ganzini et al. 2005). Until recently, the consensus was that they are neither identical nor synonymous. In the last decade, however, researchers have disputed the utility of distinguishing between the terms and are now suggesting using them interchangeably (Moye and Marson 2013), as they will be used in this chapter in order to allow for a better intersection between the ethico-legal and the practical clinical debate.

Both terms being associated with a person's ability to make deliberatively responsible and balanced decisions, *competence* was used as a legal term and was determined by a court of law, whereas *capacity* was used to refer to a clinical assessment (Alvaro 2012; Ganzini et al. 2005). As such, capacity referred to a person's performance regarding decision-making abilities, while competence referred to a judgment about an individual's capacity to make decisions (Karlawish, Casarett, and James 2002).

Indeed, it is possible to identify some shared assumptions of both terms. First, they are both associated with the ethical principles of respecting personal autonomy, self-determination, and dignity. Autonomy and self-determination are often used interchangeably in practical-ethical contexts and refer to a person's right to make a voluntary choice (Kapp 2007; Beauchamp and Childress 2013). For some philosophers, only a deontological notion of self-responsible, rational, well-informed decision-making justifies using the term 'autonomy' (Christman 1989), while self-determination covers any voluntary choice – even without sufficient information assessment. 'Dignity' refers to the intrinsic worth of every human being, simply by virtue of being human (Jacobson 2007), and serves as a legal-philosophical term for protecting any human being against instrumentalization by others, independent of that person's current capacities or cognitive abilities, but based on the general assumption that only human beings have capacities for autonomous decision-making – albeit in terms of potentiality.

Second, since both terms, 'capacity' and 'competence,' are associated with decision-making, they are both based on the assessment of similar decisional capabilities, including:

1 understanding – the ability to comprehend information and demonstrate that comprehension, including the ability to attend, encode, store, and retrieve newly presented words and phrases;
2 appreciation – the ability to determine the significance of the information, relative to one's own situation, including insight, judgment, and foresight;

3 reasoning – the process of comparing alternatives in light of consequences, through integrating, analyzing, and manipulating information; the ability to provide rational reasons for the decision, to manipulate information rationally;
4 expressing a choice – the ability to communicate and justify a decision.

(Alvaro 2012)

Since decisions vary in complexity according to their nature and context, there is no point in assessing general competence or capacity in the area of dementia; instead, there is rather a need to specifically examine the person's capacity and competence in relation to each individual decision. Indeed, it has been shown that while some decisions are intuitive and based on personal preferences, habits, values, and emotions, others require extensive information-seeking as well as logical and careful deliberation (Smebye, Kirkevold, and Engedal 2012). Obviously, greater capacity and competence are required for more complex decisions. Hence, the assessment of competence and capacity must be task-specific to be meaningful.

The relationship between cognitive deterioration and competence

Dementia is a syndrome characterized by progressive deterioration in cognition, function, and behavior, with Alzheimer's disease (AD) being the most prevalent type of dementia. *Mild cognitive impairment* (MCI) is defined as a condition characterized by newly acquired cognitive decline, to an extent that is beyond that expected by age or educational background, yet not causing significant functional impairment. The prodromal stage of dementia encompasses the spectrum of presymptomatic autosomal dominant mutation carriers; asymptomatic biomarker-positive older individuals at risk for progression to MCI, MCI due to AD, and AD dementia; and biomarker-positive individuals who have demonstrated a subtle decline from their own baseline, exceeding what is expected in typical ageing, but would not yet meet criteria for MCI and progresses up to Alzheimer's disease and complete cognitive deterioration (Sperling et al. 2011).

According to the leading current hypothesis, the clinical trajectory of cognitive deterioration is characterized by a stage of 'preclinical' asymptomatic AD, which precedes 'symptomatic' mild cognitive impairment and converts in certain cases into early dementia and then late-stage dementia (NIA www.nia.nih.gov; Dubois et al. 2014; Sperling et al. 2011).

Thus, because cognitive deterioration is progressive and gradual, the loss of capabilities that might interfere with the person's competence to make decisions in different realms is also gradual and progressive. This has raised a great deal of ethical challenges surrounding decision-making capacity (or the lack thereof) in the context of neurodegenerative diseases. Indeed, a bibliographic analysis of keywords used during the years 1980–2000 found 1,297 items (474 major items and 823 minor items) published on the topic of 'ethics' and 'dementia' (Baldwin et al. 2003). Almost two-thirds (65%) of the items dealt with four main ethical areas:

end of life; professional care; treatment; and decision-making, which included in its coding the sub-categories of surrogate, proxy, substituted judgment, and clinical/medical decision-making. What was missing then was an in-depth analysis of existing literature focusing mainly on competence/capacity and dementia. This is the aim of the following review.

Review and summary of studies assessing competence and cognitive deterioration

An Internet-based literature search relevant to the topic of competence and cognitive deterioration was conducted. The search was undertaken by using online databases including PubMed, PsycINFO, Sociological Abstracts, and CINHAL, and it was supplemented by hand-checking reference lists in relevant articles not otherwise retrieved through online sources. The key terms used in the search were (i) 'dementia' OR 'Alzheimer's disease (AD)' OR 'cognitive deterioration' AND (ii) 'competenc*' OR 'capacity.' Articles were included in the review if they (i) were published in English and in peer-reviewed journals between January 1, 1995, and December 31, 2015, and (ii) identified the defined key terms in their title, abstract, or text. Abstracts, letters to editors, conference proceedings, books, book chapters, reports, and dissertations were excluded from the review.

After deleting duplicates and publications that did not adhere to the inclusion criteria, a total of 48 studies were identified.[1]

The vast majority of the studies (n = 26) were conducted in English-speaking countries, mostly the US (Allaire et al. 2009; Appelbaum, Bonnie, and Karlawish 2005; Berry et al. 2015; Boyle et al. 2012; Griffith et al. 2005; Hirschman et al. 2005; Jefferson et al. 2008; Jefferson et al. 2012; Karlawish, Casarett, and James 2002; Kim et al. 2011a, 2011b; Lai et al. 2008; Marson et al. 1995; Marson et al. 2000; Marson et al. 2009; Menne et al. 2008; Menne & Whitlatch 2007; Mittal et al. 2007; Moye et al. 2004; Okonkwo et al. 2007; Okonkwo et al. 2008a, 2008b; Palmer et al. 2013; Seaman et al. 2015; Sherod et al. 2009; Triebel et al. 2009; Triebel et al. 2010) and the UK (Boyle 2014; Roked and Patel 2008; Samsi and Manthorpe 2013; St-Amant et al. 2012; Whelan et al. 2009). A few studies were conducted in Sweden (Stormoen et al. 2014; Tallberg et al. 2013), Germany (Hamann et al. 2011; Vollmann et al. 2003), and other countries.

Our review of the literature revealed that only four of the studies were longitudinal (Boyle et al. 2012; Okonkwo et al. 2008b; Samsi and Manthorpe 2013; Triebel et al. 2009), and all of them demonstrated that competence in different domains declines over time and is associated with cognitive deterioration. Samsi and Manthorpe (2013), who conducted the only qualitative longitudinal study, demonstrated that as cognitive functioning deteriorates, family caregivers gradually take over decision-making for the person with dementia.

In terms of the type of competence that was examined, various domains of decision-making were assessed. Fourteen studies examined competence associated with medical decision-making (Griffith et al. 2005; Hamann et al. 2011; Hirschman et al. 2005; Lui et al. 2009; Lui et al. 2012; Marson et al. 1995; Moye et al. 2004; Okonkwo et al. 2007; Okonkwo et al. 2008a, 2008b; St-Amant et al.

2012; Stormoen et al. 2014; Tallberg et al. 2013; Vollmann et al. 2003), eight examined competence to consent to research (Duron et al. 2013; Jefferson et al. 2008; Jefferson et al. 2012; Karlawish, Casarett, and James 2002; Kim et al. 2011a, 2011b; Mittal et al. 2007; Seaman et al. 2015; Whelan et al. 2009), seven examined financial competence (Lui et al. 2013; Marson et al. 2000; Marson et al. 2009; Pachana et al. 2014; Sherod et al. 2009; Triebel et al. 2009; Triebel et al. 2010), three examined voting decision-making (Appelbaum, Bonnie, and Karlawish 2005; Irastorza, Corujo, and Bañuelos 2011; Tiraboschi et al. 2011), one checked testamentary competence (Roked and Patel 2008), one investigated driving competence (Frittelli et al. 2009), and one investigated legal capacity (Giannouli and Tsolaki 2014). The rest of the studies (n = 10) assessed general decision-making in a variety of areas (Allaire et al. 2009; Berry et al. 2015; Boyle 2014; Boyle et al. 2012; Lai et al. 2008; Menne et al. 2008; Menne and Whitlatch 2007; Samsi and Manthorpe 2013; Smebye, Kirkevold, and Engedal 2012; Werner 2006).

The vast majority of the studies (n = 38) were quantitative and used structured or semi-structured instruments such as short questionnaires to assess competence. The most frequently used instruments were the MacArthur Competence Assessment Tool for Treatment (MacCat-T, Grisso and Applebaum 1998), the Financial Capacity Instrument (FIC, Marson et al. 2000), and the Capacity to Consent to Treatment Instrument (CCTI, Marson et al. 2000). Although assessing different domains of competence, most of these instruments are based on the assumption that competence requires the basic capacities of understanding, appreciation, reasoning, and the ability to express a choice.

In sum, the body of knowledge in the area of competence and cognitive deterioration has increased in the last 20 years. A wider array of competence areas is being evaluated, and more structured methods are being used. Researchers can now detect shifts and differences of competence more sensitively than before, thus supporting a detailed understanding of how decision-making capabilities deteriorate over the trajectory of AD, but the latest instruments also sensitize for the huge differences between decision-making domains (such as driving, voting, care planning, research consent, appointing proxies). Despite these methodological advancements, the area is still theoretically limited, as it does not relate to the ethical implications of the topic at all.

Main assumptions underlying the topic of competence and cognitive deterioration today

This limitation stems from three main underlying assumptions. By critically reassessing these assumptions, we identify ethical and philosophical aspects that can and should be addressed more appropriately.

The current understanding of competence and cognitive deterioration relies on the biomedical model

Although the biomedicalization of dementia has been criticized for many years (Lock 2013; Lyman 1988), research on competence and cognitive deterioration continues to be based on the main assumptions of the biomedical model. According to this model, limitations are directly caused by health conditions and reversed by medical treatment and management. Indeed, most studies we reviewed present cognitive deterioration as progressive, irreversible, and incurable; they focus mainly on loss and on the costs and burden of care. As such, they largely ignore personal constructions of the disease and subjective experiences of the person with cognitive deterioration.

Diagnostic labeling is associated with (in-)competence

Diagnostic labels serve several goals. They provide an efficient way for clinicians and researchers to understand a large amount of information; they also suggest etiology, as well as point the way toward specific interventions that may prevent or ameliorate the consequences of a condition. Moreover, diagnostic labels are often sought by affected persons to reduce uncertainty, to locate their subjective experiences of change (Mol 2008; Samsi et al. 2014), or to gain access to public healthcare (Blendon et al. 2012). However, a diagnostic label of dementia is often also accompanied by negative consequences, such as increasing fear and uncertainty, and it serves as a cue for stereotypes and stigma (Garand et al. 2009; Werner 2014).

The negative effects of diagnostic labeling of dementia might increase, in light of the current focus on preclinical diagnosis and especially on MCI. Indeed, MCI has generated numerous ethical discussions regarding the legitimate need of the diagnosis (Werner and Korczyn 2008). Graham and Ritchie (2006) have even called MCI a potentially spurious human invention, stating that it was created to give hope to patients and physicians and to provide pharmaceutical companies with additional markets and profits. Others argue that MCI is a valuable diagnosis as long as it is clearly characterized and has been empirically validated as a precursor to AD (Sperling et al. 2011) and clinical treatments are available. But as long as MCI is rather a 'risk prediction,' the value of knowing needs to be questioned, and social risks of mis- or over-interpretations weigh seriously.

In sum, the literature on competence and cognitive deterioration relies too heavily on diagnostic labeling, ignoring the heterogeneity and progressive nature of the conditions, especially in regard to the prodromal stages of dementia or MCI. Currently, this field concentrates more on asking whether a diagnosis is present than on whether the person has the mental ability required to make decisions in a meaningful way, the equivalent of a diagnosis of a lack of competence.

The limits of the current concept of competence

Competence in the area of cognitive deterioration is defined as a static concept and ignores the importance of personal values. As stated, the vast majority of studies in the area of competence and cognitive deterioration are cross-sectional rather than longitudinal and relate to capacity as a global concept that extends over time and irrespective of context. This assumption ignores the well-established statement by Brock and Buchanan (1987) that decision-making capacity is decision-relative and must be evaluated and re-evaluated over time and place.

Moreover, although, as previously stated, not all decisions are based on logical argumentation and a sense of consistency, research on competence and cognitive deterioration relies mainly on the use of structured instruments; thus, decision-making is based on rational choices and disregards the importance of feelings, intuition, and values.

Ethical aspects complementing the current debate of competence and cognitive deterioration

Overall, the ethical and philosophical aspects associated with competence and cognitive deterioration should be expanded. Only a richer view of these aspects will lead to a full and balanced understanding of the topic. We would like to make three proposals on how to advance the interdisciplinary research on competence and cognitive deterioration in the context of dementia.

An excellent starting point is the ethical framework for dementia provided by the Nuffield Council on Bioethics (2009), which emphasizes the values of autonomy and personhood. We elaborate below on three of these proposals.

Proposal 1 – move from a biomedical model to a biopsychosocial model

A more encompassing understanding of the relationships between competence and cognitive deterioration will require a critical move from the biomedical model toward the biopsychosocial model. This latter model states that a better understanding of health and related quality of life needs a broad view comprising biological, psychological, and social factors rather than purely biological aspects as the biomedical model (Borrell-Carrio, Suchman, and Epstein 2004). The biopsychosocial model has been accepted as the best model for the understanding of illness/disease in general by the World Health Association and has been supported lately in the area of dementia specifically (Spector and Orrell 2010). It should be noted that the biopsychosocial model does not ignore the main areas of the biomedical model (i.e., pathology and biology) but rather adds psychological (i.e., thoughts, emotions, and behaviors) and social (i.e., socio-economical, socio-environmental, and cultural) factors. In this way, it allows a more holistic understanding of human behavior and thus of decision-making. As such, it will enable clinicians and researchers to pronounce incompetence not on the basis of diagnosis of a specific pathology (i.e., dementia), but rather on the basis of an individual evaluation of each case and of each situation. Hence, it can also bridge the gap between the perspectives of professionals and those of affected persons (and their closely related partners) who, despite some challenges or changes, stress their agency. Thus, a diagnosis of dementia would not automatically imply an inability to make decisions. Rather, dementia would be seen as a process comprising various stages of development, with early mental deficits not necessarily implying incompetence, and with moderate and advanced mental deterioration not implying total incompetence in all areas. Instead of generalizing incompetence of the affected persons, in unclear cases, healthcare professionals should implement supportive tools to maintain or enhance decision-making capacity. As of now, tools that enhance communication and empower decision-making in dementia patients are missing. Such tools might have concrete implications for lay-professional interactions (e.g., for decisions about diagnosis, treatment, care, or research participation). For example, the informed-consent procedure should meet requirements such as use of simple language, repetition of explanation, rehearsals by affected persons and family members, and provision of visual presentations for increasing the patient's understanding of risks and benefits (Schicktanz et al. 2014). Additional means of empowerment should be explored – this might include family members functioning as mediators (not as legal proxies) or instruments such as advance care or advance research directives (Jongsma and van de Vathorst 2015).

Proposal 2 – move from ignoring emotions, values, and preferences to considering them

The use of the biopsychosocial model calls for allowing emotions, preferences, and values to be included in the process of defining decision-making and competence. This approach includes comparing each specific situation with similar situations without ignoring important moral differences between seemingly similar cases. It is at this point that attention to the person's values comes into play. This is also important for persons with cognitive deterioration, since it was demonstrated for mild and moderate stages that these persons are able to consistently express their preferences and values regarding decisions about daily living (Feinberg and Whithlatch 2001). One way to attain this goal may be by complementing the use of traditional instruments to assess competence as described on page 93 with the concept of moral sensitivity, which takes into account emotions and preferences (Jaeger 2001). Identification and integration of affected persons' preferences and values, even if those are sometimes hidden, unclear, or not easy to express, should be a major normative aim to overcome biased or paternalistic approaches in medical practice. Non-affected persons do not necessarily take the perspectives of those affected (Schicktanz, Schweda, and Franzen 2008; Schicktanz, Schweda, and Wynne 2011); thus, such a perspective might require expanding healthcare professionals' knowledge and education about moral sensitivity and ethics in general in order to help them deal with situations characterized by ethical challenges.

Proposal 3 – understand competence as a relative concept

Finally, a decision-specific and task-specific understanding and evaluation of competence should be favored. This view relies on the assumption that the ability to perform certain tasks may be affected while other abilities remain completely unaltered, therefore disregarding the possibility of declaring a global and static decision of incompetence due to a diagnosis. Moreover, we assume that competence may fluctuate, and evaluations must therefore be continuous and procedural instead of one-time. Even a seemingly absurd decision constitutes no basis for declaring a person incapable. Rather, the decision needs to be contextualized in view of the affected person's emotions, values, and expressed preferences. Thus, the outcome of the decision cannot be a basis for judging the individual's capacity.

Summary and conclusions

As societies worldwide age, the number of people with cognitive deterioration will rise accordingly. This will be accompanied by an increase in the need to assess and identify difficulties regarding these individuals' capacity to make decisions. Although a great number of studies are being published in the area, and many are suggesting and examining new measures and structured scales to assess competence by either clinicians or researchers, discussion of the ethical aspects associated with the topic is surprisingly scant. Thus, the answer to the question posited in the title of this chapter is 'no' – not enough attention is being paid to ethical issues, and an answer is required regarding how we can best expand our knowledge of this subject.

A first step is being taken by several recent worldwide initiatives (Nuffield Council on Bioethics 2009; World Health Organization 2002) that concentrate on examining the topic of the ethics of dementia. However, there is clearly more work to be done in investigating the principles that can guide ethical decisions in the area of competence and cognitive deterioration. This chapter has tried to delineate some ideas and initial steps in this direction.

Note

1 Detailed information about the studies is available from the authors upon request.

References

Papers marked (*) report the reviewed studies on competence and cognitive deterioration.

* Allaire, J. C., A. Gamaldo, B. J. Ayotte, R. Sims, and K. Whitfield. 2009. "Mild Cognitive Impairment and Objective Instrumental Everyday Functioning: The Everyday Cognition Battery Memory Test." *Journal of the American Geriatrics Society* 57 (1):120–125. doi: 10.1111/j.1532-5415.2008.02054.x.

Alvaro, L. C. 2012. "Competency: General Principles and Applicability in Dementia." *Neurologia* 27 (5):290–300. doi: 10.1016/j.nrleng.2011.12.001.

* Appelbaum, P. S., R. J. Bonnie, and J. H. T. Karlawish. 2005. "The Capacity to Vote of Persons with Alzheimer's Disease." *American Journal of Psychiatry* 162 (11):2094–2100. doi: 10.1176/appi.ajp.162.11.2094.

Baldwin, C., J. Hughes, T. Hope, R. Jacoby, and S. Ziebland. 2003. "Ethics and Dementia: Mapping the Literature by Bibliometric Analysis." *International Journal of Geriatric Psychiatry* 18 (1):41–54. doi: 10.1002/gps.770.

Beauchamp, T. L., and J. F. Childress. 2013. *Principles of Biomedical Ethics*. Oxford: Oxford University Press.

* Berry, J. M., H. L. Williams, K. D. Thomas, and J. Blair. 2015. "Perceptions of Competence: Age Moderates Views of Healthy Aging and Alzheimer's Disease." *Experimental Aging Research* 41 (2):157–176. doi: 10.1080/0361073x.2015.1001653.

Blendon, R. J., J. M. Benson, E. M. Wikler, K. J. Weldon, J. Georges, M. Baumgart, and B. A. Kallmyer. 2012. "The Impact of Experience with a Family Member with Alzheimer's Disease on Views about the Disease across Five Countries." *International Journal of Alzheimer's Disease*. doi: 10.1155/2012/903645.

Bloom, D. E., S. Chatterji, P. Kowal, P. Lloyd-Sherlock, M. McKee, B. Rechel, L. Rosenberg, and J. P. Smith. 2014. "Macroeconomic Implications of Population Ageing and Selected Policy Responses." *The Lancet* 385 (9968):649–657. http://dx.doi.org/10.1016/S0140-6736(14)61464-1.

Borrell-Carrio, F., A. L. Suchman, and R. M. Epstein. 2004. "The Biopsychosocial Model 25 Years Later: Principles, Practice, and Scientific Inquiry." *Annals of Family Medicine* 2 (6):576–582. doi: 10.1370/afm.245.

* Boyle, G. 2014. "Recognising the Agency of People with Dementia." *Disability & Society* 29 (7):1130–1144. doi: 10.1080/09687599.2014.910108.

* Boyle, P. A., L. Yu, R. S. Wilson, K. Gamble, A. S. Buchman, and D. A. Bennett. 2012. "Poor Decision Making Is a Consequence of Cognitive Decline among Older Persons without Alzheimer's Disease or Mild Cognitive Impairment." *PLoS One* 7 (8). doi: 10.1371/journal.pone.0043647.

Brock, D. W., and A. E. Buchanan. 1987. "The Profit Motive in Medicine." *Journal of Medicine and Philosophy* 12 (1):1–35. doi: 10.1093/jmp/12.1.1.

Christman, J. P., ed. 1989. *The Inner Citadel: Essays on Individual Autonomy*. New York/Oxford: Oxford University Press.

Dubois, B., H. H. Feldman, C. Jacova, H. Hampel, J. L. Molinuevo, K. Blennow, S. T. DeKosky, S. Gauthier, D. Selkoe, R. Bateman, S. Cappa, S. Crutch, S. Engelborghs, G. B. Frisoni, N. C. Fox, D. Galasko, M.-O. Habert, G. A. Jicha, A. Nordberg, F. Pasquier, G. Rabinovici, P. Robert, C. Rowe, S. Salloway, M. Sarazin, S. Epelbaum, L. C. de Souza, B. Vellas, P. J. Visser, L. Schneider, Y. Stern, P. Scheltens, and J. L. Cummings. 2014. "Advancing Research Diagnostic Criteria for Alzheimer's Disease: The IWG-2 Criteria." *The Lancet Neurology* 13 (6):614–629. doi: 10.1016/S1474-4422(14)70090-0.

* Duron, E., M. Boulay, J. S. Vidal, J. El Bchiri, M. L. Fraisse, A.-S. Rigaud, and L. Hugonot-Diener. 2013. "Capacity to Consent to Biomedical Research's Evaluation among Older Cognitively Impaired Patients: A Study to Validate the University of California Brief Assessment of Capacity to Consent Questionnaire in French among Older Cognitively Impaired Patients." *The Journal of Nutrition, Health and Aging* 17 (4):385–389. doi: 10.1007/s12603-012-0432-2.

Feinberg, L. F., and C. J. Whithlatch. 2001. "Are Persons with Cognitive Impairment Able to State Consistent Choices?" *The Gerontologist* 41 (3):374–382. doi: 10.1093/geront/41.3.374.

* Frittelli, C., D. Borghetti, G. Iudice, E. Bonanni, M. Maestri, G. Tognoni, L. Pasquali, and A. Iudice. 2009. "Effects of Alzheimer's Disease and Mild Cognitive Impairment on Driving Ability: A Controlled Clinical Study by Simulated Driving Test." *International Journal of Geriatric Psychiatry* 24 (3):232–238. doi: 10.1002/gps.2095.

Ganzini, L., L. Volicer, W. A. Nelson, E. Fox, and A. R. Derse. 2005. "Ten Myths about Decision-Making Capacity." *Journal of the American Medical Directors Association* 6 (3):100–101. doi: 10.1016/j.jamda.2005.03.040.

Garand, L., J. H. Lingler, K. O. Conner, and M. A. Dew. 2009. "Diagnosis and Diagnostic Labels, Stigma, and Participation in Research Related to Dementia and Mild Cognitive Impairment." *Research in Gerontological Nursing* 2 (2):112–121. doi: 10.3928/19404921-20090401-04.

Gauthier, S., A. Leuzy, E. Racine, and P. Rosa-Neto. 2013. "Diagnosis and Management of Alzheimer's Disease: Past, Present and Future Ethical Issues." *Progress in Neurobiology* 110:102–113. doi: 10.1016/j.pneurobio.2013.01.003.

* Giannouli, V., and M. Tsolaki. 2014. "Legal Capacity of the Elderly in Greece." *Hellenic Journal of Nuclear Medicine* 17 (1):2–6.

Graham, J. E., and K. Ritchie. 2006. "Mild Cognitive Impairment: Ethical Considerations for Nosological Flexibility in Human Kinds." *Philosophy, Psychology and Psychiatry* 13 (2):31–43. doi: 10.1353/ppp.2006.0039.

* Griffith, H. R., M. P. Dymek, P. Atchison, L. E. Harrell, and D. C. Marson. 2005. "Medical Decision-Making in Neurodegenerative Disease: Mild AD and PD with Cognitive Impairment." *Neurology* 65 (3):483–485. doi: 10.1212/01.wnl.0000171346.02965.80.

* Grisso, T., and P. S. Appelbaum. 1998. *Assessing Competence to Consent to Treatment: A Guide for Physicians and Other Health Care Professionals*. New York: Oxford University Press.

* Hamann, J., K. Bronner, J. Margull, R. Mendel, J. Diehl-Schmid, M. Bühner, R. Klein, A. Schneider, A. Kurz, and R. Perneczky. 2011. "Patient Participation in Medical and Social Decisions in Alzheimer's Disease." *Journal of the American Geriatrics Society* 59 (11):2045–2052. doi: 10.1111/j.1532-5415.2011.03661.x.

* Hirschman, K. B., C. M. Joyce, B. D. James, S. X. Xie, and J. H. T. Karlawish. 2005. "Do Alzheimer's Disease Patients Want to Participate in a Treatment Decision, and Would Their Caregivers Let Them?" *The Gerontologist* 45 (3):381–388. doi: 10.1093/geront/45.3.381.

* Irastorza, L. J., P. Corujo, and P. Bañuelos. 2011. "Capacity to Vote in Persons with Dementia and the Elderly." *International Journal of Alzheimer's Disease*. doi: 10.4061/2011/941041.

Jacobson, N. 2007. "Dignity and Health: A Review." *Social Science & Medicine* 64 (2): 292–302. doi: org/10.1016/j.socscimed.2006.08.039.

Jaeger, S. M. 2001. "Teaching Health Care Ethics: The Importance of Moral Sensitivity for Moral Reasoning." *Nursing Philosophy* 2 (2):131–142. doi: 10.1046/j.1466-769x.2001.00045.x.

* Jefferson, A. L., H. Carmona, K. A. Gifford, S. Lambe, L. K. Byerly, N. G. Cantwell, Y. Tripodis, and J. H. T. Karlawish. 2012. "Clinical Research Risk Assessment among Individuals with Mild Cognitive Impairment." *The American Journal of Geriatric Psychiatry* 20 (10):878–886. doi: 10.1097/jgp.0b013e318252e5cb.

* Jefferson, A. L., S. Lambe, D. J. Moser, L. K. Byerly, A. Ozonoff, and J. H. T. Karlawish. 2008. "Decisional Capacity for Research Participation in Individuals with Mild Cognitive Impairment." *Journal of the American Geriatrics Society* 56 (7):1236–1243. doi: 10.1111/j.1532-5415.2008.01752.x.

Jongsma, K. R., and S. van de Vathorst. 2015. "Beyond Competence: Advance Directives in Dementia Research." *Monash Bioethics* 33 (2):167–180. doi: 10.1007/s40592-015-0034-y.

Kapp, M. B. 2007. "Assessing Assessments of Decision-Making Capacity: A Few Legal Queries and Commentary on 'Assessment of Decision-Making Capacity in Older Adults'." *Journal of Gerontology: Psychological Sciences* 62B (1):12–13. doi: 10.1093/geronb/62.1.p12.

* Karlawish, J. H. T., D. J. Casarett, and B. D. James. 2002. "Alzheimer's Disease Patients' and Caregivers' Capacity, Competency, and Reasons to Enroll in an Early-Phase Alzheimer's Disease Clinical Trial." *Journal of the American Geriatrics Society* 50 (12):2019–2024. doi: 10.1046/j.1532-5415.2002.50615.x.

* Kim, S. Y. H., P. S. Appelbaum, H. M. Kim, I. F. Wall, J. A. Bourgeois, B. Frankel, K. C. Hails, J. R. Rundell, K. M. Seibel, and J. H. T. Karlawish. 2011a. "Variability of Judgments of Capacity: Experience of Capacity Evaluators in a Study of Research Consent Capacity." *Psychosomatics* 52 (4):346–353. doi: 10.1016/j.psym.2011.01.012.

* Kim, S. Y. H., J. H. T. Karlawish, H. M. Kim, I. F. Wall, A. Bozoki, and P. S. Appelbaum. 2011b. "Preservation of the Capacity to Appoint a Proxy Decision Maker: Implications for Dementia Research." *Archives of General Psychiatry* 68 (2):214–220. doi: 10.1001/archgenpsychiatry.2010.191.

* Lai, J. M., T. M. Gill, L. M. Cooney, E. H. Bradley, K. A. Hawkins, and J. H. T. Karlawish. 2008. "Everyday Decision-Making Ability in Older Persons with Cognitive Impairment." *American Journal of Geriatric Psychiatry* 16 (8):693–696. doi: 10.1097/jgp.0b013e31816c7b54.

Lock, M. 2013. *The Alzheimer Conundrum: Entanglements of Dementia and Aging*. Princeton: Princeton University Press.

* Lui, V. W. C., L. C. W. Lam, R. C. M. Chau, A. W. T. Fung, B. M. L. Wong, G. T. Y. Leung, K.-F. Leung, H. F. K. Chiu, J. H. T. Karlawish, and P. S. Appelbaum. 2012. "Capacity to Make Decisions on Medication Management in Chinese Older Persons with Mild Cognitive Impairment and Mild Alzheimer's Disease." *International Psychogeriatric Association* 24 (7):1103–1111. doi: 10.1017/S1041610212000129.

* Lui, V. W. C., L. C. W. Lam, R. C. M. Chau, A. W. T. Fung, B. M. L. Wong, G. T. Y. Leung, K.-F. Leung, H. F. K. Chiu, J. H. T. Karlawish, and P. S. Appelbaum. 2013. "Structured Assessment of Mental Capacity to Make Financial Decisions in Chinese Older Persons with Mild Cognitive Impairment and Mild Alzheimer Disease." *Journal of Geriatric Psychiatry and Neurology* 26 (2):69–77. doi: 10.1177/0891988713481268J.

* Lui, V. W. C., L. C. W. Lam, D. N. Y. Luk, L. H. L. Wong, C. W. C. Tam, H. F. K. Chiu, and P. S. Appelbaum. 2009. "Capacity to Make Treatment Decisions in Chinese Older Persons with Very Mild Dementia and Mild Alzheimer's Disease." *American Journal of Geriatric Psychiatry* 17 (5):428–4236. doi: 10.1097/jgp.0b013e31819d3797.

Lyman, K. A. 1988. "Bringing the Social Back in: A Critique of the Biomedicalization of Dementia." *The Gerontologist* 29 (5):597–605. doi: 10.1093/geront/29.5.597.

* Marson, D. C., K. K. Ingram, H. A. Cody, and L. E. Harrell. 1995. "Assessing the Competency of Patients with Alzheimer's Disease under Different Legal Standards." *Archives of Neurology* 52 (10):949–954. doi: 10.1001/archneur.1995.00540340029010.

* Marson, D. C., R. C. Martin, V. Wadley, H. R. Griffith, S. Snyder, P. S. Goode, F. C. Kinney, A. P. Nicholas, T. Steele, B. Anderson, E. Y. Zamrini, R. Raman, A. Bartolucci, and L. E. Harrell. 2009. "Clinical Interview Assessment of Financial Capacity in Older Adults with Mild Cognitive Impairment and Alzheimer's Disease." *Journal of the American Geriatrics Society* 57 (5):806–814. doi: 10.1111/j.1532-5415.2009.02202.x.

* Marson, D. C., S. M. Sawrie, S. Snyder, B. McInturff, T. Stalvey, A. Boothe, T. Aldridge, A. Chatterjee, and L. E. Harrell. 2000. "Assessing Financial Capacity in Patients with Alzheimer Disease: A Conceptual Model and Prototype Instrument." *Archives of Neurology* 57 (6):877–884. doi: 10.1001/archneur.57.6.877.

* Menne, H. L., S. S. Tucke, C. J. Whitlatch, and L. F. Feinberg. 2008. "Decision Making Involvement Scale for Individuals with Dementia and Family Caregivers." *American Journal of Alzheimer's Disease and Other Dementias* 23 (1):23–29. doi: 10.1177/1533317507308312.

* Menne, H. L., and C. J. Whitlatch. 2007. "Decision-Making Involvement of Individuals with Dementia." *The Gerontologist* 47 (6):810–819. doi: 10.1093/geront/47.6.810.

* Mittal, D., B. W. Palmer, L. B. Dunn, R. Landes, C. Ghormley, C. Beck, S. Golshan, D. Blevins, and D. V. Jeste. 2007. "Comparison of Two Enhanced Consent Procedures for

Patients with Mild Alzheimer Disease or Mild Cognitive Impairment." *The American Journal of Geriatric Psychiatry* 15 (2):163–167. doi: 10.1097/jgp.0b013e31802dd379.

Mol, A. 2008. *The Body Multiple: Ontology in Medical Practice*. Durham: Duke University Press.

* Moye, J., M. J. Karel, A. R. Azar, and R. J. Gurrera. 2004. "Capacity to Consent to Treatment: Empirical Comparison of Three Instruments in Older Adults with and without Dementia." *The Gerontologist* 44 (2):166–175. doi: 10.1093/geront/44.2.166.

Moye, J., D. C. Marson, and B. Edelstein. 2013. "Assessment of Capacity in an Aging Society." *American Psychologist* 68 (3):158–171. doi: 10.1037/a0032159.

Nuffield Council on Bioethics. 2009. *Dementia: Ethical Issues*. London: Cambridge Publishers Ltd.

* Okonkwo, O. C., H. R. Griffith, K. Belue, S. Lanza, E. Y. Zamrini, L. E. Harrell, J. C. Brockington, D. G. Clark, R. Raman, and D. C. Marson. 2007. "Medical Decision-Making Capacity in Patients with Mild Cognitive Impairment." *Neurology* 69 (15):1528–1535. doi: 10.1212/01.wnl.0000277639.90611.d9.

* Okonkwo, O. C., H. R. Griffith, K. Belue, S. Lanza, E. Y. Zamrini, L. E. Harrell, J. C. Brockington, D. G. Clark, R. Raman, and D. C. Marson. 2008a. "Cognitive Models of Medical Decision-Making Capacity in Patients with Mild Cognitive Impairment." *Journal of the International Neuropsychological Society* 14 (2):297–308. doi: 10.1017/S1355617708080338.

* Okonkwo, O. C., H. R. Griffith, J. N. Copeland, K. Belue, S. Lanza, E. Y. Zamrini, L. E. Harrell, J. C. Brockington, D. G. Clark, R. Raman, and D. C. Marson. 2008b. "Medical Decision-Making Capacity in Mild Cognitive Impairment: A 3-Year Longitudinal Study." *Neurology* 71 (19):1474–1480. doi: 10.1212/01.wnl.0000334301.32358.48.

*Pachana, N. A., G. L. Byrne, J. Wilson, C. Tilse, D. M. Pinsker, B. Massavelli, K. J. Vearncombe, and L. K. Mitchell. 2014. "Predictors of Financial Capacity Performance in Older Adults Using the Financial Competence Assessment Inventory." *International Psychogeriatrics* 26 (6):921–927. doi: 10.1017/s1041610214000209.

* Palmer, B. W., K. A. Ryan, H. M. Kim, J. H. T. Karlawish, P. S. Appelbaum, and S. Y. H. Kim. 2013. "Neuropsychological Correlates of Capacity Determination in Alzheimer's Disease: Implications for Assessment." *American Journal of Geriatric Psychiatry* 21 (4): 373–381. doi: 10.1016/j.jagp.2012.11.008.

Prince, M., R. Bryce, E. Albanese, A. Wimo, W. Ribeiro, and C. P. Ferri. 2013. "The Global Prevalence of Dementia: A Systematic Review and Meta-Analysis." *Alzheimer's & Dementia* 9 (1):63–75. doi: 10.1016/j.jalz.2012.11.007.

* Roked, F., and A. Patel. 2008. "Which Aspects of Cognitive Function Are Best Associated with Testamentary Capacity in Patients with Alzheimer's Disease?" *International Journal of Geriatric Psychiatry* 23 (5):552–553. doi: 10.1002/gps.1947.

* Samsi, K., C. Abley, S. Campbell, J. Keady, J. Manthorpe, L. Robinson, S. Watts, and J. Bond. 2014. "Negotiating a Labyrinth: Experiences of Assessment and Diagnostic Journey in Cognitive Impairment and Dementia." *International Journal of Geriatric Psychiatry* 29 (1):58–67. doi: 10.1002/gps.3969.

* Samsi, K., and J. Manthorpe. 2013. "Everyday Decision-Making in Dementia: Findings from a Longitudinal Interview Study of People with Dementia and Family Carers." *International Psychogeriatrics* 25 (6):949–961. doi: 10.1017/S1041610213000306.

Schicktanz, S., M. Schweda, J. F. Ballenger, P. J. Fox, J. Halpern, J. H. Kramer, G. Micco, S. G. Post, C. Thompson, R. T. Knight, and W. J. Jagust. 2014. "Before It Is Too Late: Professional Responsibilities in Late-Onset Alzheimer's Research and Pre-Symptomatic Prediction." *Frontiers in Human Neuroscience* 8:921. doi: 10.3389/fnhum.2014.00921.

Schicktanz, S., M. Schweda, and M. Franzen. 2008. "'In a Completely Different Light'? The Role of Being Affected for Epistemic Perspectives and Moral Attitudes of Patients, Relatives and Lay People." *Medicine, Health Care and Philosophy* 11 (1):57–72. doi: 10.1007/s11019-007-9074-2.

Schicktanz, S., M. Schweda, and B. Wynne. 2011. "The Ethics of 'Public Understanding of Ethics': Why and How Bioethics Expertise Should Include Public and Patients' Voices." *Medicine, Health Care and Philosophy* 15 (2):129–139. doi: 10.1007/s11019-011-9321-4.

* Seaman, J. B., L. Terhorst, A. Gentry, A. Hunsaker, L. S. Parker, and J. H. Lingler. 2015. "Psychometric Properties of a Decisional Capacity Screening Tool for Individuals Contemplating Participation in Alzheimer's Disease Research." *Journal of Alzheimer's Disease* 46 (1):1–9. doi: 10.3233/jad-142559.

* Sherod, M. G., H. R. Griffith, J. N. Copeland, K. Belue, S. Krzywanski, E. Y. Zamrini, L. E. Harrel, D. G. Clark, J. C. Brockington, R. E. Powers, and D. C. Marson. 2009. "Neurocognitive Predictors of Financial Capacity across the Dementia Spectrum: Normal Aging, Mild Cognitive Impairment, and Alzheimer's Disease." *Journal of the International Neuropsychological Society* 15 (2):258–267. doi: 10.1017/S1355617709090365.

* Smebye, K. L., M. Kirkevold, and K. Engedal. 2012. "How Do Persons with Dementia Participate in Decision Making Related to Health and Daily Care? A Multi-Case Study." *BMC Health Services Research* 12:241–252. doi: 10.1186/1472-6963-12-241.

Spector, A., and M. Orrell. 2010. "Using a Biopsychosocial Model of Dementia as a Tool to Guide Clinical Practice." *International Psychogeriatrics* 22 (6):957–965. doi: 10.1017/s1041610210000840.

Sperling, R. A., P. S. Aisen, L. A. Beckett, D. A. Bennett, S. Crafot, A. M. Fagan, T. Iwatsubo, C. R. Jack, J. Kaye, T. J. Montine, D. C. Park, E. M. Reiman, C. C. Rowe, E. Siemers, Y. Stern, K. Yaffe, M. C. Carrillo, B. Thies, M. Morrison-Bogorad, M. V. Wagster, and C. H. Phelps. 2011. "Toward Defining the Preclinical Stages of Alzheimer's Disease: Recommendations from the National Institute on Aging-Alzheimer's Association Workgroups on Diagnostic Guidelines for Alzheimer's Disease." *Alzheimer's & Dementia* 7 (3):280–292. doi: org/10.1016/j.jalz.2011.03.003.

* St-Amant, O., C. Ward-Griffin, R. T. DeForge, A. Oudshoorn, C. McWilliam, D. Forbes, M. Kloseck, and J. Hall. 2012. "Making Care Decisions in Home-Based Dementia Care: Why Context Matters." *Canadian Journal on Aging* 31 (4):423–434. doi: 10.1017/S0714980812000396.

* Stormoen, S., O. Almkvist, M. Eriksdotter, E. Sundström, and I.-M. Tallberg. 2014. "Cognitive Predictors of Medical Decision-Making Capacity in Mild Cognitive Impairment and Alzheimer's Disease." *International Journal of Geriatric Psychiatry* 29 (12):1304–1311. doi: 10.1002/gps.4114.

* Tallberg, I. M., S. Stormoen, O. Almkvist, M. Eriksdotter, and E. Sundström. 2013. "Investigating Medical Decision-Making Capacity in Patients with Cognitive Impairment Using a Protocol Based on Linguistic Features." *Scandinavian Journal of Psychology* 54 (5):386–392. doi: 10.1111/sjop.12068.

* Tiraboschi, P., E. Chitò, L. Sacco, M. Sala, S. Stefanini, and C. A. Defanti. 2011. "Evaluating Voting Competence in Persons with Alzheimer Disease." *International Journal of Alzheimer's Disease.* doi: 10.4061/2011/983895.

* Triebel, K. L., R. Martin, H. R. Griffith, J. C. Marceaux, O. C. Okonkwo, L. E. Harrell, D. G. Clark, J. C. Brockington, A. A. Bartolucci, and D. C. Marson. 2009. "Declining Financial Capacity in Mild Cognitive Impairment: A 1-Year Longitudinal Study." *Neurology* 73 (12):928–934. doi: 10.1212/WNL.0b013e3181b87971.

* Triebel, K. L., O. C. Okonkwo, R. Martin, H. R. Griffith, M. Crowther, and D. C. Marson. 2010. "Financial Capacity of Older African Americans with Amnestic Mild Cognitive Impairment." *Alzheimer Disease and Associated Disorders* 24 (4):365–371. doi: 10.1097/WAD.0b013e3181e7cb05.

* Vollmann, J., A. Bauer, H. Danker-Hopfe, and H. Helmchen. 2003. "Competence of Mentally Ill Patients: A Comparative Empirical Study." *Psychological Medicine* 33 (8):1463–1471. doi: 10.1017/s0033291703008389.

* Werner, P. 2006. "Lay Perceptions Regarding the Competence of Persons with Alzheimer's Disease." *International Journal of Geriatric Psychiatry* 21 (7):674–680. doi: 10.1002/gps.1546.

Werner, P. 2014. "Stigma and Alzheimer's Disease: A Systematic Review of Evidence, Theory, and Methods." In *The Stigma of Disease and Disability: Understanding Causes and Overcoming Injustices*, edited by P. W. Corrigan, 223–244. Washington, DC: American Psychological Association.

Werner, P., and A. D. Korczyn. 2008. "Mild Cognitive Impairment: Conceptual, Assessment, Ethical, and Social Issues." *Clinical Interventions in Aging* 3 (3):413–420.

* Whelan, P. J. P., J. Oleszek, A. Macdonald, and F. P. Gaughran. 2009. "The Utility of the Mini-Mental State Examination in Guiding Assessment of Capacity to Consent to Research." *International Psychogeriatrics* 21 (2):338–344. doi: 10.1017/S1041610208008314.

World Health Organization. 2002. "*Ethical Choices in Long-Term Care: What Does Justice Require?*" Geneva: World Health Organization. www.who.int/chp/knowledge/publications/ethical_choices.pdf?ua=1.

7 Opt in or opt out? Rethinking the provision of life-sustaining medical technology to the 'old old'

Hsiu-I Yang

We know that we will all die one day. But we do not know whether we will be fortunate enough to live to old age and to then have a peaceful, timely death – a desirable situation described by an old Chinese idiom as "End a long life and die straight in your own bed" (壽終正寢). Thanks to public-health measures and a higher standard of living, men and women in developed countries nowadays have an average life expectancy of around 80 years. According to WHO (2015) estimates, the global population aged 60 today can expect to live an average of 20 more years. For persons aged 80 and over (hereinafter the old old), having completed a full life, it is rational to presume that they as well as their families wish for a death that is peaceful.

Nonetheless, such a wish toward what can be perceived as a 'good death' is often thwarted by the well-established paradigm of saving lives. Following ethical and legal principles, decisions concerning potentially life-prolonging treatment must start from the presumption in favor of prolonging life unless the patient explicitly 'opts out.' This 'life-first paradigm' normally requires doctors to take all reasonable steps to prolong a patient's life, no matter how old he or she is. Patients who are 80 years or over currently constitute between 8.9 and 13.8 percent of large national ICU registries (Andersen et al. 2015). Australia and New Zealand show 5.6 percent annual increases in the numbers of octogenarians entering the ICU (Bagshaw et al. 2009); in Denmark, an 18 percent increase was observed from 2005 to 2011 (Nielsson et al. 2014). In the United States, the proportion of older Americans utilizing intensive care in the last month of their life has steadily increased over the past two decades (Teno et al. 2013). At the same time, more and more evidence shows that acute critical care increases neither survival nor quality of life for the old old patients (Ehlenbach et al. 2010; Frezza, Squillario, and Smith 1998; Gill et al. 2010; Stapleton et al. 2014; Teno et al. 2005). Nonetheless, because of the fear of malpractice lawsuits, enthusiasm toward medical technology, and the moral imperative to save lives, doctors tend to overtreat terminal patients (Smith et al. 2012; Knaus and The SUPPORT Principal Investigators 1995). Consequently, it is not uncommon for the old old to spend their final days or months unconscious in hospital beds, hooked to various life-support devices. There have been reports among clinicians in Europe, Israel, and the United States of disproportionately aggressive treatment for patients who are unlikely to benefit (Huynh et al. 2013; Piers et al. 2011).

This chapter boldly suggests that in the era of global ageing, the law as a norm-guiding instrument should take a determined step to prevent the provision of unwanted and unnecessary life-sustaining medical technology (hereinafter LSMT) to patients over 80 unless they explicitly demand otherwise. The new 'opt in' model is based on a paradigm shift from presumption of life to presumption of peaceful death for people aged 80 and older. To elaborate my thesis, I begin with an exploration of the attitudes of the old old toward death and dying and conclude that a peaceful death is a common ideal. I then examine the current opt-out model and analyze the socio-psychological causes for the failure of advance directives in achieving the goal of a 'good death.' I propose that the law should take a lead to counterbalance the prevailing medical utopian culture against death and ageing by drawing an age-oriented borderline at 80 years as a signpost of the 'end stage of life.' Everyone who passes that legal age will be seen to have lived a full life, and the preselected end-of-life care will be palliative care rather than LSMT in order to assure a peaceful death. I discuss the advantages and ethical concerns of this new opt-in model and conclude by inviting more debate and reflection on the relation of modern medicine, death, and long life.

Attitudes of the old old toward death, dying, and LSMT

Death and dying belong to the natural course of life. Seeing the end of one's life and accepting the coming of death has long been regarded as an appropriate attitude of being old (Cicero 1923). According to Erikson's theory of lifespan development (Erikson, Erikson, and Kivnick 1986), the last phase of life has to do with coming to terms with integrity versus despair and, if successfully resolved, results in 'wisdom.' Aiken's (1995) research suggests "that the elderly are more likely to see themselves as having had their day and to view death in old age as only fair" (Aiken 1995, 366–398) and that older people are better able to cope with the approaching death, partly because of their life experience, their failing health, and the loss of people close to them.

Is this general observation of death and old age applicable to the old old? Hallberg (2003) found that there were few studies focusing solely on old old individuals and their view of death and dying, but among those few, he did identify that death and dying were commonly viewed with an accepting attitude, as something unavoidable, as the completion of the life cycle, but also with very different emotions of anger, sadness, or confidence, as well as not worrying or even looking forward to death (Hallberg 2003). Fleming et al.'s (2016) investigation on the oldest old (95 years or more) also found that most of them were worried not about death itself but about the process of dying and the impact on those who would be left behind; a peaceful and pain-free death was a common ideal.

It is worth pointing out that the elderly may be emotionally prepared for death but not for dying. A lot of empirical evidence has shown that fear and anxiety about one's own death may actually decrease with age (Gesser, Wong, and Reker 1988; Kastenbaum 1996; Neimeyer 1985; Robinson and Wood 1984; Thorson and Powell 1989). Older people may have accepted the finiteness of life but still fear dying (Thomé 2003). They are more concerned about issues of dignity, self-sufficiency, and a sense of losing control (Cicirelli 2002; Hallberg 2003; Thorson and Powell 1994). A 2013 book written by the former prime minister of Singapore, Lee Kuan Yew, expressively reflects on the fear of a slow death. Lee says:

> Life is better than death. But death comes eventually to everyone. It is something which many in their prime may prefer not to think about. But at 89, I see no point in avoiding the question. What concerns me is: How do I go? Will the end come swiftly, with a stroke in one of the coronary arteries? Or will it be a stroke in the mind that lays me out in bed for months, semi-comatose? Of the two, I prefer the quick one. Some time back, I had an Advance Medical Directive done which says that if I have to be fed by a tube, and it is unlikely that I would ever be able to recover and walk about, my doctors are to remove the tube and allow me to make a quick exit. I had it signed by a lawyer friend and a doctor.
>
> (Lee 2013)

Lee is not alone in his preference. Studies have found that older patients are less likely to elect life-supporting interventions in the final stage of life. Two decades ago, the American landmark SUPPORT study revealed that older patients were less likely to elect CPR than similar younger patients (Phillips et al. 1996). A more recent study also confirms the relation of old age and limitation of LSMT (Turnbull et al. 2014).

The opt-out model: pitfalls of advance directives

Death is an inevitable biological phenomenon, and death at old age is indeed a plausible ending of a finite life. With the invention and intervention of various LSMT, however, modern society has replaced the ancient 'tame death' with a 'wild death' in which people often die alone in ICUs, wrapped in a harsh cocoon of tubes and wires (Callahan 2012). A fifth of elderly Americans die in intensive care, and of these patients, about half undergo mechanical ventilation, and a quarter undergo cardiopulmonary resuscitation in the days before their death (Angus et al. 2004; Prendergast, Claessens, and Luce 1998).

In the past 40 years, many jurisdictions in the developed countries have agreed that every individual has the legal right to refuse LSMT (Annas and Glantz 1986; Knouse 1991; Otlowski 1997). Since such a right is based on the established ethical principle of respecting patient autonomy, its implementation asks for the patient's expressive instruction to refuse (opt out). To resolve the practical problem that many patients on LSMT may have become incompetent, the focus of the right-to-die legislation is on advance directives (ADs) – documents that allow individuals to designate their preferences for medical care in the event that they cannot communicate these wishes at a future time (Andorno, Biller-Andorno, and Brauer 2009; McLean 1991).

Two decades after its implementation and following strong policy advocating, the traditional approach to creating ADs has to be considered a failure (Fagerlin and Schneider 2004). The most obvious disappointment is the poor completion rate. In the US, a national nursing home survey revealed that 14 years after the passage of the *Patient Self-Determination Act*, the most widely used ADs for elderly nursing-home residents (age 65 and over) is the do-not-resuscitate order (59.7% of residents) (Fissell et al. 2005; Voltz et al. 1998). Only 19.7 percent have a living will and even fewer a LSMT limitation (Jones et al. 2009, 5, 29). It is estimated that the number of completed ADs in the US ranges from 5 percent to 15 percent (Jones, Moss, and Harris-Kojetin 2011). In Germany, use of ADs varies between patient groups (0.3% to 62%) and is low among the general population, rising to around 10 percent in two surveys carried out in 2007 (Evans et al. 2012). In Taiwan, the idea to link ADs with the National Health Insurance (NHI) IC Card was put into effect in 2006. Despite strong media promotion, only 5,074 of the total 23 million NHI IC Card holders registered their ADs in 2006. The Department of Health then mandated all hospitals to provide a sample AD to all hospitalized patients. In addition, the *Hospice and Palliative Care Act* 2013 enacted a new article to validate the NHI IC Card register. After all these endeavors, the numbers of the NHI IC Card AD register gradually rose to 145,921 by the end of 2012 (Lee et al. 2013, 282). Among them, 13,304 (9.12%) are aged 80 or over, constituting 0.7 percent of the old old population in Taiwan in 2012. In contrast, a national survey conducted in 2011 revealed that as many as 76.5 percent of Taiwanese people aged 80 or over would sign a form to forgo aggressive treatment upon diagnosis of an incurable terminal disease (Chang, Tu, and Liao 2013).

The discrepancy between the old old people's preference of comfort care in the end-of-life stage and their reluctance to put their opt-out intention in writing is not unusual. In a German study, more than 75 percent of adult people aged 20 and 90 expressed agreement with the statement that they would like to decide when and how to die, but only 10.9 percent had signed a living will (Lang, Baltes, and Wagner 2007). A UK study found that the oldest old are willing to discuss dying and end-of-life care but seldom do (Fleming et al. 2016). High's (1993) study suggests that most participants in interventions prefer to defer to family surrogates and to avoid executing ADs. This family-surrogate-decision model is especially prevalent Japan, Taiwan, and other Asian countries. In Japan, there is a high prevalence of entrusting all decisions to the family (Voltz et al. 1998). Hsin's (2006) study also confirmed that a very important factor for the Taiwanese elderly's unwillingness to document their wishes is to prevent trouble for their adult children at such time as they have to make relevant decisions.

Such well-intentioned ideas about surrogate decision-making often have the opposite effect. Given the uncertain nature of the line between living and dying, having to make decisions about end-of-life care for beloved family members is a great burden. Without adequate guidance, people tend to choose more LSMT for their family members than they would for themselves (Wendler and Rid 2011). In a survey of attitudes toward good death in 2014, respondents exhibited a more conservative attitude to withdrawal of treatment for family members than for themselves (Tang and Lan 2014, 24–25). This discrepancy often leads to a tragic outcome: The patients suffer a slow death, the surrogates suffer bereavement and depression, and the health system suffers high costs for futile treatment. This is in stark contrast to what appears to matter most to patients: They do not want to be a burden on their loved ones at the end of their life (Mead et al. 1995; Singer et al. 1998; Steinhauser et al. 2000). Evidence shows that end-of-life discussions are associated with lower rates of ventilation, resuscitation, and ICU admission, as well as earlier hospice enrollment, and that more aggressive medical care is associated with a decrease in patients' quality of life as well as a higher risk of major depressive disorder in bereaved caregivers, whereas longer hospice stays are associated with an increase in patients' quality of life. Better patient quality of life is associated with better caregiver quality of life at follow-up (Vandervoort et al. 2014; Wright et al. 2008).

The failure of ADs has resulted in serious discussions on the psychosocial and psycho-cultural difficulties surrounding end-of-life care decision-making (Evans et al. 2012; Fagerlin and Schneider 2004; Tulsky 2005). The common theme of reform is directed toward advance care planning (ACP) to strengthen joint participation in a refined communication process (Halpern 2012; Lund, Richardson, and May 2015; Perkins 2007; Tulsky 2005; Waldrop and Meeker 2012; see Jox in this volume). A fundamental question, however, remains unanswered: how to effectively start an ACP process under the prevailing medical utopian belief that pain and suffering associated with disease, ageing, and death can eventually be eliminated by medical technology (Callahan 2012). Undoubtedly, society has witnessed increasing vitality and activity in old age, generating positive expectations about longevity and quality of life. Nonetheless, a lot of the good news from recent ageing research applies to the 'young old' or 'third age' (Baltes and Smith 2003). As Callahan (1993) points out, success in curing an illness may in fact set the stage for the advent of a different disease, perhaps a much more agonizing one. There are more and more findings about the calamities of the 'fourth age': loss of cognitive and mental fitness, high prevalence of dementia, physical frailty, and multi-morbidity (Baltes and Smith 2003; Jacobs et al. 2011; Singer et al. 2003).

A new approach: the opt-in model

The conventional 'presumption of life' paradigm suggests that a bad life is better than a good death, as there is always hope associated with life. Likewise, LSMT was originally invented to serve as a 'halfway technology' to temporarily assist a patient in critical condition so that he or she might have a chance to return to normal functions as basic as communicating, eating and drinking, or at the very least breathing. Given the uncertainty of how an illness will develop, it is very much appropriate for doctors to start by choosing to save a patient's life in a case of emergency and then change the protocols when a fatal prognosis becomes apparent. In such a case, when the continued use of LSMT does little to improve quality of life but rather extends dying, it is time to change the paradigm of presumption of life to presumption of peaceful death (Callahan 1993).

Thanks to the Hospice Care Movement, more and more people accept the idea of having palliative care instead of aggressive treatment at the 'end of life' stage.

However, the most troubling practical problem lies in identifying the borderline. How can we know for certain that a seriously ill patient is entering the 'end of life' stage and has reached the point where futile fighting needs to be replaced with preparing for a peaceful death? Modern society tends not to draw such a line but to rely on a case-by-case judgment made by medical professionals. I suggest that we supplement the medically oriented and professionally defined uncertain concept of the 'end of life' stage with a societal consensus and legally defined concept of 'end stage of life.' To do this, we should implement a definite age limitation of 80 years to define entering into the 'end stage of life,' in which a peaceful death constitutes an indispensable part of a good life. The law could and should encourage people to accept their biological lifespan by formally acknowledging that by living to the age of 80, they have accomplished a 'full life.' Accordingly, should an emergency occur and should an old old person be unable to make a competent medical decision, the legal default should be comfort care. No LSMT should be continued to be given to permanently unconscious old-old people without their written consent in ADs. There are three important components in this new opt-in model.

1. A prima facie age limitation of 80 years denoting completion of a 'full life'

The proposed age-based limitation represents a minimum social consensus of a 'full life,' so different societies can set their own specific age limitation according to their prospective demographic characteristics – which can be as high as age 85 or as low as age 75. The average life expectancy in most developed countries is around 80 years, and there are studies showing that people's desired lifetime falls within 81 to 85 years (Lang, Baltes, and Wagner 2007; Mirowsky and Ross 2000). However, chronological age does not necessarily reflect health status. 'End stage of life' does not equal 'end of life.' I want to stress that this age limitation is *prima facie* in a sense that any and every individual is allowed to re-define his or her own 'full life' age. American bioethicist Ezekiel Emanuel set an inspiring example when he published an article in 2014 declaring that he (58 years old at the time) hopes to die at 75. The age limitation helps him make decisions about his own healthcare. By choosing 75 as his 'full life' age, Emanuel says that he will refuse procedures such as flu shots and antibiotics. He will say no to any cancer treatment, cardiac stress test, pacemaker or implantable defibrillator, heart valve replacement or bypass surgery (Emanuel 2014).

This 'full life' age limitation has nothing to do with ageism, because individuals can choose to change it according to their own changing health conditions, life experiences, and reflections on death and dying. It is possible to be content with the law's interpretation of a full life and stick with the default care plan. It is also possible to choose a younger age as the 'full life' age and to implement an absolute 'no medical treatment' policy. The others, especially those who are over 80, may want to postpone the 'full life' age by expressing their desire for life-extending care (Lang, Baltes, and Wagner 2007). No matter which situation, defining an exact time will eliminate the fuzziness of the perspective of maximal life prolongation. Its specificity can motivate people to think about the end of life, to engage with existential questions, and to ponder what they want to leave behind for their children and grandchildren, their community, their fellow people, and the world.

2. Pursuing a peaceful death in the end stage of life

I argue that a presumption of peaceful death should replace the presumption of life as the guiding ethical paradigm in deciding whether to give an incompetent old old person LSMT. According to Callahan (1993), a peaceful death means accepting human fate – seeing death at old age not as an accident to prevent, but as nature's course to come. Thus, the main characteristic of a peaceful death is acceptance – accepting the inevitability of death, accepting a certain degree of pain and suffering associated with advanced age, and accepting loss of control in the dying process (Callahan 1993). In Callahan's ideal, a peaceful death merges personal, medical, and social strands, including the relief of pain, being remembered and respected, and preventing undue burden for loved ones. To a great extent, this matches a recent empirical finding on old old people's actual wishes for a good death. Hallberg's (2003) study revealed that people did not necessarily share the same view of how they want their end-of-life phase to unfold or to be handled. Even so, the most uniform directions were those emphasizing no life prolongation, being respected, the importance of integrity, being approached as a whole person, living one day at a time, having the opportunity to be involved with others, caring for others, and the balance between having loved ones close by but not being a burden to them.

Callahan (1993) expresses very clearly that a peaceful death should have both an individual and a public face. For the individual, it can bring life to a fitting close, marked by the connection to the self through reason and self-consciousness and by connection to others through dying – within the circle of human companionship and caring. For the public, death is peaceful in the sense that its control and management should not consume an undue share of resources. We should be willing, Callahan says, to bear what nature and human mortality bring us. Still, there is no reason why we should have to bear an artificially extended death (Callahan 1993).

3. Change of default in ADs

How would such presumption of peaceful death be implemented? Without an opt-in AD, should an incompetent patient over 80 be excluded from ICU care? Should octogenarians not be offered coronary bypass surgery? Should the ER doctor withhold reasonable and necessary emergency treatment before confirming how old an incompetent patient is? The inhumanity of such suggestions is self-evident. I am neither advocating age rationing nor claiming that elderly people who are terminally ill have a duty to die. Instead, it is my intention to use the law to help old old people maximize their well-being. A feasible option is to design a well-structured standard 'comfort-default AD' to be linked to every 65-year-old patient's electronic medical record. Healthcare providers would then be obliged to inform their elderly patients of the new law and to hand such comfort-default AD out to them. Should an old old patient be uncomfortable with the comfort-default AD, he or she would be advised on how to easily change it by replacing the legal age of 80 with his or her 'desired' age. Of course, it will be welcome and even encouraged if the elderly patient wants to modify the default AD to better reflect his or her own preferences and values in end-of-life care. Eventually, this strategy will result in a universal distribution of ADs among octogenarians, either as a comfort-default AD or as a modified AD.

Clearly, this plan requires a lot of institutional competency. We would need more empirical studies to support the design of an age-sensitive default AD; we would need more trained, experienced, and skilled professionals in providing advance care planning (ACP) counseling; and we would need to develop a procedure to resolve conflicts in case family members disagree. Luckily, all of the above-mentioned matters are currently being furthered. What I propose is not something unimaginable but a policy strategy to accelerate moving toward the realization of a peaceful death.

Advantages and ethical concerns

There are two major advantages of the new 'opt in' model. The first and foremost is the facilitation of a conversation about ACP between the old old and their caretakers. Under the current opt-out model, ACP discussion is difficult and disconcerting, because the topic is death and 'giving up.' Ottosson's (1999) Swedish study shows that doctors hesitate to bring up matters related to death and dying, yet patients appreciate it if they do – even though they sometimes find it emotionally upsetting (Ottosson 1999, 282–308). German physicians fear that patients associate discussion of ADs with an imminent death and therefore will reject a routine discussion (Burchardi et al. 2005). A survey of patients, physicians, nurses, and healthy controls revealed tension surrounding the widely held belief that physicians should initiate discussion about ADs. It also showed that most physicians prefer to delegate the task to patients' families and friends, with only a minority (39%) ever having discussed an AD with a patient (Sahm, Will, and Hommel 2005).

Kastenbaum (1996) states that stereotypes and negative societal attitudes toward death and dying – especially in old people – influence those in touch with older people, as well as older persons themselves. Fleming's study found that death is rarely talked about between the oldest old and their proxies (Fleming et al. 2016). Because the prospect of creating an AD is unpleasant, the future benefits of having completed an AD must be viewed as substantial to sufficiently motivate a person to actually fill out an AD. Otherwise, there is the tendency to discount future benefits in order to avoid present pain (Halpern 2012). Once the law draws a clear line at the age of 80 and sets the default to no LSMT when there is no opt-in AD, as I propose, the dynamics of the conversation will change. Because the law will have pre-selected a comfort-default AD for people over 80, it will become appropriate for adult children to inquire about their old old parents' actual wishes or to initiate a conversation by persuading the octogenarians to sign an opt-in AD. The sooner the conversation between old old people, their families, and their physicians begins, the better chance there is for a peaceful death.

Another advantage of the opt-in model is that it empowers physicians to perform good medicine on their old old patients by not having to provide painful and futile LSMT. Medical practice is value-loaded. Physicians' ethical concerns include respect for autonomy, nonmaleficence, beneficence, and justice. When the medical intervention most likely will not benefit the patient (quantitative futility) and when the intervention will produce an outcome of poor quality of life (qualitative futility) (Jecker 2014), physicians' ethical duty is to stop the futile treatment. Unfortunately, under the current opt-out model and without an effective AD, such ethical duty to stop futile treatment is often hindered by the family's hope for a miracle. Under my opt-in scheme, futile treatment is expected to decrease greatly, but it will not be eliminated completely, as many old old people might still choose a life-extension AD or still entrust the decision to their families.

Two potential ethical concerns need to be clarified further. Does this age-oriented opt-in model imply an elderly person's duty to die? How are we to deal with those old old people who do not know about the change of presumption and have no chance to opt in? Would the implementation result in some form of neglect of the elderly?

The concept of 'duty to die' was first broached by Margaret Battin (1987) in the context of global justice, and it was brought up again in 1997 by John Hardwig. Hardwig (1997) argues that an individual who is terminally ill or in need of extensive care may have a duty not only to decline this care but to die in order to avoid imposing excessively heavy burdens of care and support on family members or loved ones. According to him, this duty is stronger for people who are older and who have already lived full lives (especially if they are facing a degenerative disease such as Alzheimer's or Huntington's), whose loved ones have had difficult lives or have already had to make sacrifices for them, and who can no longer hope to make significant contributions to the lives of their loved ones. Clearly, Hardwig's thesis operates under the paradigm of presumption of life, so he tries to create a 'duty to die.' In contrast, the focus of my proposal is that old old people have a 'right to a natural death,' so that the paradigm in guiding the provision of LSMT should be shifted to presumption of peaceful death. There is no need to impose a 'duty to die' on old old people in my model, because the concept of death has been aligned with the concept of life in the old old population, and the withholding or withdrawing of LSMT presumably fits their true wishes and best interest.

Still, my proposal might be seen as a duty to make an AD choice. For anyone who passes the age of 80, the new paradigm will presume that he or she wishes to exercise the right to a peaceful death by forgoing LSMT should he or she end up in an unconscious state, needing medical attention. Those who do not share the same view will have to sign a will-to-extend-life AD to execute their own choices. In an educated society, decisions about end-of-life care are among the most personal choices any human being will ever make. While some might prefer forgoing extreme measures and letting nature take its course, there are certainly others who wish to exhaust every available resource to prolong their life as long as possible. Both of these wishes should be honored. However, although all people should have the right to decide how they want their lives to end, it does not necessarily follow that they have to be able to avoid confronting such a choice. We will all die, whether we bother to think about it or not. Considering the enormous costs – both emotional and economic – of end-of-life interventions, society has every right to expect its members to make their wishes regarding such care clear in advance. Providing LSMT to all old old people as a default – in the absence of an AD – does not make any more sense than making early termination the default. Hopefully, the new opt-in model will nudge old old people to effectuate their genuine desires for end-of-life care by communicating about ACP with their families and physicians.

But what about those old old people who are socially the least advantaged, who live alone with no family or have been abandoned by their family, and who have no idea about the change of law and therefore have no AD at all? Let us imagine a neglected old old person is sent to a hospital by neighbors, and, after emergency interventions, he or she ends up on LSMT, unconscious. Without family members, without loved ones, and without hope the patient will regain his or her competence, removal of the LSMT is an action safeguarding and facilitating his or her peaceful death, in order to relieve his or her pain and suffering and to preserve final dignity. It is by no means an act of neglect toward the elderly. Furthermore, forgoing LSMT does not mean the patient receives no treatment or no care. The preset comfort-default AD will direct the care to maintain the patient's integrity and dignity.

Conclusion

As early as 1981, Phillip Aries criticized modern medicine for stealing away the 'old tame death' by implementing a technology-controlled 'wild death.' And as early as 1993, Daniel Callahan proclaimed we should pursue a peaceful death. Two decades have passed, and mounting studies and literature on the subject have consistently revealed that we are still far away from the goal.

My proposal for a paradigm shift from presumption of life to presumption of peaceful death for those who have lived a 'full life,' defined as having reached the age of 80, may seem bold and revolutionary. In fact, its scope is very limited and conservative. It covers only a certain population (the old old), only in extreme situations (permanent unconsciousness), and only concerning specific end-of-life care (LSMT). My humble wish is to use the law as an effective nudging instrument to stimulate a more open and more honest public policy on death and dying at old age and to eventually develop a mature culture of death, in which old people can live longer and healthier and die quicker and fitter.

Being able to live to old age should be a blessing, not a burden. Autonomy for the old old should be calm and self-constrained, and death for the old old should be peaceful and serene. Simply giving an individual the right to die does not really solve any problems. The society and the law should honor their obligation to bring conceptual and institutional change by helping people plan their later life. Back in ancient times, the great Roman orator Seneca gave a lot of thought to old age and death:

> I will not relinquish old age if it leaves my better part intact. But if it begins to shake my mind, if it destroys its faculties one by one, if it leaves me not life but breath, I will depart from the putrid or tottering edifice. I will not escape by death from disease so long as it may be healed, and leaves my mind unimpaired. I will not raise my hand against myself on account of pain, for so to die is to be conquered. But I know that if I must suffer without hope of relief, I will depart, not through fear of the pain itself, but because it prevents all for which I would live.
>
> (Seneca 1969, letter 58)

References

Aiken, L. R. 1995. *Aging: An Introduction to Gerontology*. Oxford: Sage.

Andersen, F. H., H. Flaatten, P. Klepstad, U. Romild, and R. Kvåle. 2015. "Long-Term Survival and Quality of Life after Intensive Care for Patients 80 Years of Age or Older." *Annals of Intensive Care* 5:13. doi: 10.1186/s13613-015-0053-0.

Andorno, R., N. Biller-Andorno, and S. Brauer. 2009. "Advance Health Care Directives: Towards a Coordinated European Policy?" *European Journal of Health Law* 16 (3):207–227. doi: 10.1163/157180909X453053.

Angus, D. C., A. E. Barnato, W. T. Linde-Zwirble, L. Weissfeld, R. S. Watson, T. Rickert, and G. D. Rubenfeld. 2004. "Use of Intensive Care at the End of Life in the United States: An Epidemiologic Study." *Critical Care Medicine* 32 (3):638–643. doi: 10.1097/01.CCM.0000114816.62331.08.

Annas, G. J., and L. H. Glantz. 1986. "The Right of Elderly Patients to Refuse Life-Sustaining Treatment." *The Milbank Quarterly* 64 (2):95–162. doi: 10.2307/3349961.

Bagshaw, S. M., S. A. Webb, A. Delaney, C. George, D. Pilcher, G. K. Hart, and R. Bellomo. 2009. "Very Old Patients Admitted to Intensive Care in Australia and New Zealand: A Multi-Centre Cohort Analysis." *Critical Care* 13 (2):R45. doi: 10.1186/cc7768.

Baltes, P. B., and J. Smith. 2003. "New Frontiers in the Future of Aging: From Successful Aging in the Young Old to the Dilemmas of the Fourth Age." *Gerontology* 49 (2):123–135. doi: 10.1159/000067946.

Battin, M. P. 1987. "Age Rationing and the Just Distribution of Health Care: Is There a Duty to Die?" *Ethics* 97 (2):317–340. doi: 10.1086/292841.

Burchardi, N., O. Rauprich, M. Hecht, M. Beck, and J. Vollmann. 2005. "Discussing Living Wills: A Qualitative Study of a German Sample of Neurologists and ALS Patients." *Journal of the Neurological Sciences* 237 (1–2):67–74. doi: 10.1016/j.jns.2005.05.013.

Callahan, D. 1993. "Pursuing a Peaceful Death." *The Hastings Center Report* 23 (4):33–38. doi: 10.2307/3562588.

Callahan, D. 2012. "Death, Mourning, and Medical Progress." In *The Roots of Bioethics: Health, Progress, Technology, Death*, edited by D. Callahan, 87–100. Oxford: Oxford University Press.

Chang, Y.-H., S.-H. Tu, and P.-S. Liao. 2013. *2011 Taiwan Social Change Survey (Round 6, Year 2): Health*. Available at Center for Survey Research, RCHSS, Academia Sinica: https://srda.sinica.edu.tw. doi: 10.6141/TW-SRDA-C00222_2-1.

Cicero. 1923. *De Senectute De Amicitia De Divinatione*, translated by W. A. Falconer. Cambridge, MA: Harvard University Press.

Cicirelli, V. G. 2002. "Fear of Death in Older Adults: Predictions from Terror Management Theory." *The Journals of Gerontology, Series B: Psychological Sciences and Social Sciences* 57 (4):358–366. doi: 10.1093/geronb/57.4.P358.

Ehlenbach, W. J., C. L. Hough, P. K. Crane, S. J. Haneuse, S. S. Carson, J. R. Curtis, and E. B. Larson. 2010. "Association between Acute Care and Critical Illness Hospitalization and Cognitive Function in Older Adults." *The Journal of the American Medical Association* 303 (8):763–770. doi: 10.1001/jama.2010.167.

Emanuel, E. J. 2014. "Why I Hope to Die at 75: An Argument That Society and Families – and You – Will Be Better Off if Nature Takes Its Course Swiftly and Promptly." *The Atlantic*, September 17 (online).

Erikson, E. H., J. M. Erikson, and H. Q. Kivnick. 1986. *Vital Involvement in Old Age: The Experience of Old Age in Our Time*. New York: W.W. Norton.

Evans, N., C. Bausewein, A. Meñaca, E. V. Andrew, I. J. Higginson, R. Harding, R. Pool, M. Gysels, and On Behalf of Project PRISMA. 2012. "A Critical Review of Advance Directives in Germany: Attitudes, Use and Healthcare Professionals' Compliance." *Patient Education and Counseling* 87 (3):277–288. doi: 10.1016/j.pec.2011.10.004.

Fagerlin, A., and C. E. Schneider. 2004. "Enough: The Failure of the Living Will." *The Hastings Center Report* 34 (2):30–42. doi: 10.2307/3527683.

Fissell, R. B., J. L. Bragg-Gresham, A. A. Lopes, J. M. Cruz, S. Fukuhara, Y. Asano, W. W. Browon, M. L. Keen, F. K. Port, and E. W. Young. 2005. "Factors Associated with 'Do Not Resuscitate' Orders and Rates of Withdrawal from Hemodialysis in the International DOPPS." *Kidney International* 68 (3):1282–1288. doi: 10.1111/j.1523-1755.2005.00525.x.

Fleming, J., M. Farquhar, Cambridge City over-75s Cohort (CC75C) Study Collaboration, C. Brayne, and S. Barclay. 2016. "Death and the Oldest Old: Attitudes and Preferences for End-of-Life Care: Qualitative Research within a Population-Based Cohort Study." *PLoS One* 11 (4): e0150686. doi: 10.1371/journal.pone.0150686.

Frezza, E. E., D. M. Squillario, and T. J. Smith. 1998. "The Ethical Challenge and the Futile Treatment in the Older Population Admitted to the Intensive Care Unit." *American Journal of Medical Quality* 13 (3):121–126. doi: 10.1177/106286069801300303.

Gesser, G., P. T. P. Wong, and G. T. Reker. 1988. "Death Attitudes across the Life-Span: The Development and Validation of the Death Attitude Profile." *Omega* 18 (2):113–128. doi: 10.2190/0DQB-7Q1E-2BER-H6YC.

Gill, T. M., H. G. Allore, E. A. Gahbauer, and T. E. Murphy. 2010. "Change in Disability after Hospitalization or Restricted Activity in Older Persons." *The Journal of the American Medical Association* 304 (17):1919–1928. doi: 10.1001/jama.2010.1568.

Hallberg, I. R. 2003. "Death and Dying from Old People's Point of View: A Literature Review." *Aging Clinical and Experimental Research* 16 (2):87–103. doi: 10.1007/BF03324537.

Halpern, S. D. 2012. "Shaping End-of-Life Care: Behavioral Economics and Advance Directives." *Seminars in Respiratory and Critical Care Medicine* 33 (4):393–400. doi: 10.1055/s-0032-1322403.

Hardwig, J. 1997. "Is There a Duty to Die?" *The Hastings Center Report* 27 (2):34–42. doi: 10.2307/3527626.

High, D. M. 1993. "Why Are Elderly People Not Using Advance Directives?" *Journal of Aging and Health* 5 (4):497–515. doi: http://dx.doi.org/10.1177/089826439300500405.

Hsin, H.-C. 2006. "Effects of Family-Centered Values in Elder's End-of-Life Decision Making: Perspectives of Seniors in Taiwan and Compared to Seniors in New Zealand." *Formosan Journal of Medical Humanities* 7 (1–2):179–190.

Huynh, T. N., E. C. Kleerup, J. F. Wiley, T. D. Savitsky, D. Guse, B. J. Garber, and N. S. Wenger. 2013. "The Frequency and Cost of Treatment Perceived to be Futile in Critical Care." *The Journal of the American Medical Association: Internal Medicine* 173 (20):750–754. doi: 10.1001/jamainternmed.2013.10261.

Jacobs, J. M., A. Cohen, E. Ein-Mor, Y. Maaravi, and J. Stessman. 2011. "Frailty, Cognitive Impairment and Mortality among the Oldest Old." *The Journal of Nutrition, Health and Aging* 15 (8):678–682.

Jecker, N. S. 2014. "Medical Futility: Ethical Topic in Medicine." Accessed April 11, 2008. https://depts.washington.edu/bioethx/topics/futil.html.

Jones, A. F., A. J. Moss, and L. D. Harris-Kojetin. 2011. "Use of Advance Directives in Long-Term Care Populations." *National Center for Health Statistics: Data Brief* 54. www.cdc.gov/nchs/data/databriefs/db54.pdf.

Jones, A. L., L. L. Dwyer, A. R. Bercovitz, and G. W. Strahan. 2009. "The National Nursing Home Survey: 2004 Overview." *National Center for Health Statistics: Vital and Health Statistics* 13 (167):1–155. www.cdc.gov/nchs/data/series/sr_13/sr13_167.pdf.

Kastenbaum, R. 1996. "Death and Dying." In *Encyclopedia of Gerontology: Age, Aging and the Aged*, edited by J. E. Birren, V. W. Marshall, and A. Svanborg, 361–381. San Diego: Academic Press.

Knouse, J. N. 1991. "Cruzan: The Supreme Court and the Right to Die." *Loyola Law Review* 36 (4):1111–1124.

Lang, F., P. Baltes, and G. Wagner. 2007. "Desired Lifetime and End-of-Life Desires across Adulthood from 20 to 90: A Dual-Source Information Model." *The Journals of Gerontology, Series B: Psychological Sciences and Social Sciences* 62 (5):268–276.

Lee, K. Y. 2013. *One Man's View of the World*. Singapore: Straits Times Press.

Lee, Y. F., S. Q. Cheng, R. B. Zhong, Y. Y. Du, H. W. Chen, and J. K. Fong. 2013. "Executive Report Regarding the Advance Directives on Palliative Care and NIH IC Card Registry: 2006–2012." *Journal of Hospice Care* 18 (3):279–291.

Lund, S., A. Richardson, and C. May. 2015. "Barriers to Advance Care Planning at the End of Life: An Explanatory Systematic Review of Implementation Studies." *PLoS One* 10 (2): e0116629. doi: 10.1371/journal.pone.0116629.

McLean, E. D. 1991. "Living Will Statutes in Light of Cruzan v. Director, Missouri Department of Health: Ensuring That a Patient's Wishes Will Prevail." *Emory Law Journal* 40 (4):1305–1341.

Mead, G. E., S. T. O'Keeffe, C. I. Jack, A. M. Maèstri-Banks, J. R. Playfer, and M. Lye. 1995. "What Factors Influence Patient Preferences Regarding Cardiopulmonary Resuscitation?" *Journal of the Royal College of Physicians of London* 29 (4):295–298.

Mirowsky, J., and C. E. Ross. 2000. "Socioeconomic Status and Subjective Life Expectancy." *Social Psychology Quarterly* 63 (2):133–151. doi: 10.2307/2695888.

Neimeyer, R. A. 1985. "Actualization, Integration and Fear of Death: A Test of the Additive Model." *Death Studies* 9:235–250.

Nielsson, M. S., C. F. Christiansen, M. B. Johansen, B. S. Rasmussen, E. Tønnesen, and M. Nørgaard. 2014. "Mortality in Elderly ICU Patients: A Cohort Study." *Acta Anaesthesiologica Scandinavica* 58 (1):19–26. doi: 10.1111/aas.12211.

Otlowski, M. F. A. 1997. *Voluntary Euthanasia and the Common Law*. Oxford: Oxford University Press.

Ottosson, J.-O., ed. 1999. *Patient-läkarrelationen: läkekonst på vetenskaplig grund*. Stockholm: Natur och Kultur.

Perkins, H. S. 2007. "Controlling Death: The False Promise of Advance Directives." *Annals of Internal Medicine* 147 (1):51–57. doi: 10.7326/0003-4819-147-1-200707030-00008.

Phillips, R. S., N. S. Wenger, J. Teno, R. K. Oye, S. Youngner, R. Califf, P. Layde, N. Desbiens, A. F. Connors Jr., and J. Lynn. 1996. "Choices of Seriously Ill Patients about Cardiopulmonary Resuscitation: Correlates and Outcomes." *The American Journal of Medicine* 100 (2):128–137. doi: 10.1016/S0002-9343(97)89450-8.

Piers, R. D., E. Azoulay, B. Ricou, F. D. Ganz, J. Decruyenaere, A. Max, A. Michalsen, P. A. Maia, R. Owczuk, F. Rubulotta, P. Depuydt, A.-P. Meert, A. K. Reyners, A. Aquilina, M. Bekaert, N. J. Van Den Noortgate, W. J. Schrauwen, and D. D. Benoit. 2011. "Perceptions of Appropriateness of Care among European and Israeli Intensive Care Unit Nurses and Physicians." *The Journal of the American Medical Association* 306 (24):2694–2703. doi: 10.1001/jama.2011.1888.

Prendergast, T. J., M. T. Claessens, and J. M. Luce. 1998. "A National Survey of End-of-Life Care for Critically Ill Patients." *American Journal of Respiratory and Critical Care Medicine* 158 (4):1163–1167. doi: 10.1164/ajrccm.158.4.9801108.

Robinson, P. J., and K. Wood. 1984. "Fear of Death and Physical Illness." In *Personal Meanings of Death*, edited by F. Epting and R. A. Neimeyer, 127–142. Washington, DC: Hemisphere.

Sahm, S., R. Will, and G. Hommel. 2005. "What Are Cancer Patients' Preferences about Treatment at the End of Life, and Who Should Start Talking about It? A Comparison with Healthy People and Medical Staff." *Support Care Cancer* 13 (4):206–214. doi: 10.1007/s00520-004-0725-z.

Seneca. 1969. *Letters from a Stoic*, translated by R. Campbell. Harms: Penguin.

Singer, P. A., D. K. Martin, J. V. Lavery, E. C. Thiel, M. Kelner, and D. C. Mendelssohn. 1998. "Reconceptualizing Advance Care Planning from the Patient's Perspective." *Archives of Internal Medicine* 158 (8):879–884. doi: 10.1001/archinte.158.8.879.

Singer, T., P. Verhaeghen, P. Ghisletta, U. Lindenberger, P. B. Baltes, J. M. Jacobs, A. Cohen, E. Ein-Mor, and Y. Maaravi. 2003. "The Fate of Cognition in Very Old Age: Six-Year Longitudinal Findings in the Berlin Aging Study (BASE)." *Psychology & Aging* 18 (2):318–331. doi: 10.1037/0882-7974.18.2.318.

Smith, A., E. McCarthy, E. Weber, I. S. Cenzer, J. Boscardin, J. Fisher, and K. Covinsky. 2012. "Half of Older Americans Seen in Emergency Department in Last Month of Life; Most Admitted to Hospital, and Many Die There." *Affairs* 31 (6):1277–1285. doi: 10.1377/hlthaff.2011.0922.

Stapleton, R. D., W. J. Ehlenbach, R. Deyo, and J. R. Curtis. 2014. "Long-Term Outcomes after In-Hospital CPR in Older Adults with Chronic Illness." *Chest* 146 (5):1214–1225. doi: 10.1378/chest.13-2110.

Steinhauser, K. E., N. A. Christakis, E. C. Clipp, M. McNeilly, L. McIntyre, and J. A. Tulsky. 2000. "Factors Considered Important at the End of Life by Patients, Family, Physicians, and Other Care Providers." *The Journal of the American Medical Association* 284 (19):2476–2482. doi: 10.1001/jama.284.19.2476.

Tang, K. J., and Z. Y. Lan. 2014. *Report on the Futile Treatment Before Dying*. www.393citizen.com/report/php.

Teno, J. M., V. Mor, N. Ward, J. Roy, B. Clarridge, J. E. Wennberg, and E. S. Fisher. 2005. "Bereaved Family Member Perceptions of Quality of End-of-Life Care in U.S. Regions with High and Low Usage of Intensive Care Unit Care." *Journal of the American Geriatrics Society* 53 (11):1905–1911. doi: 10.1111/j.1532-5415.2005.53563.x.

Teno, J. M., P. L. Gozalo, J. P. Bynum, N. E. Leland, S. C. Miller, N. E. Morden, T. Scupp, D. C. Goodman, and V. Mor. 2013. "Change in End-of-Life Care for Medicare Beneficiaries: Site of Death, Place of Care, and Health Care Transitions in 2000, 2005, and 2009." *The Journal of the American Medical Association* 309 (5):470–477. doi: 10.1001/jama.2012.207624.

Thomé, B. 2003. "Living with Cancer in Old Age: Quality of Life and Meaning." *Bulletin No. 14*. Lund University, Faculty of Medicine (Thesis), Lund.

Thorson, J. A., and F. C. Powell. 1989. "Death Anxiety and Religion in an Older Male Sample." *Psychological Reports* 64 (3):985–986. doi: 10.2466/pr0.1989.64.3.985.

Thorson, J. A., and F. C. Powell. 1994. "A Revised Death Anxiety Scale." In *Death Anxiety Handbook: Research, Instrumentation, and Application*, edited by R. A. Neimeyer, 31–44. Philadelphia: Taylor & Francis.

Tulsky, J. A. 2005. "Beyond Advance Directives: Importance of Communication Skills at the End of Life." *The Journal of the American Medical Association* 294 (3):359–365. doi: 10.1001/jama.294.3.359.

Turnbull, A. E., B. M. Lau, A. P. Ruhl, P. A. Mendez-Tellez, C. B. Shanholtz, and D. M. Needham. 2014. "Age and Decisions to Limit Life Support for Patients with Acute Lung Injury: A Prospective Cohort Study." *Critical Care* 18 (3):R107. doi: 10.1186/cc13890.

Vandervoort, A., D. Houttekier, R. Vander Stichele, J. T. van der Steen, and L. Van den Block. 2014. "Quality of Dying in Nursing Home Residents Dying with Dementia: Does Advanced Care Planning Matter? A Nationwide Postmortem Study." *PLoS One* 9 (3):e91130. doi: 10.1371/journal.pone.0091130.

Voltz, R., A. Akabayashi, C. Reese, G. Ohi, and H. M. Sass. 1998. "End-of-Life Decisions and Advance Directives in Palliative Care: A Cross-Cultural Survey of Patients and Health-Care Professionals." *Journal of Pain and Symptom Management* 16 (3):153–162. doi: 10.1016/S0885-3924(98)00067-0.

Waldrop, D. P., and M. A. Meeker. 2012. "Communication and Advanced Care Planning in Palliative and End-of-Life Care." *Nursing Outlook* 60 (6):365–369. doi: 10.1016/j.outlook.2012.08.012.

Wendler, D., and A. Rid. 2011. "Systematic Review: The Effect on Surrogates of Making Treatment Decisions for Others." *Annals of Internal Medicine* 154 (5):336–346. doi: 10.7326/0003-4819-154-5-201103010-00008.

WHO. 2015. "Global Health Observatory." Accessed June 27, 2016. www.who.int/gho/mortality_burden_disease/life_tables/en/.

Wright, A. A., B. Zhang, A. Ray, J. W. Mack, E. Trice, T. Balboni, S. L. Mitchell, V. A. Jackson, S. D. Block, P. K. Maciejewski, and H. G. Prigerson. 2008. "Associations between End-of-Life Discussions, Patient Mental Health, Medical Care Near Death, and Caregiver Bereavement Adjustment." *The Journal of the American Medical Association* 300 (14):1665–1673. doi: 10.1001/jama.300.14.1665.

The Writing Group for the SUPPORT Investigators. 1995. "A Controlled Trial to Improve Care for Seriously Ill Hospitalized Patients." *The Journal of the American Medical Association* 274 (20):1591–1598. doi: 10.1001/jama.1995.03530200027032.

8 Not growing old – gracefully

Søren Holm

Research into the prevention of ageing or the delay of ageing processes is making steady progress (see Olshansky in this volume). The average life expectancy in wealthy countries is continuing to increase, as is the average number of healthy life years that people can expect. Some are suggesting that we are at a tipping point where human beings will soon live very long lives (more than 1,000 years) and will thereby effectively become post-human (de Grey 2003; de Grey and Rae 2007). This has sparked some philosophical interest in whether immortality or near immortality[1] is a desirable goal for human beings (Glannon 2002a, 2002b; Harris 2002, 2004; Overall 2003).

This chapter is more moderate in its ambition. It considers the ethical implications of more limited but still significant life extension. What would happen if most people lived to be 200?[2] Would such more limited life extension be a goal we ought to pursue as a society, and how should we balance the pursuit of life extension with other worthwhile societal endeavors? This is still a rather bold futuristic situation to consider. Significant increases in the human lifespan have been predicted many times in the past, but these predictions have not come true.

As we see from post-humanist and science-fiction writing, there are many ways in which life extension could happen (e.g., uploading of our minds to computers), so there is a need to specify what kind of life extension is being contemplated. In this chapter, we will consider a situation in which life extension has been achieved primarily by biological means, in which it has been achieved gradually; a situation in which people still age but at a slower rate and many people still die following a short or long period of physical decline and illness. The scenario discussed is thus a scenario in which life expectancy has not suddenly increased dramatically, in which old-age morbidity has not been compressed any more than it is now (Fries 1989), and in which the entities who have had their life extended are still recognizably human and not post- or transhuman.

The reasons for focusing on this particular scenario and not on more radical scenarios are twofold. First, I think it is a more realistic scenario than the near-immortality scenarios, at least insofar as they involve the immortality of biological beings. Second, I think that the non-biological immortality scenarios are simply so far removed from any of our current experiences that they become very difficult to evaluate ethically, whatever ethical framework we try to apply

(Holm 2007). Is it, for instance, ethically valuable to double the processing speed of an uploaded mind? And if so, how much value does it add? The non-biological immortality scenarios also involve radical changes in our technological abilities, which by themselves may change society fundamentally in ways we cannot currently predict. For instance, would the developments in information technology necessary to support mind uploading actually lead to mind uploading and a happy society of uploaded minds, or would they lead to a world dominated by non-human artificial intelligence (Bostrom 2014)? The analysis could also have focused on a less radical scenario in which most people lived to be 120, as some people do today. The main reason to analyze a slightly more radical life extension than to 120 is that life extension to 120 can probably be accommodated relatively easily within the rather uninteresting 'more of the same' scenario outlined on page 122. In the analysis, it is also necessary to make some assumptions about the society in which life extension takes place. In this chapter, the analysis will assume that life extension takes place in a well-ordered, reasonably affluent democratic society.

There is little doubt that life extension is a *pro tanto* desirable goal for (most) individuals. Most people would like to have more healthy life years and would be willing to engage in some trade-off between healthy and unhealthy life years. The ratio of the trade-off would differ from person to person, but most would for instance be willing to accept some unhealthy life extension in order to gain ten more healthy life years. However, it is important to remember that even though life extension is a desirable goal for a given individual, it is not necessarily that individual's only or most important goal, and people may be willing to trade-off length of life against the fulfillment of other important goals they want to pursue (e.g., this is a trade-off that persons preferring a sedentary lifestyle are engaged in). The problem in extending this individual analysis to the societal level is that it ignores the fact that society and social arrangements will change in response to developments in life expectancy, and a societal or all-things-considered analysis will have to take these changes into account. Thus, the societal analysis will to a considerable extent depend on a prediction of changes in social arrangements caused by changes in life expectancy.

How do we go about developing such predictions? In the following, I will first briefly summarize the developments in life expectancy since accurate records began and even more briefly outline the societal response to the rise in life expectancy during the last 170 years. Second, I will outline how a lifespan may look with a life expectancy of 200 – first in a 'more of the same scenario' and then in a 'portfolio scenario.' Third will be a brief summary of the extant ethical arguments in life-extension literature, followed by an extended elaboration of a possible alternative, which I will term 'growing old gracefully.' The conclusion of the analysis will be that a median life expectancy of 200 years does not threaten our ability to grow old gracefully but that all our conclusions about the ethical desirability or otherwise of life extension and life-extension technologies are predicated on rather uncertain predictions of the kind of society in which we will live in the future.

The past as a guide to the future?

One way to predict what will happen if life expectancy increases in the future is to investigate what happened in the past when life expectancy increased rapidly.

Figure 8.1 shows average life expectancy at birth and at different ages for England and Wales for the time period 1700 to 2013 (for the period 1845 to 2013, it also shows age-related average life expectancy; see Roser 2016). There is a long period of stable life expectancy lasting almost 150 years, and then life expectancy starts to climb. One important feature to note is that for people who survive infancy and live to the age of five, average life expectancy has been pretty good for a long time. And, if we look at median life expectancy for men (the age at which 50 percent of a cohort has died, corresponding to the middle line of the graph below), we see that it has increased approximately 35 years since 1841 (Office for National Statistics 2012). We also see that the modal age of death (i.e., the most common age at death) was stable for a very long time and has begun to increase only very recently.

How did societies historically adapt to the increase in life expectancy? Here, we have to distinguish two different possible causal drivers of societal change: (1) the decreasing infant, child, and maternal mortality, and (2) the increase in life expectancy after early childhood.

The rapid decrease in infant and child mortality led directly to the so-called demographic transition, since families no longer needed to sustain high birth rates in order to ensure that at least some of their children survived into adulthood

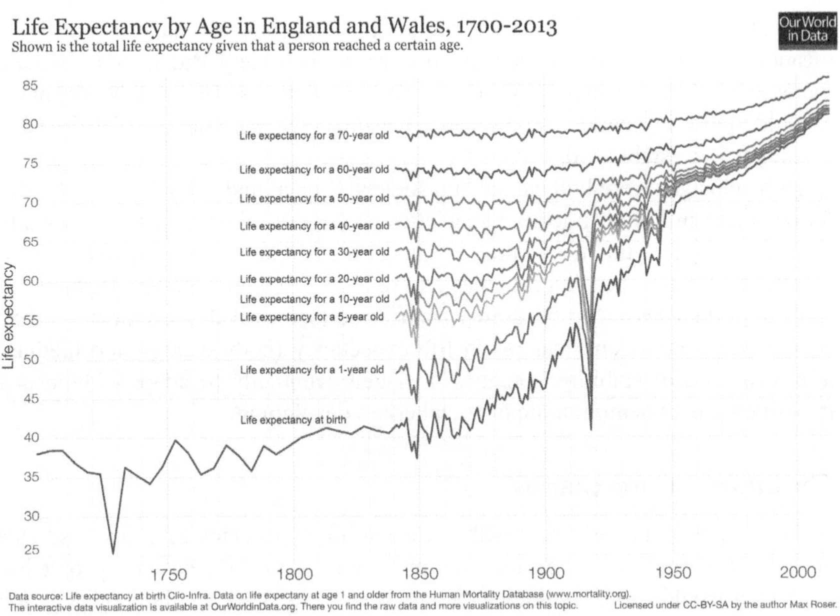

Figure 8.1 Life expectancy by age in England and Wales, 1700–2013

Source: Courtesy of Our World in Data (https://ourworldindata.org/life-expectancy/).

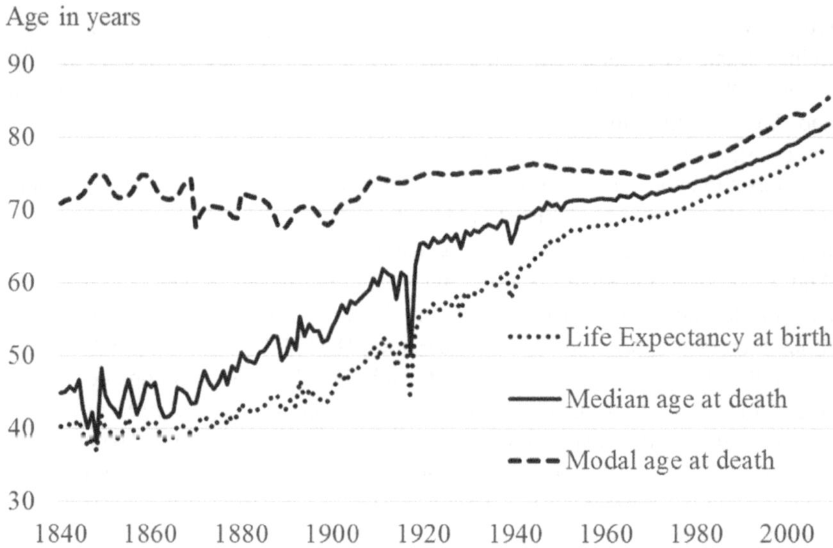

Figure 8.2 Changes in male life expectancy in the UK

Source: Office for National Statistics.

(Chesnais 1992; Lee 2003). The reduction in number of pregnancies and births meant that women were freed to take up new roles in society. But the more general increase in life expectancy also had very important effects. The period recognized as childhood was extended, adolescence was invented, and the role of retiree and pensioner was established.

These changes were both social and societal. Social understandings of the different stages in life changed, and societies had to put in place new structures to enable and support the new reality. For instance, school systems had to be reconfigured, and public pension schemes had to be devised and revised. Perhaps the most important lesson to be drawn from these historical developments is that, despite very significant changes in life expectancy (both average and median) after centuries of stability, societies managed eventually to adapt without any major permanent demographic or social crises developing.

The future – two scenarios

So, what future can we expect with a median life expectancy of 200 years? One possible scenario is what we could call 'more of the same.' Because the people living longer would still be biological beings, they would have a childhood, a period of adulthood, and a period of old age. It is likely that the childhood/adolescence segment would be expanded, but not by very much unless our life-extension technology slowed down childhood development, and any technology that did so would be undesirable. The old-age segment would be somewhat expanded, but in the 'more of the same' scenario, most of the extra lifetime would be spent in an adult phase of life that looked like adult life today – a period of work, family building, and saving enough for a private or public pension fund to last through a longer period of old age.

Another possible scenario, which I will call the 'portfolio scenario,' involves more significant changes to the period of adulthood. Being an adult for more than 100 years would allow people much more freedom to have a portfolio career, to have periods of retirement/breaks from work interspersed throughout adult life, and to have a succession of sexual and reproductive partners and families. The freedoms created by a much longer adult life would also plausibly enlarge the range of realistically pursuable life plans and therefore lead to greater diversity in society. Some 120-year-olds would be at work; others would be retraining for a new profession; others would be having their second or third family; others would be taking five years off to see the wonders of the world. Instead of having one overarching arch of life with a clearly defined direction and segmentation, some people might have a long period of life in which they participate in a number of consecutive 'cycles' of work or family-making. If this is the scenario that comes about, then a person's starting point in life might become even more important than it is now, because being able to invest financial and social capital will be crucial for upward mobility during life.

It is likely that both scenarios significantly underestimate how different society will be if/when we reach a life expectancy of 200 years, since many other technological and social developments will occur that will also impact on society and on people's possible life courses. Many of the main differences between society at the time of this writing (2016) and society 150 years ago (1866) are not the result of the rather impressive increase (more than 30 years) in median life expectancy during that period but the result of completely unrelated technological developments. Just one example of a simple development with far-reaching implications is the invention of the bicycle, which geneticist Steve Jones has called "the most important event in recent human evolution" (Jones 2000, 294–295) because it increased the possibilities of human genetic mixing by increasing the distance that people could easily travel every day.

Ethical analysis

How should we evaluate life extension to 200 years from a societal perspective? The standard 'liberal' approach to this question proceeds along the following lines (Cutas 2008; Harris 2002, 2004):[3]

1 Claim life extension to be an all-purpose good, directly linked to the ability to obtain other goods in life.
2 Claim life extension to be desired by everyone because of (1).
3 Conclude that (1) and (2) are sufficient to show that life extension to 200 years is a good that should be pursued.

4 Rebut counterclaims concerning:

 a how life extension may be bad for (some) individuals (Glannon 2002a, 2002b; Moore 2006; Williams 1973);

 b how life extension may lead to large-scale social problems (overpopulation, social segmentation, social injustice, etc.) (Overall 2003);

 i Accept counterclaims in principle, but deflect their force through liberal/libertarian arguments showing that individuals have a right to pursue life extension.

 ii Deny the 'social' counterclaims – for example, by reference to predicted future technological development that will fix the problem.

Both the argument and the counterarguments are well rehearsed in the literature, and there is not much I can add to them. In relation to (1)–(3), it is important to remember that even if (1) and (2) can be established (or established when a few people with deviating preference structures have been excluded from consideration), this does not in itself tell us how important life extension is. The possession of a fifth finger, a hand, and an arm all fulfill (1) and (2) in being all-purpose goods desired by everyone with normal preference structures, but they are not equally important, and their importance varies from person to person depending on their life plan. We therefore need further arguments specifying exactly how important life extension is, absolutely and compared to other important goods. And only when we have those further arguments will we be in a position to say whether society ought to spend resources on promoting life extension. With regard to the rebuttals in (4), the deflection strategy through an appeal to individual rights can work only outside of a consequentialist framing. If the argument for pursuing life extension is consequentialist, then it is no answer to those who claim that there are negative consequences that need to be taken into account to posit non-consequentialist individual rights.

Another way in which we could approach the analysis is what I will term 'growing old gracefully,' which is roughly equivalent to the overarching obligation to acquire and display the relevant virtues, or to discharge your moral obligations and duties, in each particular segment of your life. If you reach old age and can look back and say 'Yes, I have discharged my moral duties well throughout my life, I have lived my life as someone in my position should lead a life,' then you have grown old gracefully in an ethical sense. If we apply this perspective to life extension, then a future with life extension will be *pro tanto* as good as or better than the present, if the chance of growing old gracefully in the future is at least as good as or better than it is presently. The 'growing old gracefully' approach has some affinities with Aristotle's derivation and definition of virtue in his *Nicomachean Ethics*, where virtue is defined as follows:

> So virtue is a purposive disposition, lying in a mean that is relative to us and determined by a rational principle, and by that which a prudent man would

use to determine it. It is a mean between two kinds of vice, one of excess and the other of deficiency.

(Aristotle 1976, 101–102)

Aristotle further claims that someone is truly virtuous only if he integrates in his character all those virtues that are appropriate to him and his role in life. For Aristotle, someone would presumably have grown old gracefully if he could look back at his life and say that he had first acquired the appropriate virtues and then lived a virtuous life according to those virtues.[4] The point at which the 'growing old gracefully' approach departs from Aristotle is primarily in not requiring a static set of virtues but being open to the idea that these may change dramatically over the life course.

In the following, I will primarily analyze 'growing old gracefully' in terms of duties and obligations, but a parallel argument can be developed in terms of virtues. It is unlikely that the duties and obligations of the very young and the very old are going to change significantly in any of the two scenarios outlined above, and it is also unlikely that their ability to discharge those duties is going to change very much. What we therefore need to concentrate our attention on is 'the expanded middle,' the considerably extended segment of adult life. What are the duties and obligations during this segment of life, and how can we fulfill them if we live much longer than we do currently?

Before attempting an answer to this question, it is necessary to discuss whether the question makes sense, since it could be claimed that people cannot have positive moral obligations that they have not themselves chosen to have. We can have unchosen negative moral obligations, such as obligations not to harm other people, but not unchosen positive moral obligations. If this is true, it makes little sense to discuss the positive obligations of adults, since these will purely be a matter of individual choice. In discussions about whether adult children have any moral obligations in relation to their parents, such as obligations to support them in old age, it is, for instance, claimed by some that adult children can have such obligations only if they have themselves chosen to have them. The mere fact that they are the children of particular parents does not create obligations (Blustein 1982; Daniels 1988; English 1992).

This argument is, I think, partly true, but it obscures an underlying complex moral landscape where obligations can be generated and extinguished by actions and events that may involve some kind of choice, but where it is not the obligations themselves that are the main focus of the choice. People can assume or accept a particular social role whether or not they fully understand the moral and social obligations that come with it. The role of parent is a prime example. If someone chooses to become a parent through reproduction or adoption, they thereby acquire a complex set of obligations toward their child, obligations which will change over time as the child develops and matures. Parents have in some sense chosen to have the obligations they have toward their 14-year-old daughter, but at the time they chose the role, they probably had only a vague idea of what the exact obligations would be 14 years and nine months later. Nevertheless, the role obligations are binding. Many other social roles, such as the role of university teacher or police officer, also come with inbuilt moral obligations.

Obligations may also plausibly be generated by reciprocity, either in one-on-one relationships or in larger networks of reciprocity. Children who have been loved and supported by their parents through childhood and adolescence may simply by that fact have acquired a defeasible but nevertheless real moral obligation to support their parents if their parents need support. And, to take another example, someone who has been living in a supportive and friendly local community may over time acquire moral obligations toward members of that community. On the other hand, obligations that people have voluntarily assumed may be extinguished or defeated by events that are outside of their control.

The issues discussed here can perhaps be handled more directly within a virtue theoretical framework. The virtues are not innate; they are learned and developed by people living in and learning from particular social roles, so it follows straightforwardly that (1) the virtues of a parent are virtues that a parent ought to develop to fulfill the parent role in a morally good way and (2) insofar as some of these virtues are specific to the parent role, you only start developing them once you assume the role. You do not choose the virtues; the virtues are inherent in the role, and the morally excellent person will develop them.

This entails that it is still meaningful to ask what moral duties and obligations adults would have, and what virtues they should possess, in a society where the adult segment of life had expanded radically. But how would we go about answering those questions? The introduction of an expanded middle of life would create new social roles, with their own sets of obligations and virtues, and would require us to map out revised obligations for already existing roles. There would, for example, be many more great-great-grandparents than there are now, but what obligations (if any) would they have toward their great-great-grandchildren? And, how would those obligations be influenced by the fact that those great-great-grandparents also had children at various stages of life from two or three subsequent relationships? And, what obligations would 147-year-old well-established academics have toward eager, newly minted PhDs trying to step onto the academic career ladder?

Raising these questions immediately shows that if the portfolio scenario is the more likely scenario, then our abilities to intuit or provide an analytic justification for a particular set of obligations or virtues become limited. Parents would still have a set of obligations toward their non-adult children that will be similar to the ones they have now, simply because children need parents to discharge those obligations in order to have a chance at a good life. But other obligations may change and mutate beyond recognition if we enter a situation in which there is no particular overarching arch to life that most people follow, a situation in which each individual is somewhere in one of the 'cycles' of adulthood, in or out of sync with those who were partners, collaborators, or co-constructors in or results of their previous cycle(s). Whereas intra-cycle obligations and virtues are likely to be similar to current general adult and role obligations, it is much more difficult to predict the shape of inter-cycle obligations and virtues. To what extent can old role- or reciprocity-based obligations just be jettisoned and new ones assumed?

Given that there would be no change in personal identity occurring even though persons pursued a portfolio life, obligations could be fully extinguished only if (a) they had been fully discharged, (b) they had been justified in ongoing social interaction and reciprocity and the social interaction had ceased, or (c) the persons to whom the obligations were owed had released the duty holder. The duty holders could not themselves renounce the duties. This means that in the portfolio scenario, people would likely accumulate a larger set of obligations than they currently accumulate in adult life. But given that we all already hold a large and probably inconsistent set of obligations of varying strengths, this does not in itself show that we would not be able to grow old gracefully even with a 200-year-long portfolio life. It also seems to indicate that persons living through a portfolio life would have to develop a 'meta-virtue' akin to Aristotelian *phronesis*, enabling them to choose rightly when weighing the obligations and virtues inherent in their current role and cycle against the obligations and virtues fitting their previous roles and cycles. This may involve something like an aesthetic appreciation of how a complicated life fits together as a whole.

Life extension as a societal goal

Should society allocate resources to anti-ageing research, and, if so, how important is it to pursue this goal compared to other important goals? This issue has been discussed within the health context – for instance, by Daniel Callahan and his opponents (Callahan 2000, 2003), but here we will consider it more broadly. In this context, it is important to note that the increases in life expectancy we have seen so far have come as (desirable) side effects of medical, public health, educational, and other developments and inventions that have not had life extension as a primary goal. This process is likely to continue into the future. New drugs will, for instance, be developed to treat specific diseases and conditions, and it will be found that they also have a life-extending effect (e.g., statins). New life-extending technologies will therefore continue to be developed even if resources are not allocated to anti-ageing research directly.

So, how important is the direct pursuit of life extension if we accept that life extension is a *pro tanto* good? In one sense, it could be claimed to be very important. Most of us do not want to die, and if asked at any given time whether we would like someone to develop a technology that extended our life by ten years, we would probably say 'yes' and state that this goal should have high societal priority. And we would give this answer every time we were asked the question, thereby seemingly accumulating evidence of the direct pursuit of life extension having an enormous importance. There is, however, a problem here with double-counting, since it is not obvious that the fact that I continually think something is important, and state it every time I am asked, provides cumulative evidence of importance. The mere fact of repeatedly asking, stating, and counting cannot make life extension either more or less important.

In another comparative sense, life extension may not be so important. As long as there are many people dying unnecessarily in childhood or early adulthood from preventable or treatable conditions, it could be argued that life extension for them should take priority over life extension for those who already have had a long life. Similarly, many people currently live lives that could be much better – that is, they could have a much higher level of welfare if societal resources were expended on housing, education, and so forth, and it is again arguable that we would do better as a society by focusing on their problems rather than on anti-ageing research. None of these considerations are conclusive, because they are essentially comparative along a number of parameters. If anti-ageing research realistically promised significant, simple, and cheap life extension,[5] it might on balance outweigh what would otherwise be more pressing, current needs. However, assessing the realistic promise of anti-ageing research is not a philosophical task.

Conclusion

One thread running through this chapter is that we know much less about a possible future society with radical life extension than is often assumed in ethical argument. This is a serious problem for any and all analyses of the ethics of life extension, whether those analyses are triumphalist or skeptical, insofar as the analysis relies on positive or negative predictions about the future as premises. The problem arises partly because we tend to perform our ethical analysis *ceteris paribus*, but in the case of life extension we have good reasons to believe that everything else will not be equal. The very technologies that would enable us to achieve the life extension that we analyze would also lead to many other changes in society. But the nature of these changes would depend on the particular technologies, and we cannot currently predict with any certainty which technology, or more plausibly which combination of technologies, will emerge as the 'winner.' So, a society with a given number of life-extended cyborgs is likely to look very different to a society with the same number of life-extended fully biological humans, not because the ethical issues facing the two populations will be different *ceteris paribus*, but because the other possible uses of the enabling technologies are very different and will lead to the development of very different social formations. This is a significant problem for all ethical evaluations, irrespective of the underlying ethical theory, because there are no knockout arguments showing conclusively that life extension is in itself either morally good or bad available within any of the standard ethical theories. And, appealing to risk-aversiveness or decision-making principles, such as the precautionary principle, is not going to be of much help either. We know for certain that some life extension will come about as a side effect of developments that are not aimed at life extension, and we cannot rule out that some intervention aimed at solving a problem occurring in old age, such as myo- or osteopenia, will not turn out to have significant life-extending 'side effects.' So, there is nowhere for our precaution to bite. The research and development will be pursued with *bona fide* therapeutic or preventative aims, and it is only later that we will come to realize that the intervention developed also has significant life-extending effects.

I have argued in this chapter that we have no reason to believe that life extension in itself (*ceteris paribus*) would make growing old gracefully more difficult than it is now and that life extension is therefore a *pro tanto* good. That conclusion is, however, dependent on an assumption of relative social stability and a degree of inequality similar to what we have in current societies. If life-extension technologies are introduced into societies with much greater degrees of inequality, they might have social effects that are not benign, leaving the affluent part of society free to pursue a portfolio lifestyle while the other part of society is tied to a longer life of drudgery.

However, the one lesson we can learn from history is that societies will muddle through and would likely eventually find ethically acceptable ways of handling the new challenges created by radical life extension.

Notes

1 A biological organism that was biologically immortal and had an infinite lifespan would still be physically destructible and therefore susceptible to catastrophic accidents and only 'nearly immortal.'

2 The situation I refer to is a society with a median life expectancy of 200 years. Such a society could still have an average life expectancy below 200 years, since early deaths (e.g., deaths in infancy) detract more from the average than from the median in this scenario.

In this chapter, 'life expectancy' is used with the slightly unusual meaning of 'median life expectancy' unless specifically qualified.

3 The main disagreements in the literature could equally well have been outlined with a skeptical approach as the starting point.

4 I am here ignoring Aristotle's stated view in his *Rhetoric* that the old cannot be virtuous (Aristotle 2004).

5 That is, the intervention in itself is cheap, and it does not create significant downstream costs.

References

Aristotle. 1976. *Ethics*, translated by J. A. K. Thomson and H. Tredennick. London: Penguin Classics.

Aristotle. 2004. *Rhetoric*, translated by W. R. Roberts. Dover: Dover Thrift Editions.

Blustein, J. 1982. *Parents and Children: The Ethics of the Family*. New York: Oxford University Press.

Bostrom, N. 2014. *Superintelligence: Paths, Dangers, Strategies*. Oxford: Oxford University Press.

Callahan, D. 2000. *The Troubled Dream of Life: In Search of a Peaceful Death*. Washington, DC: Georgetown University Press.

Callahan, D. 2003. *What Price Better Health? Hazards of the Research Imperative*. Berkeley: University of California Press.

Chesnais, J.-C. 1992. *The Demographic Transition: Stages, Patterns, and Economic Implications: A Longitudinal Study of Sixty-Seven Countries Covering the Period 1720–1984*. Oxford: Clarendon Press.

Cutas, D. E. 2008. "Life Extension, Overpopulation and the Right to Life: Against Lethal Ethics." *Journal of Medical Ethics* 34 (9):e7. doi: 10.1136/jme.2007.023622.

Daniels, N. 1988. *Am I My Parents' Keeper? An Essay on Justice between the Young and the Old*. New York: Oxford University Press.

English, J. 1992. "What Do Grown Children Owe Their Parents?" In *Aging and Ethics*, edited by N. Jecker, 147–154. Clifton, NJ: Humana Press.

Fries, J. F. 1989. "The Compression of Morbidity: Near or Far?" *The Milbank Quarterly* 67 (2):208–232. doi: 10.2307/3350138.

Glannon, W. 2002a. "Identity, Prudential Concern, and Extended Lives." *Bioethics* 16 (3):266–283. doi: 10.1111/1467-8519.00285.

Glannon, W. 2002b. "Extending the Human Life Span." *Journal of Medicine and Philosophy* 27 (3):339–354. doi: 10.1076/jmep.27.3.339.2978.

Grey, A. D. de 2003. "The Foreseeability of Real Anti-Aging Medicine: Focusing the Debate." *Experimental Gerontology* 38 (9):927–934.

Grey, A. D. de, and M. Rae. 2007. *Ending Aging: The Rejuvenation Breakthroughs That Could Reverse Human Aging in Our Lifetime*. New York: St. Martin's Griffin.

Harris, J. 2002. "Intimations of Immortality: The Ethics and Justice of Life-Extending Therapies." *Current Legal Problems* 55 (1):65–95. doi: 10.1093/clp/55.1.65.

Harris, J. 2004. "Immortal Ethics." *Annals of the New York Academy of Sciences* 1019 (1):527–534. doi: 10.1196/annals.1297.098.

Holm, S. 2007. "Naturalness and Anthropology in Modern Bioethics, with a Special View to Trans- and Post-Humanism." In *Theology and Science: Issues for Future Dialogue*, edited by H. Kragh, 17–29. Aarhus: University of Aarhus Press.

Jones, S. 2000. *The Language of Genes* (Revised edition). London: Flamingo.

Lee, R. 2003. "The Demographic Transition: Three Centuries of Fundamental Change." *The Journal of Economic Perspectives* 17 (4):167–190. doi: 10.1257/089533003772034943.

Moore, A. W. 2006. "Williams, Nietzsche, and the Meaninglessness of Immortality." *Mind* 115 (458):311–330. doi: 10.1093/mind/fzl311.

Office for National Statistics. 2012. *Mortality in England and Wales: Average Life Span*. http://webarchive.nationalarchives.gov.uk/20160105160709/ and www.ons.gov.uk/ons/dcp171776_292196.pdf.

Overall, C. 2003. *Aging, Death, and Human Longevity: A Philosophical Inquiry*. Berkeley: University of California Press.

Roser, M. 2016. "Life Expectancy." Published online at OurWorldInData.org. https://ourworldindata.org/life-expectancy/.

Williams, B. 1973. "The Makropulos Case: Reflections on the Tedium of Immortality." In *Problems of the Self: Philosophical Papers 1956–1972*, edited by B. Williams, 82–100. Cambridge: Cambridge University Press.

9 How to think about age-group justice

The capabilities approach

Nancy S. Jecker

Introduction[1]

As individuals, we are accustomed to growing older. Yet not just individuals, but also societies age. A society is said to age when its number of older people increases relative to its number of younger people. Ageing societies pose ethical challenges for healthcare systems, because older people use more healthcare resources on average than younger people do, and they tend to present with relatively higher rates of chronic healthcare problems. The task of this chapter is to critically reflect on the twin challenges of rising healthcare costs and the shifting nature of healthcare needs. My goal will be to offer an ethics framework appropriate to the subject matter. The framework I propose is referred to in the literature as a 'capabilities approach' to justice. It places emphasis on the respect and recognition we owe to the elderly. The capabilities account is at variance with the dominant emphasis of autonomy that characterizes much of contemporary Western philosophy and bioethics. For this reason, I will try to show throughout the chapter why a capabilities account has advantages over autonomy-based accounts for addressing ethical issues raised by ageing societies.

Background

Industrialized nations have been ageing for as long as demographic records have been kept. In 1800, for example, the demographic makeup of developed countries was similar to that of many developing countries in the early 1990s, with roughly half the population under the age of 16 and very few people living beyond age 60. Since that time, increases in life expectancy combined with declines in fertility rates have dramatically increased the proportion of older people in developed nations. Although the age profile of many developing countries remains heavily weighted toward younger age groups, the same demographic ageing that has occurred over more than a century in the developed world is predicted to occur much more rapidly in developing countries without the benefit of an extended period of economic growth to ensure older people's financial security and provide for their health and social care. Moreover, the sheer number of people entering older age groups in the world's most populated countries, such as India and China, is daunting. India's older population is forecast to increase nearly 280 percent from its current level of 60 million today to 227 million by 2050, and China's older population will increase from 110 million today to 330 million by 2050 (WHO and National Institute on Aging 2011).

What future societies will regard as distinct about the ageing of societies during the 20th and 21st centuries is the *rapid pace* at which it is occurring. In the US, the percentage of people aged 65 and over increased from 4 percent in 1900 to 12 percent in 2000 and it is projected to reach 20 percent in 2050. Rapidly ageing societies raise unprecedented ethical challenges for healthcare systems globally. One challenge is the increasing demand for and cost of healthcare. People 65 and over consume, on average, a far greater share of healthcare resources than those under the age of 65. The average healthcare expense for elderly people is $11,089 per year, compared to $3,352 per year for those ages 19 to 64 (US Department of Health and Human Services, Agency for Healthcare Research 2006). Growing demand for healthcare raises the question of what constitutes a just distribution of healthcare between younger and older age groups.

Societal ageing also creates ethical challenges for healthcare systems, because older individuals experience a far greater incidence of chronic, disabling conditions than younger persons do. Defined as a health problem that persists over time and requires some degree of health management (Whelan 2002), 'chronic disease' includes conditions such as diabetes; cancers; cardiovascular disease; depression; asthma; and respiratory diseases, such as chronic obstructive pulmonary disease. The shift to chronic health problems presents challenges for health systems around the world, because these systems were developed primarily to treat acute conditions, rather than the kind of chronic problems facing the elderly. In contrast to acute health conditions, chronic health problems cannot be fixed and become worse over time. One challenge will be to develop healthcare infrastructures to serve the growing population of chronically ill elderly people. Whereas acute problems are generally managed in hospitals, chronic conditions are typically managed in outpatient settings, such as nursing homes, assisted living facilities, and group homes, or by home healthcare aids in the patient's or caregiver's residence. A related challenge is to determine the scope and limits of society's ethical obligation to support elderly individuals who require assistance with activities of daily living due to declines in cognitive or physical functioning. To what extent does this obligation rest with society as a whole, and to what extent should it be considered a private responsibility – for example, the responsibility of individuals and families (see ter Meulen in this volume)?

Meeting the challenges of ageing societies requires rethinking and retooling the methods and principles of ethical and bioethical analyses. The daily work of caring for the chronically ill, which has been compared to the "tedious, grinding labor of Sisyphus" (Jennings, Callahan, and Caplan 1988), tends to lack the excitement that characterizes acute care medicine. People caring for chronically ill patients are less likely to face life-or-death decisions and more likely to encounter ethical decisions related to mundane activities of daily living, such as toileting, transfer, and feeding. Although everyday ethics may appear at first glance to be less ethically significant, the cumulative impact of such decisions can be life altering for caregivers and care recipients alike. Thus, over time, chronic disease has large impacts on quality of life for patients and caregivers.

Although the dominant trend in Western bioethics is to emphasize the value of respect for patient autonomy, this value may become less relevant as the population becomes increasingly geriatric, increasingly dependent, and increasingly vulnerable to physical decline and cognitive disabilities. 'Autonomy' is the ability to govern oneself, to choose the principles and goals that one lives by. Autonomy presupposes that a person possesses the intellectual capacity to assess and choose her own values and goals. Yet, as people age, their ability to function autonomously tends to decline. For example, with increasing age, risk of dementias, such as Alzheimer's, increases. Whereas prevalence of dementia is very low at younger ages, it nearly doubles with every five years of age after age 65 (National Institute on Aging and World Health Organization 2011). According to one recent study by the Organization for Economic Cooperation and Development, dementia affects fewer than 3 percent of those aged 65 to 69, but almost 30 percent of those aged 85 to 89 (Oxley 2009). Although early-stage dementia may interfere only mildly with cognitive tasks, its final stages cause loss of memory, reasoning, speech, and other cognitive functions. Due to the relatively high prevalence of dementia, the oldest old are frequently unable to live autonomously or to understand and consent on their own behalf to medical treatment.

In ageing societies, ideals such as human dignity and self-respect, which are intimately linked to human relationship and community, may assume greater significance than autonomy. By 'human dignity,' I follow the Kantian tradition and refer specifically to that which has value in itself, rather than having value merely in relation to some outside end or to an observer's judgments. Although not all elderly people possess decision-making capacity and autonomy, all possess human dignity that merits respect. 'Respect' comes from the Latin *respicere*, which means 'to look back at' or 'to look again.' Common to the various definitions of respect is a perceptual element in which "the person who respects something pays attention to it and perceives it differently from someone who does not and responds to it in light of that perception" (Dillon 2016). In this sense, if I respect someone, I pay heed or give proper attention to them; I try to "see the object clearly, as it really is in its own right" (Dillon 2016) rather than seeing it solely through the filter of my own desires and fears or likes and dislikes. Whereas respect applies to all human beings, autonomy applies more narrowly to those human beings who possess certain cognitive abilities necessary for self-government.

A capabilities approach to justice

The idea of respect for persons is closely related to justice, for justice concerns most fundamentally the respect owed each of us. Western philosophy and bioethics tend to conceive of justice principles in terms of autonomy, as the outcome of a suitably defined rational choice. According to this approach, duties of justice consist of those duties we would agree to impose on ourselves or would hypothetically choose if we were deliberating under suitably defined conditions. Thus, Daniels argues that the way to think about age-group justice is to frame this problem in terms of a first-person prudential choice. We are to ask ourselves what distribution of resources we would choose for ourselves and how we would prefer to allocate healthcare across our own lifespan (Daniels 1988, 2001, 2008).

The capabilities approach, by contrast, begins not with individual choice of justice principles but with the more basic idea of respect for persons. Respect is object-generated, rather than subject-generated (Dillon 2016). In other words, it is elicited by the object of our respect, rather than by our own will or decision. Darwall (1977) distinguishes between appraisal and recognition respect, and it is the latter form of respect that the capabilities view draws on. Recognition respect refers to "the disposition to give appropriate weight or consideration in one's practical deliberations to some fact about the object and to regulate one's conduct by constraints derived from that fact" (Dillon 2016). By contrast, appraisal respect is based on our own favorable estimation of a person's merits and character. When we respect someone because we judge that they are honest, we are showing appraisal respect. However, if we respect an individual because of that individual's inherent worth and dignity, we are recognizing qualities persons have independent of our appraisal. Persons merit recognition respect not because we choose to show it but because of the kinds of objects they are. As Kant observes, persons have an absolute dignity and worth, in contrast to mere things, which are instruments we may use to accomplish our own subjective ends. Respect, according to Kant , is owed to persons as such, and it is not based on what persons happen to accomplish or achieve. Recognition respect expresses "deference, in the most basic sense of yielding: self-absorption and egocentric concerns give way to consideration of the object, one's motives or feelings submit to the object's reality, one is disposed to act in obedience to the object's demands" (Dillon 2016). To summarize, we can say that the worth and dignity of persons (1) is extrinsic to and independent of us, (2) constrains our actions, (3) is owed by everyone regardless of their desires or preferences, and (4) is universally applicable in the sense that "if F is a respect-warranting feature of object O, then respecting O on account of F commits us, other things equal, to respecting other things that also have feature F" (Dillon 2016).

Building on the idea of respect for human dignity, the capabilities view holds that by virtue of possessing an inherent worth and dignity, persons deserve the opportunity to choose to live a life of human dignity. This approach focuses not on the resources people are given but on what people are able to do and be. The dual importance of doing and being reflects the fact that we value both functioning and capability. In other words, we value both actual outcomes (how people are actually functioning) and people's capacity to choose various outcomes (what people are capable of doing). According to this model, what matters is not that people's current preferences are satisfied but whether a range of options is open to people – that is, whether they have the capability to do other things. For example, a woman who is staying at home caring for a frail, elderly parent may be doing what she wants to do, but the capabilities approach asks us to consider whether she has the ability to make a different choice. Does society afford her the opportunity to work outside the home and find other ways of supporting her elderly parent? What other opportunities would a just society support? To address this requires an account of the basic capabilities required for human dignity.

Let us assume that all people possess an *equal* worth and dignity; then each of us deserves an equal set of the basic capabilities required for human flourishing (Nussbaum 2003). Yet notice that capability equality does not mean the same thing as providing people with an equal share of resources, because having resources does not necessarily mean that one is able to convert those resources into capabilities and functioning. For example, someone who has health insurance may not be able to convert that benefit into capabilities and functioning if they do not know about the health services available in their community and how to access them.

What are the capabilities central to living a human life, and what level of capability is sufficient to ensure human dignity? The following have been proposed as among the central human capabilities:

(1) *Life*: being able to live to the end of a human life of normal length;
(2) *Bodily health*: being able to have good health, being adequately nourished, being able to have adequate shelter;
(3) *Bodily integrity*: being able to move freely from place to place;
(4) *Senses, imagination, thought*: being able to imagine, think, reason, and use the senses, and to do these things in a way informed and cultivated by an adequate education;
(5) *Emotions*: being able to have attachments to things and persons outside oneself, including being able to love those who love and care for one;
(6) *Practical reason*: being able to form a conception of the good and to engage in critical reflection about the planning of one's life;
(7) *Affiliation*: being able to live for and in relation to others, to recognize and show concern for other human beings, to engage in various forms of social interaction;
(8) *Other species*: being able to live with concern for and in relation to animals and the world of nature;
(9) *Play*: being able to laugh, to play, to enjoy recreational activities;
(10) *Control over one's environment*: having control over one's political and material environment, such as having the rights of free speech and freedom of association, and being able to hold property; having the right to seek employment on an equal basis with others.

(Nussbaum 2011, 33–34)

Once we have an account of the central capabilities, the next step is determining how to structure basic social institutions to support them. According to the capabilities view, a just society structures social institutions in a way that establishes a sufficient level of well-being (functioning) and capability for human dignity. The central human capabilities comprise a fundamental, pre-political entitlement based on an inalienable human dignity. As Nussbaum notes, "once we identify a group of especially important functions in human life, we are then in a position to ask what social and political institutions are doing about them" (1992, 214). For example, are healthcare institutions providing citizens with what they need in order to be capable of functioning in all of these human ways? Are citizens functioning in a minimal way? According to the capabilities approach, justice requires society to ensure that all of its members are equipped with a minimum threshold level of these central human capabilities.

Yet, one might ask why we should accept these capabilities as the important functions in human life. After all, we might come up with a different list or allow the list to vary from one society to the next. Perhaps we should, as Sen (2009) suggests, let each society decide for itself which capabilities are central. To address this, the capabilities account must provide an answer to the question of where the capabilities come from. One answer holds that the central capabilities are grounded in 'essentialism,' or the view that human life has certain central defining features. One version of essentialism (Nussbaum 1992) begins with a 'thick vague theory of the good.' The theory of good is 'thick' because it proposes that certain specific functions and ends are most important or essential for human beings; but at the same time it is 'vague' because it admits of multiple specifications in accordance with local morals and personal conceptions of the good. This form of essentialism is internalist, rather than metaphysical, because it does not purport to derive from any source external to human beings and human history (Nussbaum 1992, 215). Internalist essentialism starts with the observation that we can identify which individuals and groups are human in different times and places and across diverse cultures. Such recognitions point to a shared understanding of the essential features of a human form of life, the features that make a life human wherever and whenever we find it. The Kantian notion of human dignity noted on page 133 does not include a shared understanding of the central features of a human form of life. For this, capability theorists draw on other philosophers, such as Aristotle. Aristotle derives morality from his account of human flourishing (the good life) and from closely related ideas of the function and ends of a human being. Working in this tradition, Nussbaum offers an account of the central human capabilities as including the following:

(1) *Mortality*: All human beings face death, know that they face it, and have an aversion to death.
(2) *The human body*: All human beings live their entire lives in bodies of a certain sort, with physical needs, desires, and vulnerabilities.
(3) *Pleasure and pain*: The capacity for pleasure and pain is common to all human life.
(4) *Cognitive capability*: All human beings have the ability to perceive, imagine, and think; a group of individuals who totally lacked sensory perception or thinking capacity would not be one we identified as human.
(5) *Early infant development*: All human beings begin helpless, hungry, and dependent on others; this early experience, which varies with different social arrangements, shapes the formation of future desires and complex emotions.

(6) *Practical reason*: All human beings try to plan and manage their own lives and a being that altogether lacks this ability would probably not be considered fully human.
(7) *Affiliation with other human beings*: All humans need to be recognized and felt by other human beings; we regard a life not lived in affiliation with others to be a life not worth living.
(8) *Relatedness to other species and to nature*: All human beings are dependent on other living things, such as plants and animals, and we regard the natural order with some measure of respect and concern.
(9) *Humor and play*: All human beings use forms of recreation and laughter as a mode of mutual recognition in the sense that if a child is never able to play or laugh, we consider this a deep disturbance and question whether the child is capable of leading a fully human life.
(10) *Separateness*: Each and every human being, despite living in affiliation with others, is one in number and proceeds on an individual path from birth to death.

(Nussbaum 1992, 216–220)

These universal human features represent one possible source of the central capabilities. To illustrate, we can consider the fact that humans everywhere live in bodies of a certain sort, with physical needs, desires, and vulnerabilities; because of this, bodily health is a central human capability. Likewise, human beings perceive, imagine, and think; as a result, one of our central capabilities is being able to imagine, to think, to reason, and to use the senses and do these things in a way informed and cultivated by an adequate education. In this way, the capabilities are grounded on an essentialist account of the human being.

If we accept the central capabilities, the next step is to determine how to structure social and political institutions to support them. The goal is not to identify the lowest possible threshold, beneath which a life will be so impoverished that it will not be human at all, but a somewhat higher threshold, beneath which those characteristic functions are available in such a reduced way that although it is a human life, it is not a *good* human life. Taken together, the basic capabilities, such as life, health, affiliation, practical reason, and control over one's environment, tell us what social and political institutions are required to do to enable human beings to function well. The capabilities approach is practical and Aristotelian in the sense that it focuses on the proper function (*ergon*) of a thing. Just as an eye is a 'good eye' only when it can perform its function of seeing, Aristotelian ethics holds that there is a function specific to humans and that a human being can be said to be 'functioning well' when it can perform that function. According to the capabilities view, since a life that lacked any one of the basic capabilities would not be a life we recognized as human, "it would be reasonable to take these things as a focus for concern, in asking how public policy can promote the good of human beings" (Nussbaum 1992, 222). Moreover, since each item on the list of functional capabilities is vital to human functioning, we must proceed with caution when considering trade-offs among the various capabilities. To be acceptable, a trade-off cannot result in people falling below a minimal threshold with respect to any of the central capabilities.

What is the minimum level of capabilities and functioning? Answering this question requires moving beyond the anthropologically-based description of human capabilities to offer a normative account of justice and of what people deserve or are entitled to receive. As already suggested, a just society will establish a sufficient level of well-being (functioning) and capability (capacity to choose functionings) for human dignity. This approach draws on the idea of recognition respect described on page 134. It also draws on the idea of respect for human dignity associated with philosophers such as Kant. Kant places respect for persons, including oneself, at the front and center of his moral theory, although he was not the first to do so. Classic Roman thinkers such as Cicero identified *dignitas* to refer to the dignity of human beings as such, independent of any particular status or role (McCrudden 2008). During the Middle Ages, human beings were thought to have dignity by virtue of being made in the image of God. Enlightenment thinkers insisted on a broader conception of human dignity, independent of God and other outside sources. Thus, Kant held that people are ends in themselves and merit respect regardless of external factors, such as how we are inclined to treat them. For Kant, the dignity and worth of individuals is absolute, not relative.

Drawing on this family of ideas, the capabilities approach includes a sufficiency requirement, which demands that everyone be brought up to the minimum level required to show respect for human dignity. While other approaches to justice share an emphasis on sufficiency (Powers and Faden 2006), the capabilities view is unique in applying this principle not only to outcomes, such as well-being, but also to the more complex concept of capability. According to the capabilities framework, the aspiration of justice is not simply that people in fact achieve a certain level of functioning or well-being, but rather that people achieve some threshold level of choice and capacity. On this analysis, when thinking about limits in any particular situation, such as healthcare services, we have a reasoned basis for limiting justice obligations: We can ask ourselves whether doing less still succeeds in bringing everyone up to the floor of human dignity that individuals deserve.

The account we are considering thus combines an Aristotelian capabilities approach with a Kantian notion of dignity and human rights. The Aristotelian element sets out the basic capabilities and functioning unique to human beings. The Kantian element introduces a normative component that identifies the minimum level of functioning or well-being that society is required to ensure in order to demonstrate the proper respect for human dignity. The complicated relation between these quite heterogeneous theoretical frameworks deserves more extensive consideration than I can provide here. For the purposes of this chapter, we will set aside many unanswered questions so that we may apply the framework we are delineating to the task at hand – namely, allocating scarce healthcare resources in ageing societies.

Ethical and social implications

How might the capabilities account of justice help us think about the kinds of ethical problems that arise for healthcare systems in a rapidly ageing society? One place to start is with the question "Which kinds of resources are subject to justice requirements according to the capabilities view?" Addressing this question requires looking at the effects that various resources have on the basic capabilities outlined on page 135. Healthcare in general will be one of the goods that are distributed by justice, because it is a central means for the exercise and realization of people's basic capabilities. The two most relevant capabilities in this regard are *life* and *bodily health.* Bodily health not only supports life but also contains value in itself since it implies the absence of the suffering associated with physical disease or injury. Bodily health, or a certain degree of bodily health, is also associated with other capabilities, such as physical and intellectual activity, which can be eroded when a person experiences illness or injury. We can say that health, along with life, constitutes a basic foundational necessity for individual and social flourishing. These capabilities exert moral and political claims upon us to provide the means for their actualization. This does not entail that it is a society's responsibility to maximize individual or social flourishing; instead, societies should "equip individuals with the opportunity to avail themselves of the tools, with which they are already naturally endowed but may be hampered through disease or disabling injury, to be able to choose for themselves which fulfilling activities they will engage in for their own and others' benefit" (Eberl, Kinney, and Williams 2011, 551). Equipping individuals with the ability to choose requires doing somewhat more than the minimum necessary to sustain a human form of life. It calls upon society to bring individuals up to a level where a good life becomes possible.

If we assume that all people possess an equal worth and dignity, each of us deserves an equal set of the basic capabilities required for human flourishing. Yet, notice that capability equality does not mean the same thing as giving everyone equal access to a basic level of healthcare resources. As noted already, people possess varying abilities to convert resources into functioning. For example, as noted above, older individuals experience relatively higher rates of chronic illness and disability than other age groups; thus, it may take more resources for them to achieve the same level of basic functioning. For example, an older, or more disabled, or more seriously ill person may need more income (for assistance, for prosthetics, for treatment) to achieve the same functionings as younger or non-handicapped individuals (Sen 2009). Generally speaking, a fair share of resources for chronically ill and disabled people will require a larger share of resources, because medical conditions and associated treatments are ongoing. A system that looks only at lifetime costs of care or only at the goal of equality in the distribution of resources might miss the unique features of caring for the chronically disabled. The capabilities approach outlined here drills down to the core capabilities people possess, rather than looking merely at what resources people have at their disposal. It requires society to ensure that everyone is brought up to a level of capability required by human dignity, which is distinct from the requirement to ensure that everyone has a minimum floor of resources at their disposal.

In addition to health status, many other factors influence people's ability to convert resources into real functioning and capability. Social determinants play an integral role. For instance, an elderly person living in poverty may be unable to afford her share of costly medications, even when health insurance covers a portion of the cost. Likewise, an elderly person who cannot drive and who lacks access to public transportation may be unable to participate in rehabilitation services provided outside the home, even when such services are available in her community. A capabilities approach offers us a broader view of justice in the sense that it takes into account myriad factors that influence health, not just the specific resources associated with the provision of healthcare services (Jecker 2008).

Rising healthcare costs

Older individuals consume on average a greater share of healthcare resources. At a population level, there is some debate in the literature as to exactly what impact this will have on the health economy and overall healthcare costs. Two competing views are the medicalization thesis and the compression thesis (Schmidt 2012).

The medicalization thesis: Increasingly longer life expectancies will in fact lead to higher levels of morbidity, care needs, and health-related costs.

The compression thesis: Increasingly longer life expectancies will not in fact lead to higher levels of morbidity, care needs, and health-related costs. Instead, the period in which care is needed will be condensed over a relatively shorter period of time than it previously was.

Although this debate is empirical in nature, important normative questions about distributive justice are inextricably tied to it. Thus, pressure to limit costs and ration care will be greater or lesser, depending on which of these empirical predictions is borne out.

The compression thesis imagines a future in which medical research brings real progress in preventing, curing, and treating the symptoms of chronic conditions more prevalent in old age, such as Alzheimer's disease, cancer, stroke, and cardiovascular disease. Should this occur, the compression thesis will be validated. However, at least for the foreseeable future – that is, until such progress occurs – the reality is that as societies age, the cost of healthcare rises. The rising cost of healthcare currently associated with population ageing raises the question of what limits we can ethically impose. How much of society's resources should be devoted to old age? Are we ever justified in limiting healthcare based on age? What is a just distribution of healthcare among age groups? One response to such questions is to propose that healthcare should be rationed on the basis of old age. Bioethicists such as Daniel Callahan (1987, 2012), Norman Daniels (1985, 1988), Richard Lamm (1987), and Samuel Preston (1984) support old age-based rationing of healthcare. Callahan, for example, proposes rationing publicly funded life-extending care based on old age. Such a proposal might be implemented once society comes to accept the idea that "government has a duty, based on our collective social obligation, to help people live out a natural life span, but not actively to help extend life beyond that point" (Callahan 1987, 137). Both Lamm and Preston favor directing fewer resources to older age groups and more to younger persons as a necessary condition of meeting duties to younger and future generations. They maintain that unless society limits healthcare expenditures for the old, it will eventually impoverish health services and other social goods for the young. In addition to rationing, Lamm and others have argued that the elderly have a positive duty to die so that resources may be invested elsewhere for the benefit of younger age groups (Jecker 2014a). Finally, Daniels urges one to think about justice between the young and old from a first-person point of view. According to him, when we succeed in viewing our lives as a whole, rather than from a particular point in time, it will sometimes be prudent for us to prefer a healthcare plan that distributes fewer services to us in old age in exchange for more services earlier in life.

Yet, when it comes to actually implementing such proposals, the social and political mandate to do so has been lacking. Thus, resistance to age-based limits on healthcare can be found among international groups, such as the European Union (2007, Article 21); the World Health Organization (2002); and the United Nations (1948, Preamble). In the scholarly literature, critics of age-based rationing object, for example, to the implications of age-based rationing for women (Jecker 1991); to the violation that age-based rationing implies of the moral thrust of both Judaism and Christianity (Post 1991); and to the message that age-based rationing conveys about the meaning and worth of the lives of aged persons (Jecker 2014a; Murray 1991). Finally, critics cast doubt on the prediction that age-based rationing would yield large financial savings in healthcare expenditures. They point out that the amount of money that would be saved by old age-based rationing would be negligible if these dollars were simply spent elsewhere in the healthcare system.

What light can a capabilities approach shed on this debate? Are we ever justified in age-based rationing of healthcare according to this approach? We can begin by noting that the capabilities view rejects any form of rationing that results in anyone, young or old, falling below the minimal threshold of capability and functioning. However, maintaining everyone at a threshold level of the first capability, life, does not necessarily require society to pay for life-extending care regardless of age; it requires ensuring that everyone can reach the end of a human life of normal length. It might be consistent with the sufficiency requirement set by the capabilities approach to impose age-based limits on publicly funded healthcare, such as kidney transplantation, which is currently funded in the United States without age restriction. From a practical standpoint, the notion of a 'normal' length of human life is a changing, rather than a fixed, idea. This implies that the actual age or age range for limiting publicly funded life-extended care must remain open to revision.

The shift to chronic disease

As noted on page 132, in addition to increasing healthcare costs, societal ageing will increase the number of disabled persons and the need for long-term care, including adult day care, in-home services, and care in resident facilities, convalescent homes, and intermediate and skilled nursing facilities. What are the justice concerns related to caring for patients with chronic disease? And who should pay for and provide this care? For example, if an elderly person requires assistance with activities of daily living due to declines in cognitive or physical functioning, what is society's obligation to support such services? Compared with acute interventions, such as a hospital stay, the support services required to assist people with activities of daily living are much less costly. Yet, is there a social obligation to provide or pay for such services? According to the capabilities view, long-term care is a social obligation if it is required in order to bring people up to the basic capabilities level that is required for human dignity. The basic capabilities at stake include not only bodily health and life, which we have already discussed, but also bodily integrity, which includes the ability to move freely from place to place. So, for example, ensuring that the disabled elderly have assistance with transfer from bed to wheelchair is a requirement of justice, because this activity is integral to the central capabilities. When people lose the ability to live independently, society is required to ensure access to basic caregiving services necessary to prevent falling below a threshold level needed for human dignity.

But what are the limits of society's obligation in this area? Although the cost of individual services may be minimal, the growing population of older adults means that these costs will quickly add up and cumulatively strain healthcare and social-support systems globally. Are societies justified in limiting publicly funded basic caregiving on the basis of age? For example, once individuals live beyond a normal lifespan, may society ethically shift the cost of basic caregiving to private individuals and families? According to the capabilities view that I have set out, there is no justification for age-based limits on basic caregiving. Instead, societies ethically must ensure that healthcare and social arrangements are structured in such a way that the dependent elderly have access to caregiving services necessary for the threshold level of functioning and capability required for human dignity. This point contrasts with the conclusion reached on page 141, which allows for the possibility of limiting publicly funded life-extending services beyond a certain age. Unlike life-extending services, caregiving emphasizes quality of life, and it attempts to guarantee that people can live out their final days in an environment that recognizes their dignity and worth as persons.

Egalitarianism

The central line of argument suggested by the approach I am delineating is egalitarian. The capabilities view as I interpret it underscores the importance of equality in our basic functioning capabilities. It sets for everyone the goal of attaining an adequate level of human capabilities to the extent possible. According to this view, what matters is not that everyone has an equal amount of resources; instead, what matters is people's ability to convert resources into capabilities and functioning. The capabilities view emphasizes the question of whether people can effectively achieve what they want to achieve and be what they want to be. Although not all capability theorists set the goal of attaining capability equality, the interpretation of the capabilities approach I am proposing does (Jecker 2014b). My account seeks to establish a set of basic capabilities required for human flourishing and it argues for equality with respect to these basic capabilities. Expressed differently, each and every person should be sustained in each of his or her basic capabilities at a threshold level.

Although the capabilities framework represents an egalitarian approach, it applies requirements of equality only to the basic floor of a healthcare system. Thus, it is consistent with the capabilities view to allow a two-tier system that tolerates inequalities beyond the basic level of healthcare. Whereas everyone is treated equal in the sense of being brought up to a certain floor, those who can afford it may purchase private insurance and obtain better or more extensive care. Allowing inequalities beyond the basic level is consistent with the requirement of equal respect for persons. It is consistent with showing equal respect for human dignity to allow some, but not others, to (for example) purchase expensive cosmetic procedures. However, it would not meet the requirements of equal respect for persons to allow some, but not others, to have access to childhood vaccines or emergency medical care (Gutmann 1983).

Conclusion: advantages of a capabilities approach

Throughout this chapter, I have argued that a capabilities approach is particularly well-suited for thinking about ageing populations. In contrast to dominant approaches to justice that emphasize autonomy and rational choice, the philosophical starting point of the capabilities approach is to ask what supports people's basic functionings and capabilities at a level sufficient to maintain human dignity. Rather than asking whether or not individuals rationally agree to accept certain distributive principles, the capabilities view asks what is required for individuals to be capable of functioning well. This starting point carries distinct advantages. First, it allows us to give an account of what we owe to persons who cannot rationally deliberate. Since elderly individuals are more likely than members of other age groups to experience cognitive impairments that interfere with decisional capacity, this represents an important advantage. The capabilities approach can do for us what autonomy-based approaches to justice cannot – namely, justify a set of basic entitlements for everyone. It does not create outliers of those who lack cognitive capacities. Instead, it recognizes the equal worth and dignity of all human beings (Jecker 2013).

Second, a capabilities approach makes evident that bringing everyone up to a threshold level of the central capabilities is not simply a matter of providing everyone access to basic resources. Since individuals possess varying abilities to convert resources into functioning and capabilities, those with less ability may require a greater share of resources. Elderly people experience higher rates of chronic illness and disability; as a result, they may require more resources, such as income, to achieve the same functioning and capabilities as younger people. A justice approach that looks only at the goal of equality in the distribution of resources may miss this important point (Sen 2009).

Finally, the capabilities view offers a more robust account of justice by grounding justice principles on important facts about human beings. By contrast, autonomy-based views seek to eliminate all sources of morality that are outside human will and agency. As a result, autonomy-based approaches tend to offer procedural, not substantive, analyses of justice. Thus, Kant offers a test for moral principles without actually generating any moral principles. The capabilities view has the advantage of offering more. It identifies the source of dignity to be species membership. The functioning that is characteristic for a species is what establishes the central capabilities and associated obligations for each species member (Jecker 2013). By contrast, autonomy-based accounts tend to see species membership as morally irrelevant and focus instead on rational agency as being our most salient feature. Yet, focusing on rationality alone leaves out many of the central functionings and capabilities that merit recognition and respect.

In conclusion, the capabilities approach rejects the idea that justice principles are the outcome of a suitably defined rational choice. Instead, it proposes an Aristotelian-style analysis to identify the central functionings and capabilities of human beings, making this the source of justice principles. Drawing on the Kantian notion of recognition respect, owed to human beings by virtue of the kind of beings they are, the capabilities view requires supporting people at a level of functioning and capability required for human dignity. In practical terms, respecting elderly persons may be at variance with what we want to do or how society prefers to invest its resources. Yet, such respect is morally required. Doing less violates the minimal obligations we owe the elderly. Even if we live in a youth-focused culture, one that emphasizes activity and independence, we have an obligation to behave in ways that show dependent elderly persons the respect they deserve.

Note

1 Acknowledgments: The sections on age-based rationing and long-term care are a condensed version of my more detailed analysis provided in "Justice between Age Groups: An Objection to the Prudential Lifespan Approach" (Jecker 2013).

References

Callahan, D. 1987. *Setting Limits*. New York: Simon and Schuster.

Callahan, D. 2012. "Must We Ration Health Care for the Elderly?" *Journal of Law, Medicine and Ethics* 40 (1):10–16. doi: 10.1111/j.1748-720X.2012.00640.x.

Daniels, N. 1985. *Just Health Care*. New York: Cambridge University Press.

Daniels, N. 1988. *Am I My Parents' Keeper? An Essay on Justice between the Young and the Old*. New York: Oxford University Press.

Daniels, N. 2001. "Justice, Health, and Healthcare." *American Journal of Bioethics* 1 (2):2–16. doi: 10.1162/152651601300168834.

Daniels, N. 2008. "Justice between Adjacent Generations: Further Thoughts." *Journal of Political Philosophy* 16 (4):475–494. doi: 10.1111/j.1467-9760.2008.00320.x.

Darwall, S. 1977. "Two Kinds of Respect." *Ethics* 88 (1):36–49.

Dillon, R. S. 2016. "Respect." In *The Stanford Encyclopedia of Philosophy* (online), edited by E. N. Zalta. http://plato.stanford.edu/archives/fall2015/entries/respect/.

Eberl, J. T., E. D. Kinney, and M. J. Williams. 2011. "Foundation for a Natural Right to Health Care." *Journal of Medicine and Philosophy* 36 (6):537–557. doi: 10.1093/jmp/jhr047.

European Union. 2007. *Charter of Fundamental Rights of the European Union*. Accessed September 27, 2012. http://eur.lex.europa.eu/LexUriServ/LexUriServ.do?uri=OJ:C:2007:303:0001:0016:EN:PDF.

Gutmann, A. 1983. "For and against Equal Access to Health Care." In *President's Commission for the Study of Ethical Problems in Health Care and Biomedical and Behavioral Research*. Washington, DC: US Government Printing Office.

Jecker, N. S. 1991. "Age-Based Rationing and Women." *Journal of the American Medical Association* 266 (25):3012–3015. doi: 10.1001/jama.1991.03470210080037.

Jecker, N. S. 2008. "A Broader View of Justice." *The American Journal of Bioethics* 8 (10): 2–10. doi: 10.1080/15265160802478412.

Jecker, N. S. 2013. "Justice between Age Groups: An Objection to the Prudential Lifespan Approach." *American Journal of Bioethics* 13 (8):3–15. doi: 10.1080/15265161.2013.802061.

Jecker, N. S. 2014a. "Against a Duty to Die." *Virtual Mentor: American Medical Association Journal* 16 (5):390–394.

Jecker, N. S. 2014b. "Justice." In *Encyclopedia of Bioethics* (4th edition), edited by B. Jennings, 1774–1784. New York: Cenage Learning.

Jennings, B., D. Callahan, and A. L. Caplan. 1988. "Ethical Challenges of Chronic Illness." *Hastings Center Report* 18 (1):1–16.

Lamm, R. D. 1987. "Ethical Care for the Elderly: Are We Cheating Our Children?" In *Should Medical Care Be Rationed by Age?*, edited by T. M. Smeeding, M. P. Battin, L. P. Francis, and B. M. Landesman, xi–xv. Totowa, NJ: Rowman & Littlefield.

McCrudden, C. 2008. "Human Dignity and Judicial Interpretation of Human Rights." *The European Journal of International Law* 19 (4):655–724. doi: 10.1093/ejil/chn043.

Murray, T. 1991. "Meaning, Aging, and Public Policy." In *Too Old for Health Care? Controversies in Medicine, Law, Economics, and Ethics*, edited by R. H. Binstock and S. G. Post, 164–179. Baltimore, MD: Johns Hopkins University Press.

National Institute on Aging and World Health Organization. 2011. "Global Health and Aging." Accessed November 13, 2012. www.who.int/ageing/publications/global health/en/index.html.

Nussbaum, M. C. 1992. "Human Functioning and Social Justice: In Defense of Aristotelian Essentialism." *Political Theory* 20 (2):202–246.

Nussbaum, M. C. 2003. "Capabilities as Fundamental Entitlements: Sen and Social Justice." *Feminist Economics* 9 (2–3):33–59. doi: 10.1080/1354570022000077926.

Nussbaum, M. C. 2011. *Creating Capabilities: The Human Development Approach*. Cambridge, MA: Harvard University Press.

Oxley, H. 2009. "Policies for Healthy Ageing: An Overview." *Organization for Economic Cooperation and Development Health Working Papers* 42. Accessed August 20, 2016. www.oecd-ilibrary.org/social-issues-migration-health/policies-for-healthy-ageing 226757488706.

Post, S. G. 1991. "Justice for Elderly People in Jewish and Christian Thought." In *Too Old for Health Care?*, edited by R. H. Binstock and S. G. Post, 120–137. Baltimore, MD: Johns Hopkins University Press.

Powers, M., and R. Faden. 2006. *Social Justice: The Moral Foundations of Public Health and Health Policy*. New York: Oxford University Press.

Preston, S. H. 1984. "Children and the Elderly in the U.S." *Scientific American* 251 (6):44–57.

Schmidt, H. 2012. "Personal Responsibility for Health: A Proposal for a Nuanced Approach." In *Accountability and Responsibility in Health Care: Issues in Addressing an Emerging Global Challenge*, edited by B. Rosen, A. Israeli, and M. Shortell, 431–462. Singapore: World Scientific Publishing Company.

Sen, A. K. 2009. *The Idea of Justice*. Cambridge, MA: Harvard University Press.

United Nations General Assembly. 1948. *The Universal Declaration of Human Rights*. Accessed September 27, 2012. www.un.org/en/documents/udhr/index.shtml.

U.S. Department of Health and Human Services, Agency for Healthcare Research. 2006. "The High Concentration of U.S. Health Expenditures." *Research in Action* 19:1–9.

Whelan, J. 2002. "WHO Calls for Countries to Shift from Acute to Chronic Care." *British Medical Journal* 324 (7348):1237.

World Health Organization. 2002. *Active Ageing: A Policy Framework*. Accessed August 20, 2016. www.who.int/ageing/publications/active_ageing/en/.

Part 3

Individual provisions and public policies in ageing societies

10 Final decisions for the final crisis

Hopes and hypes regarding the advance directive in Germany

Kai Brauer

After recent legislation on advance healthcare directives (in short: advance directives (AD)) in Germany, it has become possible to make legally binding decisions regarding one's end of life before actually being affected by the 'final crisis' to which such a decision normally refers. It was hoped that problematic treatment situations in hospitals could be prevented that way. However, it has often been remarked that each AD constitutes a paradox: The way a terminal crisis plays out, as well as its actual influence on the patient, cannot be grasped without having experienced such crisis. Thus, on one hand, a written expression of will cannot be ignored once a problematic treatment situation at the end of the life has occurred. On the other hand, however, there are doubts on whether a written AD is really necessary or helpful, redundant because of other rules and institutions, or even superfluous. This may be one of the ethical problems becoming more relevant due to the development of modern medicine (Schweda and Schicktanz 2012). Yet, not only experts or professionals have to deal with these questions. On the contrary, everybody has to find their own solution. Which conditions and ideas confront those who are currently preparing themselves for a 'final crisis' by drafting an AD?

This chapter explores the views of those who are interested in the possibility of an AD. Sociologically, this is interesting from the perspective of individualization theory, life-course theory, and biographical research (Beck 1986; Kohli 1985). The process of preparing an AD functions as an attempt to increase personal autonomy and self-determined decision-making regarding a phase in a person's life that would not permit communicating actual decisions and desires. In this sense, ADs are another symptom of the fundamental social processes of individualization and institutionalization of personal biographies. Beyond that, the legal system itself has long called for a regulation of the matter. The new law has not only reinforced the rights of patients at the end of life. It has also furthered critical discussion regarding patients' rights in general. Against this backdrop, this chapter presents findings from a qualitative study on dealing with ADs in Germany and identifies four distinct types of action emerging in the context of planning for end-of-life decisions.

Hype: the making of the AD

The legal regulation of ADs in Germany was a comparatively speedy and at the same time intensively discussed process (Hahn 2009). After controversial debates in the German parliament (Bundestag), fueled by a statement of the Association of German Jurists (Deutscher Juristentag) in 2006 about the legalization of assisted suicide and driven by accordant reactions from the churches, the *Third Law on the Rights of Terminally Ill Persons* finally passed in September 2009, converting the AD into a legally recognized institution. Disregarding an AD in clinical practice can now constitute a punishable assault. Hence, the AD is of considerable significance for medical personnel treating a patient – assuming that a sufficient number of patients already have a legally binding written will outlining their wishes for final medical treatment and death. The law has provided a legal instrument for laypersons, although it may still be new and unfamiliar to most of them.

The moral and legal principles underpinning the AD are by no means new. Similar documents, such as so-called 'patient wills,' had been in use in Germany long before the recent discussion (Borasio, Heßler, and Wiesing 2009; Hahn 2009; Kopetzki 2000). The implementation of the aforementioned law was meant to provide legal certainty and to restrict assisted suicide. Indeed, the requirement of informed consent to any medical treatment has become clearer with the legal establishment of and the discussions on this principle. However, the consequence is not only a strengthening of patients' rights in a few borderline cases (Lauter and Helmchen 2006; Stollberg 2008a). From a sociological perspective, comparatively complicated clinical constellations have been introduced to everyday thought and practice. Thus, the new rules for end-of-life treatment become relevant for individual biographies inasmuch as it is assumed to be self-evident that everybody needs a personal AD with precise medical definitions.

However, while those involved in the legislative process were eager to provide the possibility of an AD, the number of individuals making use of this possibility remains well below the expectations. Although very few[1] Germans and Austrians (who have had a similar legal development) have completed an AD, often many think that everyone should apply this form of self-care. Thus, the question of the relevance of the AD for the individual not only arises from a perceived crisis, but is also propagated by the state, medical doctors, and other stakeholders, so that it can hardly be avoided anymore. The way of thinking and planning one's own death thus receives a new institutional framing (Nassehi, Brüggen, and Saake 2002). Most institutions have supported the introduction of ADs by making relevant information available to both patients and staff. Consequently, in the case of hospitalization, the existence of an AD will be checked, or the staff will directly address the question (Nauck and Jaspers 2011). All procedures and forms have been adjusted accordingly. Questions such as "Do you already have an AD?" are printed right at the top of medical-history forms, sometimes even before the fields for gender, age, and medical results. Since, theoretically, every person may at some point need medical treatment, the logical conclusion seems to be that everyone, regardless of their health status and age, should protect themselves with an AD. Does this establish a new standard? A requirement for optimization, a regulation to be taken care of in any event, even in absence of fear of suffering and death? And why have not all citizens made use of this option, which is clearly seen as desirable? What does the new legal institution mean in sociological terms?

Hope and hype regarding the advance directive: a sociological perspective

From a sociological perspective, the AD is first and foremost a written document. As in a testament, it is intended to convey one's will for posterity, is not publicly announced, remains private, and should be read only by authorized personnel. It does not refer to material inheritance but rather to one's very physical existence. The legal definitions that determine which medical interventions are desired and which should be excluded when people find themselves in the role of the patient and are not able to express their wishes is a matter of life and death. These are areas that were previously entrusted to the will of God and subsequently to the responsible professions (medical doctors). The fact that not everyone immediately drafted an AD aggrieves the activists who fought for its implementation. They warn that considerations about an AD are possibly made 'too late' because in a situation of life-threatening disease and intensive care, there might not be enough time for an appropriate decision. Therefore, the law should advise a timely drafting, ideally just after reaching legal maturity (in Germany from the age of 18).

In fact, it is not surprising that only few have actually chosen the option of drafting an AD so far. The issues involved hardly seem imperative in everyday life. Of course, questions of chronic illness and death ought to be part of the general *life course* (or, better, of the *Life-World / 'Lebenswelt'* in terms of Alfred Schütz) but not necessarily of *everyday life*. Without special information, specific experience, and imagination, the possibility of writing an AD and the existence of legal regulations for its implementation are irrelevant to people's daily routines. The AD becomes relevant in everyday life only when direct or indirect experience of intensive care and life-threatening situations is recognized and interpreted in terms of a possible threat. This is surely not a routine day-to-day situation or a simple choice but the result of a crisis or the imagining of an existential crisis in the future. Thus, when a need for appropriate information about ADs arises, it is embedded in discourses of fear and notions of pain. The sociological analysis of the interest in ADs cannot ignore these extraordinary circumstances.

Thus, spreading the word on ADs depends on how advertising and information address the relevant stakeholders and their imaginations. Compared to other forms of prospective self-protection (such as preventive anti-ageing practices or life insurance), the technical details and monetary costs of the AD appear negligible. Therefore, it could be expected that typical aspects of inequality (income, education, gender) play only a minor role. In contrast, age distribution and the frequency of chronic disease and anticipated proximity to death suggest that the proportion of older people with corresponding requirements is higher. A review of this hypothesis by means of quantifying methods would certainly be interesting. But in view of the unclear latent structure and objective sense of the phenomenon AD for everyday life and social contexts, it would be an undemanding sociological exercise. Instead, what should actually be analyzed empirically is the impact of the practical implementation of the AD law on the decision-making processes of real people. What kind of meanings are constructed when individuals discuss the possibility of a living will?

While the views of highly informed health and care clients will mostly mirror the general scale of the educated bourgeoisie, the perception of laypersons who live in rather precarious conditions or have little contact with medical and care problems is particularly important. As Stollberg (2008b) pointed out, the 'autonomous patient' (in German: *mündiger Patient*) may be an intellectual fiction anyway. Regarding questions about the meaning of the AD and their biopolitical dimension, not only the well-informed intellectual upper class has to deal with existential decisions. The focus of research should be directed on the ways the routinization of the practice depends on specific conceptual worlds: How do practical arguments for or against the AD influence individual subjective horizons (Husserl 1986; Schütz 1971) and the structure of biographical decision-making processes? And how do prospective perspectives of biographical planning (Kohli 1981, 1985, 1994) come to include the self-determined shaping of the end of life? What forms of handling these decisions are possible; which types can be distinguished?

Empirical research: discussions on advance directive

In a four-year project, group discussions and interviews with experts and laypersons were conducted.[2] The main data corpus for the analysis were 12 group discussions performed in four German cities in 2011 and 2012. For the composition of the groups, we aimed at a balanced distribution of age (20–85 years) and gender (48 females and 28 males). Decisive for participation was the respondents' self-definition as 'interested in ADs,' regardless of the intensity of interest or the amount of prior knowledge. People who found the topic irrelevant or repellent were not included. Thus, the recruited participants were interested in ADs to a certain extent.

A conversation about the topic was stimulated in order to elicit the corresponding background experiences and life realities (Bohnsack 1997). After a general description of the research topic, the participants were invited to present themselves and their interest in ADs. Thus, they had to make a connection between their own biographical background and the topic, spontaneously formulating and interrelating contributions without precise instructions or guidance from the facilitators. This way, the scope of detail and frame of relevance remained as open as possible (Schütz 1971). The participants could contribute stories, arguments, or justifications, either seamlessly, dramatically sharpened, or neutrally reported; they could abruptly change topic or close with questions. Of course, there were manifold possible inter-subjectively comprehensible reference points (e.g., 'disease,' 'ageing,' 'dying,' 'medicine,' 'work,' 'compassion,' 'science,' 'economy'). This created a dynamic of presentation with its own inherent time and content frames ("For how long do they want me to talk? How interesting am I or is my self-presentation for the group and the researchers, and how does it connect me to the topic in a logical way?") that could not be anticipated in advance. For analysis, these introduction passages were of special interest.

The evaluation of the discussions took place in several stages. Through coding methods (following Glaser and Strauss 2009), an overview of the manifest statements, the selected contents, the thematic priority settings, and the utilized metaphors was obtained. Furthermore, according to the documentary method (Bohnsack 2007), an overview of specific discursive dynamics and courses of argumentation was attained. The analysis of text passages from the transcripts usually started with the sequential analysis of the biographical entry sequences (Pilz 2007; Wernet 2006), which allowed the adequate exploration of the aforementioned question forms. The steps of the interpretation will not be described here in detail. The process of defining different types (reconstruction) started from one case and was pursued through the maximum contrast method of theoretical sampling and an overview of all cases.

Types between hope and hype

Which types of dealing with the AD can be distinguished? Although most of the participants in the discussions did not actually have an AD, all of them were interested in the topic. Fear of physical suffering at the end of life was a strong motive for all of them. The question is in what ways the AD is believed to guarantee self-determination and to prevent the final medical treatment of a 'worst-case scenario' from culminating in a 'total meltdown.'

(a) Hype-type 'radical fiction': great feelings and crude imagination

According to the first type, such a meltdown would indeed be inevitable unless the medical professionals were given the order to terminate treatment at some point. The core slogan for this type expresses rather strong emotions: "Because of the AD, I feel really terrific!" From the 'radical fiction' perspective, the goal of writing an AD is simply to fend off suffering at the end of life. At the same time, the practice of writing and drafting the AD is already considered sufficient in order to secure a self-determined death. Hence, the demand for further, more detailed information is rather low. Descriptions of the situation in which the AD should apply remain vague and uncertain. One's own existence at the end of life is imagined as a body that is being taken care of by others. This appears as an unacceptable (or unworthy) situation. Chances of recovery are ignored. Also, the possibility that in a final agony, one would actually prefer a life of dependence to death is not considered or discussed.

From the 'radical' point of view, the central goal of an AD is the recovery of one's own future integrity for *the here and now*. One's own death is seen not as a paradoxical fate but as the consistent conclusion and radical solution of an imagined problem (inevitable suffering in intensive care). Thus, the AD creates an additional stabilization of the self – especially for individuals in precarious life situations. For this type, the writing of an AD already guarantees autonomy and self-confidence, which would otherwise be difficult to achieve. These considerations do not necessarily have to lead to the actual composition of an AD. The thought alone can spark feelings of extreme elation. By radical rejection of medical science and technology, at least the competence of the doctors can be contained. Their decisions appear as representative of all societal authorities, whose interventions in one's own life are generally experienced as an imposition.

The radical effort of self-determination at the end of life indicates an imaginative horizon shaped through precarious social positions. Writing an AD also allows the 'radical type' a subjective stabilization of his current social status. A high degree of self-care, responsibility, planning competence, and provision can be demonstrated. In individualized societies, where social position is accredited to the performance and track record of the individual, the possibility of a symbolic statement of self-determination (Soeffner 2010) is gratefully accepted. Whether the desired degree of self-determination will actually have the intended 'effect' later on cannot be controlled. The 'radical fiction' type must rely on the efficacy of the document 'my own AD.' Thus, its effect is symbolically charged.

Furthermore, the 'radical' type perceives disease per se as 'unproductive' – and hence reprehensible. He adheres to the idea that the value of one's own life (and that of others) depends on personal performance. When a healing process does not result in the recovery of productivity, thus only incurring medical expenses, it is perceived as useless. From this perspective, needing care amounts to 'social parasitism' – even if it is acknowledged that such situations can occur through no fault of one's own. Such radicalism is latently anti-humanistic and at times even explicitly inhuman. Thus, some participants use expressions such as "when you have to be fed, you're like a living piece of meat" and even "off to the gas chamber" when faced with the question of what one would do in the case of coma and feeding tube. That talk about euthanasia here flows into Nazi vocabulary is clearly a gross misstep and an exception to the rule, but structurally no coincidence.

A decisive structural feature of the 'radical type' is the demonstrative dissociation from sickness and the sick, or rather those who are hesitant regarding the preventive rejection of situations that threaten autonomy. It would be a trivial misinterpretation to dismiss this as 'uncertainty,' 'low empathy,' or even 'cognitive weakness.' Much more important is that in a precarious economic and sociocultural context, imagining an AD becomes an attractive promise of security, so that the previously described 'radical fiction' suggests itself as a form of practical risk minimization.

Alternative ways of handling a situation of vulnerability are almost inconceivable for the 'radical' type and are avoided during the group discussions. The AD provides the 'radical' with a 'smooth solution' (Thielicke 1968), one that eliminates any insecurity or ambivalence of dialectic approaches. An autonomous confrontation with questions of destiny is thus blocked, and humility becomes superfluous. The radicalism of the type finally expresses itself through the negation – or rather the drastic rejection – of any skepticism, which leads to a strong feeling of elation with and through the AD. The exclusion of skepticism and the achievement of a feeling of elation here and now with an AD are thus the constitutive attributes of the type.

(b) Hope-type 'reflective skepticism': wanting to handle uncertainty

Who is able to oppose the strong suggestive power of a 'smooth solution'? According to the theoretical sampling of Grounded Theory, types should be reconstructed through maximal contrast. Therefore, we looked for constructions of meaning that rather discourage definite decidedness, that cannot make someone drafting an AD happy, interpretations that do not comply with the shortened and drastic fictions of the state of the last treatment being the 'maximum credible accident.'

In fact, such arguments can be assigned to certain cases that constitute a type of their own. Skepticism (about the purpose and effectiveness of the AD) is its central rationale and distinctive feature. The respective participants position themselves against radical interpretations and solutions in the group discussions. They are obviously missing the rigorous control fiction of the first type. A feeling of elation toward the AD cannot be observed. In contrast, a reflected and differentiated handling of risks is displayed and sometimes extended to other areas of life. The fundamental uncertainty of the future is not denied, nor are the sensitive issues of chronic disease and death – regardless of the possibility of completing an AD. An explicit deliberation on ambivalent and incalculable future situations and conditions is therefore not avoided but critically evaluated.

The possibility that sources of insecurity and risk can generate further dilemmas and open questions is taken into account. In contrast to the 'radical' type, it is inconceivable for the 'reflective' type that an AD could actually transform the doubt and helplessness regarding the hypothetical scenario of a 'final' disease into a feeling of security. As this type acknowledges uncertainty, the new possibilities offered by the AD stimulate reflections on one's own way of life and ethical considerations on the value of life in general. Thus, in this case, the AD actually initiates and promotes the confrontation with death – just as it is supposed to end this confrontation in the case of the first type. The opposition between the types – the AD as a solution to a dramatic problem versus the problematizing of this solution – was evident in the group discussions and shaped dominant lines of argument.

The 'reflective' type looks for solutions in the same place as the 'radicals' but has very different problems in and attitudes about life. The respective participants are not completely opposed to the AD. However, even if they were to write such a disposition, their skepticism would remain. The prospective planning of the very last phase of life also provides stabilization in the here and now, but it does so through reflection and deliberation, not by simply generating a feeling of relief and happiness. Typically, this type's knowledge of the reality of intensive care is more extensive. For proponents of this type, the purpose of the AD is to promote the discussion of this reality rather than blocking it. Security is achieved through ever more knowledge, which leads to a partial or temporary decision but not to final closure. Humility toward their own (and others') final crisis constitutes the condition for the skeptics' ambivalent approval or eventual rejection of the AD.

(c) Hype-type 'bureaucratic insurance': regulated/ settled end of life

A third, intermediary way of dealing with the AD – without the radicalism of the first, but also without the uncertainty of the second group – can be described as the 'bureaucratic insurance' type. In the data material, this type, which is neither skeptical nor radical, constitutes the largest group. The respective participants see the AD as a simple but effective means of insurance. These 'insured' are similar to the 'radicals' in that they tend to show resistance to ambivalent thoughts about disease, and they perceive the loss of autonomy per se as a misfortune to be avoided. However, unlike the 'radicals,' they do not cultivate fantasies of euthanasia, nor do they achieve feelings of great elation by drafting an AD. In order to stabilize their current position, they consider it sufficient to complete an AD as neatly and correctly as possible, just like filling out an insurance form. For this purpose, legal and medical knowledge is required, something the 'insured' have in common with the 'skeptics.' It is not enough to sign just any paper that might help in some way. Instead, the AD is perceived as a bureaucratic document that should be approached in a deliberate manner and designed in a practicable way. The 'insured' also propose compiling a national registry (preferably on the Internet) in order to make all ADs available to the police and emergency-care services at all times. For the 'radicals,' this seems somewhat strange, as they find it sufficient to disclose and discuss their AD with friends (or, as some comment ironically, have it tattooed on their bodies). In contrast, the 'bureaucratic' type is particularly interested in the practical feasibility of the AD as a legal instrument. They feel reassured by having a solid and sophisticated document with an appropriate institutional or bureaucratic background. Therefore, this type explicitly draws on media discourses about the legal optimization of the AD and ridicules the situation of those without such a disposition (the 'uninsured'). Again, a sense of skepticism remains. However, in contrast to the 'skeptical' type, this skepticism is concerned not with the general ambivalence of illness and care at the end of life but with the bureaucratic implementation of the written will: "Is there someone who knows about it or knows where it is kept?" For the 'skeptics,' the 'bureaucratic' arguments and details put forward in this context are ultimately irrelevant. For the radicals, they are only of secondary importance.

In the group discussions, the 'insured' sometimes follow the views of the 'radical fiction' type and support them with their own examples. However, they do not propagate ideologies of worthy and unworthy life to increase their own feeling of elation. Instead, they underline the pressing need for improvement in order to attain the efficacy of an absolutely safe AD. They also share some of the uncertainties of the skeptics, but draw different conclusions, along the lines of 'better safe than sorry.' By completing an AD, the task of bureaucratic provision should be taken care of once and for all. The 'bureaucrats' do not want their insurance to be as open and undefined as the 'reflective' types prefer things to be. And while the form itself hardly matters for the 'radicals,' the 'insured' continue to work on their AD.

(d) Anti-type 'confident refusal': irrelevant regulation

Theoretically, there should also be stakeholders who generally reject arguments in favor of ADs and refuse the whole way of thinking. From a logical point of view, they would have to be distinguished not only from the 'radical' and 'bureaucratic' forms of agreement, but also from the uncertainty of the skeptics. However, in the group discussions, no such voices were heard, probably because people with a dismissive attitude toward the discussions held within the scope of the project did not feel compelled to participate. Therefore, it would be difficult to find empirical evidence of such a type in the data material used here. Nevertheless, a prominent opponent of the AD can be cited as representative of the 'confident refusal' type. Physician and psychiatrist Klaus Dörner, who became known in Germany in the 1970s because of his criticism of psychiatry (with slogans such as "Going insane is human" and "Open the institutions") and today actively criticizes the current methods of caring for the elderly, notably said in a talk show:

> I have nothing against advance directives. But if I completed something like that, it would be at odds with the way I have lived my life so far. Up until now, I haven't taken out any insurance for the future and I have kept an open attitude. And I actually intend to continue with this for the final life phase of dying as well.[3]

Thus, this type is by no means ignorant of the possibility of drafting an AD, but articulates a clear position against it. His confidence in the relevant institutions, individuals, and roles in the final treatment is comparatively high. His imaginativeness regarding dramatic situations in the sense of 'worst-case scenarios' at the end of life is not necessarily less powerful than that of the 'radicals.' However, the decisive specificity is practical competence, a set of life skills that is unsettled neither by dramatic fiction nor by skepticism or bureaucratic trust in insurance. Dealing with the knowledge of one's own vulnerability leads to practical solutions and concrete biographical plans (for Dörner, this could be the 'autonomous care groups' he promotes). This requires a profound confrontation with dependence and need for help, and it excludes attitudes of prospective resignation or simple bureaucratic insurance. In dealing with the AD, this type, which can remain neither skeptical nor reflective, could be identified as 'confident refusal.' For this type, although a durable power of attorney for healthcare is a consideration, an AD seems to be out of the question. This anti-type is less likely to reject the AD on ideological grounds; it appears simply irrelevant to his life practice.

Future: hope or hype as expressions of imagination and trust

How will the AD change our society? Does it strengthen individual autonomy, or does it create constraints that block alternative solutions for the end of life? Both possibilities imply a simplified idea of life planning and biographical decisions. They overlook the temporal dimension of prospection significant for all biographical planning. From within the here and now of everyday life, prospection refers to an envisaged future and to the relating of that future to one's current situation. Thereby, every decision that is written in advance has specific qualities. Biographical decisions are directed toward a specific "tomorrow"; they refer to "next year," "when I'm 65," or "a few months after retiring" (Brauer 2008; Kohli 1981, 1994). By contrast, the AD comes into effect when "it begins": when "the final illness will have become unbearable."

In practice, the AD tries to come to grips with what Alfred Schütz (2003) calls 'dealing with the future perfect.' This means that my actions are perceived in terms of things 'I will have achieved.' In planning, I seem to look back upon the imagined results of my actions in the future perfect tense; I consider them "modo futuri exacti" (Schütz 2003, 94). This way, the imagined success is independent of the actual outcomes of my future actions. This is what the term 'prospectivity' means: A meaningful plan of action directly affects my present self-image, regardless of the possibility of measuring its future success. Of course, I could, theoretically, at a later time, reflect in retrospect on how a past anticipation has become reality. This is the 'balance' aspect of biographical foresight (Kohli 1994). Only the results of completed actions – never those of still-ongoing activities – can be evaluated objectively. Nevertheless, *prospectivity*, as a temporal structure of life planning, must necessarily be based on the imagination of a desired state in the future. Thus, for decisions made in the present, ideas about the future must suffice in order to accomplish the 'future perfect.' In a way, since the actual biographical payoff of the provisions made in the present can never be estimated by the subject itself *ex post* (in the case of the AD, this would mean *post mortem*), these provisions are quite easy to make. From a secular point of view, the risk of being held accountable later on – or of experiencing the consequences of a provision – is low when these ultimately lead to death. Thus, the authors of an AD are able to make cool, 'rational' calculations (or 'radical' dispositions) because the situation to be dealt with is a phase in life that lies beyond personal experience ('after' the 'future perfect').

The surprising simultaneity of imagination and trust in the AD can unfold only because the relevant definitions refer to an indefinite date in a future located in the 'afterlife' of one's own embodied experience. This is also typical of testamentary dispositions. It is a typical prospective safety construction which in fact explicitly presupposes the individual's demise but at the same time unfolds an immense effect on current everyday life and its experience. For the 'radical fiction' type, the AD also offers an extremely practicable and obvious form of symbolizing autonomy, which has an immediate prospective effect in the experience of precarious everyday life. That it could also be possible to decide against one's own will to live is of little importance.

These analyses focused on the effects of the relatively new social institution of the AD from the perspective of everyday practice. It was explored how the possibility of the AD shifts into our awareness; which biographical experiences and perspectives are addressed; and which constructions of meaning are provoked in everyday life. For this purpose, central media and legal arguments were recalled.

This discussion, which is led both emotionally and politically, motivates individuals to think about the final treatment they want to receive. Thus, the biographical foresight of a conceived catastrophic end-of-life situation became comprehensible in group discussions. The political pressure to find a general rule for all situations at the end of life – for every conceivable situation and constellation – is mirrored in the arguments of everyday knowledge. For many, it seems absolutely necessary to draft an AD as soon as possible – at least once the final treatment situation is perceived as a permanent threat.

The easiest way to react to the pressure to decide about the AD is by denying or suppressing any ambivalence. This inevitably leads to 'radical' or 'bureaucratic' solutions. Thus, the law on ADs may promote profound reflection and debate on issues such as trust, dependence, the need for care, and death, but it can also foster the belief in structural euthanasia, which entails a differentiation of worthy and unworthy life and tends to lead to strict and simplified solutions. As the threat to one's own quality of life and will to live cannot be anticipated at the time of drafting, a vivid imagining of suffering at the end of life is necessary in order to justify the AD; illness and intensive care can become a 'worst imaginable treatment scenario,' an anticipated personal 'maximum credible accident.' This is the rationalized reason – at least for the 'radical fiction' and 'bureaucratic insurance' types – for seeking an ultimate and smooth solution of all problems. By being required to determine their treatment themselves, these cases inevitably turn not only against some medical treatments (considered useless) and the responsible professions (medicine, nursing), but possibly also against their own relatives, and eventually also their own ('chronically ill' and therefore dysfunctional) body. Structurally, the body (as an ephemeral apparatus) is legally shielded against undesired treatment, and thus the correct pace of dying, according to the individual's own free will and without long suffering, is announced to the outside world. This should be interpreted not as anticipated suicide but rather in the sense that the AD serves to stabilize the current biographical position due to the 'knowledge' or 'certainty' of a quick death. This is an imposing effect of prospectivity, which makes it possible to achieve self-confidence through the determination of a state that is imagined as a threat – even though this state will not necessarily occur and the effect of the AD can never be personally verified. Prospection through the AD works for the 'radical' type as "Now I feel good because I can decide that I'll be spared from that later on" and for the 'bureaucratic' type as "I feel safer because I have made my will clear, even for the worst-case scenario."

For the two other types, 'skeptic' and 'refusing,' the structural effect of prospectivity is also fundamental. However, for them the AD offers no real help in this regard. Skepticism toward the relevance of the AD remains. Writing instructions on "how I should be treated" for a phase of life for which personal perceptions and desires cannot be envisioned is not really considered a reasonable life plan and remains a solution that, biographically, hardly makes sense. 'Skeptics' cannot achieve a 'smooth solution' by drafting an AD, because they question its very form. Their slogan of prospection is "I feel safer now when I deal with the possible future situation in more detail and I don't decide too soon on a specific form, something that might harm me, but only when I've pondered other solutions long enough." For this type, the AD becomes a motive to intensively reflect on existential questions. This can also be a way of strengthening and stabilizing the self through biographical planning. Even representatives of the 'refusing' type can gain stability through the possibility of presenting and expressing their position of refusal. In this case, however, prospection has the stabilizing effect *without* an AD. "I can do without such a simple piece of paper, because my trust in those who'll be taking care of me is more important, and this gives me confidence now" would be this type's slogan. Thus, an activation of social ties and networks is explicitly required at a fixed point in the future, and at the same time decisions made to date are confidently confirmed. Since the 'confident' do not actively seek this effect, they usually do not have much stake in this kind of organized discussion about ADs. Their confidence makes ongoing discursive confirmation largely superfluous.

The effect of this structure in further public discussion could be striking. The critics' latent suggestion that ADs are in fact 'humbug' could undermine the supporters' self-constructed position. Therefore, the latter have to suppress or negate the refusers' point of view. The position of the 'skeptics' also confuses those who seek to gain safety from the AD. Therefore, public discourse about AD might eventually mirror what was indicated in our group discussions: While problems and arguments stimulate the 'reflective' type to confront end-of-life topics and to search for solutions, they rather confirm the 'radical' and 'bureaucratic' types' position and thus lead to the termination of considerations that are experienced as a source of insecurity and powerlessness. In a generally uncertain and precarious "society of anxiety" (Bude 2014), the AD is thankfully accepted as a possibility for self-empowerment; the refusal of this possibility remains incomprehensible to most people.

Conclusion

It has to be asked whether the prospective contribution of the AD could be significant for individual biographies and also for the future of the relationship between medical personnel, on one hand, and patients and their relatives, on the other. It becomes apparent that a regulation, although it may be helpful on a legal and bureaucratic level, cannot solve existential questions (and should never try to do so). Despite economic maximization and the dramatized call for decisions, the recognition of and dealing with the will of the incurably ill who are not able to express themselves should first and foremost remain a societal concern, especially with the existence of the AD as a new life-planning option. Notwithstanding the multiple meanings associated with the AD and the necessity of a general regulation, professional counseling on the topic, case-specific solutions, and individual reflections are indispensable.

Today, leading representatives of palliative medicine and care, who demanded and promoted the law on ADs, rather tend toward the position of the 'skeptics.' The teams for specialized outpatient palliative care, established in the course of recent legislation on palliative care, support a minimum three-stage counseling process for drafting an AD, including involving close relatives. And ethicists demand the development of a more comprehensive counseling process of 'Advance Care Planning (ACP)' (Klindtworth et al. 2013; In der Schmitten and Marckmann 2013; see Jox in this volume).

Against this backdrop, adequate debate about the 'final treatment' should be a task not only of individualized biographical foresight, but also of professional social and psychotherapeutic services. In this respect, the legal security provided by the law on ADs could indeed facilitate an adequate (and professionally supported) confrontation with one's own life and death. This is already inherent in the 'skeptic' type described above. However, those who assume that a simple document could definitely prevent suffering and the related costs will inevitably be disappointed.

Notes

1 As of June 2013, 1.7 million people had an AD on the German central register (ZVR – Zentrales Vorsorge Register), which is less than 5% of the people who had the right to do so. The interest in and knowledge of the AD were indicated by a representative Allensbach survey 2009 as being more than 90%. See also the expectations in Lang and Wagner (2007) and Van Oorschot (2008). The number of ADs not in the central register can only be guessed; it should be larger and constantly growing.

2 Joint research project "Biomedical Life Plans for Aging" (2010–2014) of the University Medical Center Göttingen and the Institute of Sociology of the Friedrich-Alexander University Erlangen-Nürnberg, as well at the Carinthia University of Applied Sciences. The research was funded by the German Ministry for Education and Research (grant no. 01GP1004). This chapter is the contribution of the author alone. These findings were also published in German by Brauer, Adloff, and Pfaller (2014).

3 WDR television talkshow *Tacheles: Sterben à la carte?* (01.11.2005) www.tacheles.net/archiv.php?id=28.

References

Beck, U. 1986. *Risikogesellschaft. Auf dem Weg in eine andere Moderne*. Frankfurt am Main: Suhrkamp.

Bohnsack, R. 1997. "Gruppendiskussionsverfahren und Milieuforschung." In *Handbuch Qualitative Forschungsmethoden in der Erziehungswissenschaft*, edited by B. Friebertshäuser and A. Prengel, 492–501. Weinheim/München: Juventa.

Bohnsack, R. 2007. "Typenbildung, Generalisierung und komparative Analyse." In *Die dokumentarische Methode und ihre Forschungspraxis. Grundlagen qualitativer Sozialforschung*, edited by R. Bohnsack, I. Netwig-Gesemann, and A.-M. Nohl, 225–253. Wiesbaden: Springer VS.

Borasio, G., H. Heßler, and U. Wiesing. 2009. "Patientenverfügungsgesetz. Umsetzung in der klinischen Praxis." *Deutsches Ärzteblatt* 106 (40):A1952–A1957.

Brauer, K. 2008. "'Was hast Du erreicht?': Höhere Lebenserwartung und höhere Erwartungen an die Biographie." In *Die Natur der Gesellschaft. Verhandlungen des 33. Kongresses der Deutschen Gesellschaft für Soziologie in Kassel 2006*, edited by K.-S. Rehberg, 1543–1555. Frankfurt am Main/New York: Campus.

Brauer, K., F. Adloff, and L. Pfaller. 2014. ". . .'Wie mit mir umzugehen ist.' Zur biographischen Relevanz und Prospektivität von Patientenverfügungen." *Soziale Welt: Zeitschrift für Sozialwissenschaftliche Forschung und Praxis* 65 (4):425–449.

Bude, H. 2014. *Gesellschaft der Angst*. Hamburg: Hamburger Edition HIS.

Glaser, B. G., and A. L. Strauss. 2009. *The Discovery of Grounded Theory: Strategies for Qualitative Research*. Piscataway, NJ: Transaction Publishers.

Hahn, E. 2009. "Die 'neue' Rechtslage zur Patientenverfügung." *KU Gesundheitsmanagement* 12:53–54.

Husserl, E. 1986. *Phänomenologie der Lebenswelt. Ausgewählte Texte II*. Stuttgart: Reclam.

In der Schmitten, J., and G. Marckmann. 2013. "Sackgasse Patientenverfügung. Neue Wege mit Advance Care Planning am Beispiel von beizeiten begleiten." *Zeitschrift für medizinische Ethik* 59 (3):229–243.

Klindtworth, K., N. Schneider, L. Radbruch, and S. Jünger. 2013. "Versorgung am Lebensende." *Zeitschrift für Palliativmedizin* 14 (1):22–28.

Kohli, M. 1981. "Zur Theorie der biographischen Selbst- und Fremdwahrnehmung." In *Lebenswelt und soziale Probleme. Verhandlungen des 20. Soziologentages*, edited by J. Matthes, 502–520. Frankfurt am Main: Campus.

Kohli, M. 1985. "Die Institutionalisierung des Lebenslaufs." *Kölner Zeitschrift für Soziologie und Sozialpsychologie* 37:1–27.

Kohli, M. 1994. "Zukunft und Erwartung aus der Sicht der Biographieforschung." In *Erwartungen an die Zukunft. Zeithorizonte und Wertewandel in der sozialwissenschaftlichen Diskussion*, edited by E. Holst, J. P. Rinderspacher, and J. Schupp, 119–138. Frankfurt am Main: Campus.

Kopetzki, C., ed. 2000. *Antizipierte Patientenverfügung. "Patiententestament" und Stellvertretung in Gesundheitsangelegenheiten*. Wien: Manz.

Lang, F., and G. Wagner. 2007. "Patientenverfügungen in Deutschland: Empirische Evidenz für die Jahre 2005 bis 2007." *Deutsche medizinische Wochenschrift* 132 (48):2558–2652.

Lauter, H., and H. Helmchen. 2006. "Vorausverfügter Behandlungsverzicht bei Verlust der Selbstbestimmbarkeit infolge persistierender Hirnerkrankung." *Der Nervenarzt* 77 (9): 1031–1039. doi: 10.1007/s00115-006-2117-8.

Nassehi, A., S. Brüggen, and I. Saake. 2002. "Beratung zum Tode. Eine neue ars moriendi?" *Berliner Journal für Soziologie* 12 (1):63–85. doi: 10.1007/BF03204043.

Nauck, F., and B. Jaspers. 2011. "Patientenverfügung als vertrauensbildende Maßnahme." In *Sterbebegleitung: Vertrauenssache. Herausforderungen einer person- und bedürfnisorientierten Begleitung am Lebensende*, edited by G. Höver, H. Baranzke, and A. Schaeffer, 175–192. Würzburg: Königshausen und Neumann.

Pilz, D. 2007. *Krisengeschöpfe: Zur Theorie und Methodologie der Objektiven Hermeneutik*. Wiesbaden: Deutscher Universitätsverlag.

Schütz, A. 1971. *Das Problem der Relevanz*. Frankfurt am Main: Suhrkamp.

Schütz, A. 2003. "Über die mannigfaltigen Wirklichkeiten." In Alfred Schütz, *Werkausgabe*, volume 1: *Theorie der Lebenswelt 1. Die pragmatische Schichtung der Lebenswelt*, edited by M. Endreß and Ilja Srubar, 181–239. Konstanz: UVK.

Schütze, F. 1981. "Prozeßstrukturen des Lebensablaufs." In *Biographie in handlungswissenschaftlicher Perspektive*, edited by J. Matthes, A. Pfeifenberger, and M. Stosberg, 66–155. Nürnberg: Verlag der Nürnberger Forschungsvereinigung e.V.

Schweda, M., and S. Schicktanz. 2012. "Das Unbehagen an der Medikalisierung. Theoretische und ethische Aspekte der biomedizinischen Lebensplanung." In *Pro-Age oder Anti-Aging. Altern im Fokus der modernen Medizin*, edited by S. Schicktanz and M. Schweda, 23–40. Frankfurt am Main/New York: Campus.

Soeffner, H.-G. 2010. *Symbolische Formung. Eine Soziologie des Symbols und des Rituals*. Weilerswist: Velbrück.

Stollberg, G. 2008a. "Informed Consent und Shared Decision Making. Ein Überblick über medizinische und sozialwissenschaftliche Literatur." *Soziale Welt: Zeitschrift für Sozialwissenschaftliche Forschung und Praxis* 59 (4):397–411. doi: 10.2307/40878613.

Stollberg, G. 2008b. "Kunden der Medizin: Der Mythos vom mündigen Patienten." In *Moderne Mythen der Medizin. Studien zur organisierten Krankenbehandlung*, edited by I. Saake and W. Vogd, 345–361. Wiesbaden: VS Verlag für Sozialwissenschaften.

Thielicke, H. 1968. "Illusion der 'glatten Lösung': Ethische Fragen der modernen Medizin." *Langenbecks Archiv für Chirurgie* 321:1–34.

Van Oorschot, B. 2008. "Patientenverfügungen aus Bevölkerungs- und Patientensicht. Eine Übersicht über empirische Studien aus dem deutschen Sprachraum." *Bulletin de la Societé des Sciences Medicales du Grand-Duche de Luxembourg* 3:443–454.

Wernet, A. 2006. *Einführung in die Interpretationstechnik der Objektiven Hermeneutik*. Wiesbaden: VS Verlag für Sozialwissenschaften.

11 Preparing existential decisions in later life

Advance healthcare planning

Ralf J. Jox

The demographic change that many high- and middle-income countries are currently undergoing has significant and long-lasting repercussions on the healthcare in these countries. As the average lifespan of citizens extends, the burden of disease and the associated healthcare activities will inevitably transform. Most people can enjoy a relatively long phase of good health after retirement from work before they are gradually affected by multiple age-related chronic disorders that can be mitigated but not cured. Despite the ever-increasing attempts of high-performing, costly healthcare systems to prevent, treat, and rehabilitate these age-related conditions with multiple drugs and interventions, these efforts do not alter and may only cloud the fact that death will eventually ensue, often as a result of these chronic disorders. All the leading causes of death – cardiovascular and respiratory diseases, cancer, neurodegenerative diseases (to name the most common) – are characterized by an inexorably progressive character that makes death foreseeable several weeks, months, or years before its actual occurrence (Murray et al. 2005; van der Heide et al. 2003). The later life of most people is therefore associated with the increasing awareness of an accumulating disease burden, death coming close, and the necessity to make vital healthcare decisions (Gruenewald and White 2006). A paradigmatic example is a person[1] who develops arterial hypertension in her sixth decade of life, type 2 diabetes and cardiovascular disease in her seventh decade, cerebrovascular events in her eighth decade, and eventually a joint vascular-Alzheimer's dementia in her ninth decade.

The multiple treatment and care options for the recurrent crises of chronic disorders, in combination with life-saving emergency and critical-care measures that are highly effective, leads to situations in which patients' lives are saved at a cost of suffering that many patients deem too high. A few decades ago, medicine was still stubbornly following the technological imperative to treat as much as was treatable; today the problem is rather incertitude of healthcare professionals, patients, and their families about when and how to treat medical conditions at the close of life. This vexing incertitude is at the root of many ethical problems in clinical practice. The ethical quandaries are complicated by the fact that many of the persons who are existentially affected by these treatment decisions – the patients themselves – are not able to participate in decision-making due to impaired cognition or consciousness. The more a chronic disorder progresses, the more likely the patient will lose decision-making capacity, and the more ethically, emotionally, and socially significant the necessary decisions will become.

It is this social and medical context that gives rise and attractiveness to the idea of advance healthcare planning. The core idea of advance healthcare planning (or the diverse practices named under this umbrella term) is to enable the individual to influence, orient, or even direct his or her future healthcare in the event of impaired decision-making capacity. The concept did not emerge in medicine itself. In the 1960s, the idea of so-called living wills (later called 'advance directives'), documenting the patient's refusal of certain forms of life-sustaining treatment for future situations (e.g., resuscitation, artificial respiration), arose in the context of the patient-rights movement regarding the end of life, originally explicated by US human-rights lawyer Luis Kutner (1969) and promoted by euthanasia societies (Benzenhöfer and Hack-Molitor 2009). In the following decades, the idea of '(medical) living wills' gathered more and more support, primarily in North America but also in Northern and Western Europe. The underlying reasons for the proliferation of this idea can be associated with fundamental changes in healthcare and in society at large. In healthcare, the rapid invention of life-sustaining technologies in the second half of the 20th century; the shift from a generalist, home-based family medicine to a fragmented, hospital-based specialist medicine with an ensuing crisis of patient-physician trust; and the replacement of medical paternalism by the new paradigm of patient autonomy have driven the rise of advance patient directives (Beauchamp and Childress 2013; Brown 2003). This development was fueled by fundamental societal changes, notably the intensification of liberal individualism in an ever more market-based society, the demise of traditional value coordinates constructed by churches and families, and the pluralization of societies in the wake of migration processes, globalization, and the Internet revolution (Lack, Biller-Andorno, and Brauer 2013; Pellegrino 1999).

It was in the 1990s, however, that a significant redirection occurred in the concept of advance healthcare directives. After the US *Patient Self-Determination Act* 1990 had raised the hopes and promises attached to advance directives (Greco et al. 1991), the disappointment was even more bitter as the large SUPPORT study revealed that the prevalence and effects of advance directives in the United States remained marginal (Knaus and The SUPPORT Principles Investigators 1995; Teno et al. 1997a). The investigators concluded that instead of the traditional advance directive as a single document, there was the need for "a more comprehensive advance care planning" (Teno et al. 1997b, 500). Such a comprehensive, communication-based model had first been pioneered in Wisconsin under the label 'Respecting Choices' (Hammes and Rooney 1998). With the publication of a sharply worded article in *The Hastings Center Report* in 2004, the failure of the traditional living will became evident to many professionals and scholars (Fagerlin and Schneider 2004).

The comprehensive systems approach that was pioneered by 'Respecting Choices' slowly influenced other pilot projects, such as the Australian project 'Respecting Patient Choices,' which began in 2002 and has since become Australian national policy (Detering et al. 2010; Detering and Silvester 2015). With the foundation of the Advance Care Planning and End of Life Society in 2010 and its ensuing conferences, these models continued to become better known and serve as role models for other regions (In der Schmitten et al. 2014; Korfage et al. 2015). Confusingly, however, the term 'advance care planning' (ACP) is increasingly being used for the traditional 'advance directive' or even as a general term for any kind of anticipatory healthcare planning (In der Schmitten and Marckmann 2015). Currently, there is a highly heterogeneous plethora of programs and offers around anticipatory healthcare planning, demonstrating the need for the clear identification of best-practice models, the formulation of quality criteria, and the publication of evidence-based consensus recommendations.

In this article, I will first recapitulate the definition and elements of comprehensive ACP models, as opposed to traditional advance directives. Then I will formulate the ethical justification for these new models. Finally, I will sketch controversial points and knowledge gaps that warrant thorough empirical research in the years to come.

What is advance care planning?

To date, there is no official or authoritative definition of ACP, but two groups of experts (an American group and a task force of the European Association of Palliative Care) are currently preparing white papers or consensus recommendations based on Delphi studies (Rietjens et al. 2015). Notwithstanding, many researchers and expert bodies have suggested definitions of ACP that may be instructive:

> Advance care planning refers to the whole process of discussion of end-of-life care, clarification of related values and goals, and embodiment of preferences through written documents and medical orders. This process can start at any time and be revisited periodically, but it becomes more focused as health status changes. Ideally, these conversations (1) occur with a person's health care agent and primary clinician, along with other members of the clinical team; (2) are recorded and updated as needed; and (3) allow for flexible decision making in the context of the patient's current medical situation.
> (Institute of Medicine 2015, 122)

> Advance care planning (ACP) is a process of communication between individuals and their healthcare agents to understand, reflect on, discuss and plan for future healthcare decisions for a time when individuals are not able to make their own healthcare decisions. This process can be facilitated by a specially trained health professional or can occur as part of routine care with the person's usual health professionals. The ACP process ideally results in the designation of a health care proxy, and in the creation of a written plan, commonly referred to as an advance directive, which accurately reflects the individual's goals, values, and wishes about future healthcare. Since goals and medical treatment decisions may change over time, especially if overall health or if a person's situation changes, planning needs to be reviewed. The

> types of planning may vary depending on whether the person is healthy, has mild to moderate chronic illness, or is likely to die in next 12 months. ACP is therefore ongoing, and is subject to continual re-evaluation and possible updating, triggered by key health or life experiences.
>
> (International Society for Advance Care Planning and End of Life 2015)

In an attempt to distill these definitions, reflecting the core consensus of ACP experts from the international scientific literature (Coors, Jox, and In der Schmitten 2015; Emanuel, von Gunten, and Ferris 2000; Hammes and Rooney 1998; In der Schmitten et al. 2011), I am proposing the following core definition of ACP:

> Advance Care Planning (ACP) is a structured communication process between an individual, his family, his healthcare agent (if existing), and facilitating healthcare professionals that consists of identifying personal values of the individual, reflecting on the meanings and consequences of anticipated illness scenarios, defining goals and preferences of care for these situations, issuing appropriate documents and legal instruments that will help direct future healthcare decisions, and reviewing these steps at adequate intervals.

The overarching aim of ACP is the same as for advance directives – namely, to enhance patient autonomy by extending it to situations where the patient does not retain decision-making capacity anymore. Although this is undeniably the primary aim, there may be secondary aims attached to ACP that will become evident from the theoretical and ethical analysis of ACP in the second part of this article.

The two cited expert definitions and my own core definition above encapsulate the crucial elements of ACP. Before examining these elements and their meaning step by step, however, I think it will be helpful to emphasize and illustrate the principal difference between the more traditional model of advance directives and the emerging model of ACP that is meant to replace this traditional model. Up to now, many people who have written advance directives (living wills) have done so more or less on their own; they have taken an advance directive form, filled it in, archived it in their personal documents, and were satisfied that they now had sufficiently prepared for the end of their life, forestalling becoming a victim of medical overtreatment (Becker et al. 2010; Nauck et al. 2014).

In contrast, the model of ACP is characterized by three distinct features: interactivity, item-plurality, and iterativity (see Figure 11.1).

(1) *Interactivity* means that the individual is not left alone to write a document on his own; he is embedded in a conducive social situation in which conversations are fostered between him, his loved ones (usually relatives), his healthcare agent (if he has already issued durable powers of attorney to a healthcare

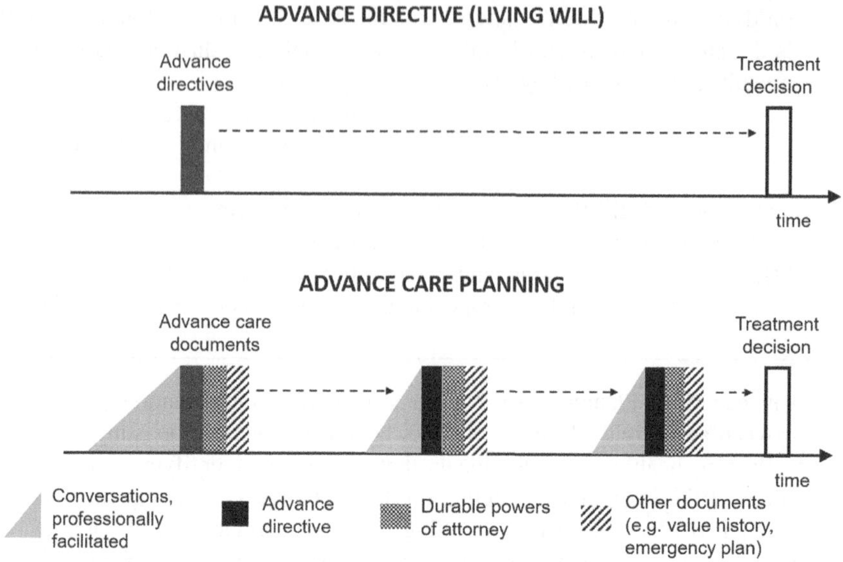

Figure 11.1 Conceptual schema contrasting the advance directive (living will) and the model of advance care planning (ACP), illustrating the ACP characteristics of (1) interactivity (gray triangles for conversations), (2) item plurality (bars with different patterns for various documents), and (3) iterativity (multiple revisions along the time scale)

agent), his general practitioner (primary care physician), and health professionals who facilitate these conversations in a structured manner.

(2) *Item plurality* refers to the fact that these conversations often result not only in a single document such as the advance directive, but in a plurality of diverse documents and legal instruments that are used to plan future care: personal value summaries or narratives, durable powers of attorney (designation of healthcare agents), emergency plans, and physician orders for life-sustaining treatment, just to name the most important ones. In addition to these written documents, the conversations are documented in the memories of those present and maybe also in written memory-protocols of the conversation partners, so that, at a future time when a decision needs to be made, this decision can rest on various forms of documentation and recollection of the patient's will.

(3) *Iterativity*, finally, is the characteristic that the conversations about values, preferences, and future care do not happen only once but are conceived as iterative steps in a longitudinal process. At personally meaningful intervals, the conversations are taken up again and deepened, a new health situation is reflected upon, and the advance care documents are reviewed and, if necessary, altered.

This characterization of ACP, however, is still incomplete. ACP is more than an approach helping the individual plan ahead. In fact, it has two foci, corresponding to the conception of ACP as a communication process: The first focus is the sender (who makes anticipatory decisions), and the second focus is the recipient (who interprets and implements these decisions at a later time). Hence, ACP tries to make sure that care plans and anticipatory documents will be understood, properly interpreted, and correctly applied in healthcare decision making (see Figure 11.2). To achieve this, ACP tries to bring the documents to the attention of the healthcare professionals who are faced with making care decisions for the individual, by way of depositing the documents at the local health partners (hospital, emergency service, health provider, etc.), including them on the patient's electronically readable health-insurance card, using quickly retrievable registries or other means to allow instant access to the documents. In addition, all parties involved in making the decisions – healthcare professionals, patient substitutes (patient-designated agents or court-appointed guardians), and even ethics consultants and courts – should be trained in reading, interpreting, and applying the advance care documents to the clinical situation, which is therefore also part of ACP. Eventually, the ACP model also includes standardized procedures, guidelines, or other material to help healthcare professionals apply advance care decisions and make patient-centered care decisions.

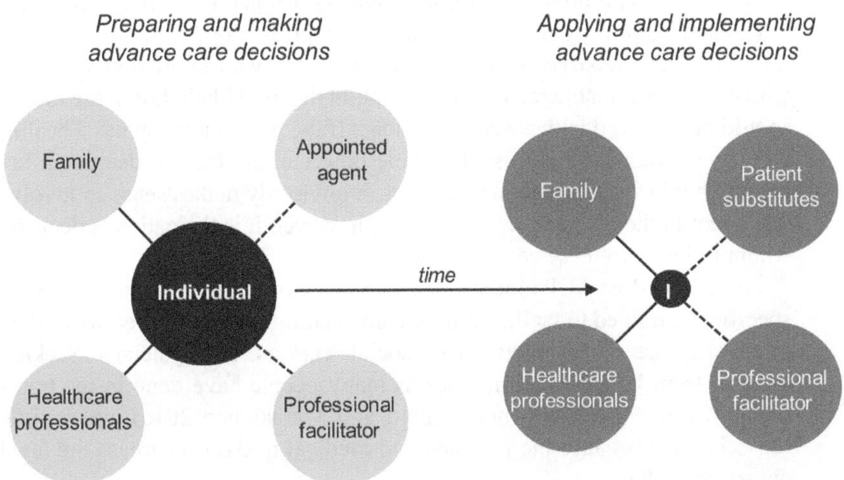

Figure 11.2 Conceptual schema depicting the roles and relations of involved parties in ACP – both at the time of preparing and making advance decisions (left cluster) and at the later time of interpreting and applying advance decisions to clinical situations (right cluster). Note: I = Individual (shown in reduced size on the right to symbolize the loss of decision-making capacity); Dotted lines: These parties need not be involved in every case of ACP.

With this general concept in mind, let us now look at the individual elements of ACP in a more concrete and practical manner:

(a) *Access*: Although ACP is practiced predominantly by individuals who are elderly, chronically ill, or even suffering from incurable progressive diseases (Ho et al. 2016; Rao et al. 2014; Wilson et al. 2013), it is generally amenable to every individual. Every human being has the risk of losing decision-making capacity due to an accident, an illness, or other events. Yet, ACP programs may have diverse tracks that are tailored to certain life situations (e.g., for the young and healthy, for the chronically ill, for the very old) (Hammes, Rooney, and Gundrum 2010). Psychiatry might be another area where specific forms of ACP are needed, which is evidenced by the increasing use of so-called joint crisis plans, which can be seen as nascent forms of ACP (Henderson et al. 2008). For individuals who suffer from chronic or severe progressive diseases, more and more disease-specific ACP programs are being developed (Brown 2015; Kirchhoff et al. 2012).

(b) *Setting*: ACP will usually encompass personal contact between the individual and his conversation partners (although it seems practicable to use telephone, televisual, or online forms of conversation) (Austin et al. 2015; Boettcher, Turner, and Briggs 2015). The conversations can occur at home, within a healthcare context, or in other locations, as long as a private and conducive atmosphere can be ensured.

(c) *Participants*: As a minimum, these conversations happen between the individual and his physician, his nurse, or another professional caregiver. Ideally, however, close relatives whom the person trusts, who know him well, and who have a sustainable relationship with him that will likely last in the future, should be involved in these conversations. If the person already has a healthcare agent whom she entrusted durable power of attorney to decide on her behalf should she become incompetent, it obviously makes sense to involve this agent in the discussions. Ultimately, however, it is the patient's decision whom to invite to these conversations.

(d) *Facilitation*: Most ACP models advocate and employ professionals who are specifically trained to facilitate these conversations in a structured way. Most often, they are nurse practitioners, social workers, or physicians. Seeking counsel from lawyers and notaries as many people have done in the traditional advance directives model (Petri and Marckmann 2016) makes little sense in ACP because the personal and medical questions surpass the legal questions by far.

(e) *Structure*: ACP conversations will commonly begin with a reflection on personal values, life stories, and meaning in life. They will then shift to the current and anticipated health situation of the person, trying to identify future scenarios that are likely to occur and/or have a special importance for the individual. The crucial step is the development of concrete preferences regarding who should decide in the case of incapacity (appointing an agent) and what should be done with regard to not only medical treatment, but also nursing care and other health-related practices.

(f) *Documentation*: From ethical and practical points of view, written documentation is not absolutely necessary and may be dispensable in some situations. Many laws, however, confer a higher authority to written advance directives compared to orally expressed advance care statements, which makes sense given the strength of evidence of written documents. There are also other arguments supporting documentation. During a longitudinal communication process, documentation makes it easier to fix results and remember them at a later meeting; it urges everyone to be more precise and concrete than in purely oral conversations; and, ultimately, it can be a significant emotional, ethical, and legal help for the healthcare professionals, patient surrogates, and family members who have to make decisions later on. Comprehensive ACP models make sure that care documents are easily retrievable when they are needed.

(g) *Application*: The specific training of healthcare professionals and institutions on how to apply advance care documents and make decisions with respect to patient autonomy is crucial for the success of ACP. This training can be supported by guidelines, policies, structures of clinical ethics support, and community outreach.

What is the ethical justification for advance care planning?

Although ACP is currently enjoying an increasing popularity and is becoming the object of numerous empirical studies, there is barely any literature on the theoretical and ethical basis of ACP (Hammes and Harter 2015). This may be explained by the fact that ACP is so obviously 'right' that no one makes an effort to justify it. Yet, if ACP is to become standard policy, it is certainly important to demonstrate the many justifications for this development. I will group these justifications according to three ethical theories that are among the most influential ones in medical ethics: principlism, care ethics, and communitarianism.

Principlist justification

The four principles of biomedical ethics – respect for autonomy, beneficence, nonmaleficence, and justice – are probably the most pervasive approach to applied medical ethics (Beauchamp and Childress 2013). Among these four principles, respect for autonomy is the first one that immediately comes to mind when one thinks of ACP. And, in fact, ACP centers on this principle and strives to give due respect to patients' autonomy. ACP is a premier way to enable patients to determine the way they want to be treated in the event of decisional incapacity. Individuals can thereby refuse certain treatment measures based on their own values and preferences. But this aspect of autonomy, the negative freedom rights, is only part of this principle. Autonomy can be strengthened and enhanced by positive actions, such as providing information to, supporting, and empowering the individual. ACP is a model that does exactly that: It enhances the ability of the person to exercise her autonomy by ensuring thorough information on pertinent medical issues, by supporting her through structured, facilitated discussions with family members and healthcare professionals, and by offering systems that allow her preferences to really have an impact on actual practice.

It is often forgotten, however, that ACP can equally be justified by the principles of nonmaleficence and beneficence. In fact, many advance refusals of treatment at the end of life guard the patient from an inappropriate overtreatment that would cause more harm than benefit to him (e.g., non-beneficial life support). In addition, ACP serves the well-being of the individual not only at the time of treatment decisions, but also well before. The very process of ACP has immediate and potentially long-lasting beneficial psychosocial effects on the person. She gains the well-founded confidence that her preferences will be respected, which may increase peace of mind for an extended period of time. She also familiarizes herself with her own health state, any existing illnesses, and likely changes in the future. Thus, she will be better prepared and suffer less if an accident, a serious disease, or a deterioration of an existing disease will hit her at a later time. Moreover, ACP can open the gate to a frank and honest communication about values, health problems, and death both within her family and between the person and her physician, which likely will have beneficial effects on the depth of these relationships. In sum, ACP enhances and deepens a real dialogue about existential issues in life, and such a dialogue is one of the keys to meaning, serenity, and happiness in life.

Even the fourth principle of biomedical ethics, justice, supports the model of ACP. This is because ACP can contribute to a fair reallocation of (limited) resources in healthcare by better aligning care with the different individuals' needs. Two systematic reviews of cost implications of ACP programs found a tendency toward significant cost savings through ACP, at least for some patients (Dixon, Matosevic, and Knapp 2015), notably by preventing overtreatment at the end of life (Klingler, In der Schmitten, and Marckmann 2015). Another systematic review found that ACP reduces the likelihood of admission to intensive-care units for patients with life-limiting diseases and a high risk of death (Khandelwal et al. 2015).

Care-ethics justification

Inspired by feminist moral philosophy, care ethics emphasizes the relevance of personal relationships, interdependency, and interpersonal responses (Gilligan 1982; Slote 2007; Tong and Williams 2014). It has some affinity to virtue ethics in that it stresses individual attitudes and emotional engagement more than universal, impartial, and agent-independent rules of action (Halwani 2003). Healthcare is obviously a practice field that is particularly subject to the lens of care ethics, given that it centers on the relationship between the caregiver and the person cared for. I want to show that care ethics (and, in a broader sense, virtue ethics) can give a very robust and convincing justification for ACP.

In its essence, ACP is a form of care. In contrast to the traditional advance directive (living will) model, ACP does not leave the person alone but places her in a net of relationships with others who support her by listening to and interpreting her wishes, exchanging ideas, and empowering decisions that are likely to be implemented in the healthcare system. ACP fulfills all four elements of care as conceptualized in the work of Joan Tronto (2005):

(1) attentiveness: ACP starts with listening to the individual, his needs, values, and goals.
(2) responsibility: ACP is a way of sharing responsibility between the individual, his loved ones, healthcare professionals, and professional facilitators. In taking over a share of responsibility, professionals ease the burden for the individual and promote sustainable decision-making.
(3) competence: ACP takes the fact seriously that talking about and preparing future care needs professional competencies, providing special ACP training for facilitators and healthcare professionals.
(4) responsiveness: The singular path of each ACP is shaped by the responses of the individual alongside a process of conversations, taking account of the vulnerable situation of the individual.

From a virtue-ethics perspective, ACP promotes numerous ethically positive attitudes that are traditionally regarded as virtues. It is a process that fosters mutual empathy and respect, because not only are healthcare professionals and family members called upon to understand and respect the wishes of the individual, but also the individual needs to develop empathy and respect for the needs, worries, and interests of his family members and professional caregivers. This enhances the likelihood that family members and healthcare agents will in fact honor the patient's preferences and will not refuse to implement them because of feeling overwhelmed, unfairly burdened, or disrespected when the preferences will have to be applied. Among the other virtues fostered by ACP is the courage to face deteriorating health changes, morbidity, suffering, and death in all people involved, as well as the modesty that flows from accepting the limits of medicine and the finitude of life.

Communitarian justification

Communitarianism is a philosophy that emphasizes the fact that individuals are shaped by their places and roles in a community, that communities are pivotal in enabling the well-being of the individual, and that communities are entities with their own interests, functions, and capacities (Callahan 2003; Etzioni 2011). Although communitarianism originated as a political philosophy opposing an extreme form of liberalism, it can also be applied to medical ethics (Callahan 2003). In emphasizing common goods of healthcare, the needs and interests of social communities, and the dependency of the patient on his family and community, communitarian bioethics counterbalances a sometimes rigid and reductive liberalist bioethics.

ACP is a prime example of an intervention that strikes a fair balance between liberal and communitarian bioethics. It follows a relational concept of autonomy and it conceives the (future) patient not as an atomistic island, but as a social being within a network of private and professional relations. The dialogue – or, rather, trialogue – between the patient, his loved ones, and professionals forms the core community that drives the success of ACP. If this trialogue works well, medical-treatment decisions can reliably, responsibly, and consensually be made within this subsidiary core community without the need for court proceedings or other involvement of higher state institutions. It has been shown that ACP significantly reduces the burden on family members and healthcare agents – it even lowers their levels of anxiety and depression (Detering et al. 2010) – and the same surely holds true for healthcare professionals. Healthcare workers benefit not only from a clearer orientation in their treatment decisions, but also in terms of improved communication with the patient. Moreover, ACP promotes common goods of healthcare. I have already outlined that ACP can increase health benefits, avoid overtreatment, and prevent a waste of resources. ACP may even have an effect on the system of healthcare as a whole, transforming it from a technocratic, supply-driven, and provider-centered business to a more humane, needs-driven, patient- and family-centered activity. This transformative effect is difficult to measure, and it may be supported by other trends of 'talking medicine' (such as palliative care and clinical ethics). ACP may even contribute to a more relaxed and serene view of human mortality, forestalling the frenzied medicalization of the end of life and allowing for a more natural death. In fostering an awareness of life's finitude, a reflective deliberation of life plans, and a critical stance toward medicine within communities and the society as a whole, ACP serves relevant interests of democratic societies.

What do we need to know about advance care planning from empirical research?

Many of the arguments that underpin the ethical justification of ACP rest upon empirical facts, such as ACP's positive impact on psychological well-being, the quality of communication, or the adherence to the patient's preferences in making treatment decisions. All of these empirical facts are grounded in the experiences of professionals developing and applying ACP, and many of them have also been corroborated in empirical studies (Austin et al. 2015; Brinkman-Stoppelenburg, Rietjens, and van der Heide 2014; Houben et al. 2014; Khandelwal et al. 2015; Klingler, In der Schmitten, and Marckmann 2015; Martin et al. 2016). Yet, given the variability of ACP practice models, it is imperative to correlate each positive consequence with specific elements in best-practice models of ACP. Thereby, we should be able to answer the question "Which elements are absolutely necessary and vital in order to accomplish the positive effects that justify ACP?" This is the first step toward ensuring and enhancing the quality of ACP. In the following I will sketch some of the questions for future research on ACP.

Timing of ACP conversations

The question of the right time to have conversations about future care and care preferences remains unresolved. Evidently, there is no one-size-fits-all answer;

the merits of each individual case must be considered. Yet, there may be certain generalizable points in different biographies when ACP may be more appropriate than at other points. Obviously, significant personal life events, such as the diagnosis of a severe or incurable disease, hospitalization, the illness or death of a loved one, or significant changes in one's dearest relationships, are good opportunities for ACP. It is less clear when to talk about ACP if there are no such life events. Moreover, the rhythm of the iterative ACP conversations is another difficult question – surely it has to be influenced by the individual characteristics of each ACP process, but to have some knowledge about meaningful intervals could nevertheless help. In order to maximize mutual understanding and thorough decision-making, it may also be prudent to have two or three shorter conversations at brief intervals rather than one long one.

Participants in ACP conversations

It is equally unclear what the ideal composition of ACP conversations is. Obviously, the individual (future patient) has to be present and be in the center of these conversations, and he or she also has the right to decide who should be present at these confidential discussions. The essence of ACP is that at least one healthcare professional should take part in these conversations – be it someone who regularly takes care of the patient (such as the primary care physician, the nurse practitioner, or the responsible social worker in a nursing home) or be it someone who is external to the patient and acts as a professional facilitator of ACP conversations. Many leading ACP models, such as 'Respecting Choices,' are built around professional facilitators who are diligently trained and prepared for their activities, and they supposedly are the major reasons for the success of these ACP models. Yet, there is also some concern that this approach may not be feasible or affordable everywhere in healthcare. People living in rural areas or poor countries, patients who have a very close relationship to their caregivers, or those who have significant cultural or language barriers may find it more appropriate to have ACP conversations without professional facilitators. Research should therefore clearly delineate the effects of best-practice ACP facilitation and conceive of ways to substitute for professional facilitation if it is not possible or not appropriate.

Supporting materials and supplementary approaches

ACP research may learn a lot from an exchange with scholars from the area of shared decision-making, who have championed written and audiovisual decision aids to facilitate autonomous healthcare decision-making (Austin et al. 2015; Lenz et al. 2012). Decision aids may be particularly helpful in conveying factual information on disease courses, complications, and treatment regimens, but they may also be instrumental in clarifying personal values and attitudes. Because a major objection against ACP is the limited capacity to imagine future states of health (Fagerlin and Schneider 2004), ACP might benefit significantly from involving narratives, testimonials, or personal contact with patients (or their family members) who already have experienced these states. For the younger generation, modern media such as the Internet and mobile apps might open up additional approaches to ACP. For other population groups, such as migrants or illiterates, specific supplementary information in their own language or in simple language might be essential. In order to offer ACP fairly to all citizens who desire to use it, it will be important not to lose sight of the often neglected subpopulations of society.

Approaches in the case of fading decision-making capacity

It is not rare that patients will become interested in ACP once they are diagnosed with a disease that threatens their cognitive capacities, such as Alzheimer's disease (Hamann et al. 2011). In such situations, they will easily become aware that treatment decisions will soon have to be made by others on their behalf. Yet, in the beginning of a dementia, they already have lost some selected cognitive abilities (Bronner et al. 2016; Hamann et al. 2011). ACP should therefore be responsive to patients with gradual or selective cognitive deficits and try to compensate for these deficits as long as possible. However, it is still unclear how to involve these patients in further treatment and care planning after they have undoubtedly lost decision-making capacity. It may be particularly difficult to keep patients involved if their current verbal or nonverbal behavior seems to contradict the preferences they had fixed in their autonomously written advance statements (Jox 2014). Another highly complicated question surfaces if patients are already in a state of decisional incapacity when the possibility of ACP is first raised and they have not expressed any anticipatory preferences so far. Some scholars argue that healthcare agents or court-appointed guardians may engage in what can be called ACP by proxy, discussing advance decisions with healthcare professionals and documenting them as orientation and preparation for future situations (In der Schmitten et al. 2015; Volicer et al. 2002; Jox 2016).

Integration in healthcare systems

Many open questions center on the integration of ACP into the healthcare system: Should there be any incentives for the insured to use ACP or for healthcare professionals to engage in ACP? Is ACP an activity that should be prioritized in the context of limited resources for healthcare, and should it be paid on a solidary basis or out of pocket? What is the best place to integrate ACP in the healthcare system: inpatient or outpatient services? Which laws are needed in order to guarantee an effective ACP? What are the best ways to ensure that anticipatory documents are readily available and are applied in a rigorous and responsible way? And what does it mean to develop culturally sensitive forms of ACP and maintain ACP as an offer and not a social obligation?

These five clusters are of course not comprehensive, but they represent some of the most urgent and evident open questions. They already underscore, however, that ACP is a field where empirical research needs to intensify in the near future to find answers to ethically and practically relevant questions. In this article, I started out by defining and explicating the emerging model of ACP in contrast to the traditional model of advance directives (living wills). In the second part of this article, I offered a pluralistic account of the ethical justification of ACP that makes a compelling case in favor of developing ACP to a standard approach in healthcare. Finally, I sketched some urgent questions for empirical research in the field of ACP. It is my firm conviction that if best-practice ACP models are expanded and integrated into healthcare systems on a wide basis, this will enormously help us make existential decisions in later life and will contribute to more humane, responsible, and respectful healthcare for vulnerable populations, especially the elderly and the people at the end of their lives.

Note

1 If general personal statements use the feminine or masculine form, the other sex is always meant as well.

References

Austin, C. A., D. Mohottige, R. L. Sudore, A. K. Smith, and L. C. Hanson. 2015. "Tools to Promote Shared Decision Making in Serious Illness: A Systematic Review." *The Journal of the American Medical Association: Internal Medicine* 175 (7):1213–1221. doi: 10.1001/jamainternmed.2015.1679.

Beauchamp, T. L., and J. F. Childress. 2013. *Principles of Biomedical Ethics*. New York: Oxford University Press.

Becker, M., B. Jaspers, C. King, L. Radbruch, R. Voltz, and F. Nauck. 2010. "Did You Seek Assistance for Writing Your Advance Directive? A Qualitative Study." *Wiener Klinische Wochenschrift* 122 (21–22):620–625. doi: 10.1007/s00508-010-1470-6.

Benzenhöfer, U., and G. Hack-Molitor. 2009. "Die Rolle von Luis Kutner bei der Entwicklung der Patientenverfügung." *Hessisches Ärzteblatt* 70 (6):411–413.

Boettcher, I., R. Turner, and L. Briggs. 2015. "Telephonic Advance Care Planning Facilitated by Health Plan Case Managers." *Palliative & Supportive Care* 13 (3):795–800. doi: 10.1017/s1478951514000698.

Brinkman-Stoppelenburg, A., J. A. Rietjens, and A. van der Heide. 2014. "The Effects of Advance Care Planning on End-of-Life Care: A Systematic Review." *Palliative Medicine* 28 (8):1000–1025. doi: 10.1177/0269216314526272.

Bronner, K., R. Perneczky, R. McCabe, A. Kurz, and J. Hamann. 2016. "Which Medical and Social Decision Topics Are Important after Early Diagnosis of Alzheimer's Disease from the Perspectives of People with Alzheimer's Disease, Spouses and Professionals?" *BMC Research Notes* 8 (9):149. doi: 10.1186/s13104-016-1960-3.

Brown, B. A. 2003. "The History of Advance Directives: A Literature Review." *Journal of Gerontological Nursing* 29 (9):4–14. doi: 10.3928/0098-9134-20030901-04.

Brown, J. 2015. "Advance Care Planning in Dementia." *The Lancet: Psychiatry* 2 (9):774–775. doi: 10.1016/s2215-0366(15)00311-9.

Callahan, D. 2003. "Individual Good and Common Good: A Communitarian Approach to Bioethics." *Perspectives in Biology and Medicine* 46 (4):496–507. doi: 10.1353/pbm.2003.0083.

Coors, M., R. J. Jox, and J. in der Schmitten. 2015. *Advance Care Planning. Von der Patientenverfügung zur gesundheitlichen Vorausplanung*. Stuttgart: Kohlhammer.

Detering, K. M., A. D. Hancock, M. C. Reade, and W. Silvester. 2010. "The Impact of Advance Care Planning on End of Life Care in Elderly Patients: Randomised Controlled Trial." *British Medical Journal* 340:c1345. doi: http://dx.doi.org/10.1136/bmj.c1345.

Detering, K. M., and W. Silvester. 2015. "Implementierung von Advance Care Planning in Australien: das Programm 'Respecting Patient Choices'." In *Advance Care Planning*, edited by M. Coors, R. J. Jox, and J. in der Schmitten, 196–208. Stuttgart: Kohlhammer.

Dixon, J., T. Matosevic, and M. Knapp. 2015. "The Economic Evidence for Advance Care Planning: Systematic Review of Evidence." *Palliative Medicine* 29 (10):869–884. doi: 10.1177/0269216315586659.

Emanuel, L. L., C. F. von Gunten, and F. D. Ferris. 2000. "Advance Care Planning." *Archives of Family Medicine* 9 (10):1181–1187.

Etzioni, A. 2011. "On a Communitarian Approach to Bioethics." *Theoretical Medicine & Bioethics* 32 (5):363–374. doi: 10.1007/s11017-011-9187-8.

Fagerlin, A., and C. E. Schneider. 2004. "Enough: The Failure of the Living Will." *The Hastings Center Report* 34 (2):30–42. doi: 10.2307/3527683.

Gilligan, C. 1982. *In a Different Voice*. Cambridge, MA: Harvard University Press.

Greco, P. J., K. A. Schulman, R. Lavizzo-Mourey, and J. Hansen-Flaschen. 1991. "The Patient Self-Determination Act and the Future of Advance Directives." *Annals of Internal Medicine* 115 (8):639–643. doi: 10.7326/0003-4819-115-8-639.

Gruenewald, D. A., and E. J. White. 2006. "The Illness Experience of Older Adults near the End of Life: A Systematic Review." *Anesthesiology Clinics* 24 (1):163–180, ix. doi: 10.1016/j.atc.2005.12.003.

Halwani, R. 2003. "Care Ethics and Virtue Ethics." *Hypatia* 18 (3):161–192.

Hamann, J., K. Bronner, J. Margull, R. Mendel, J. Diehl-Schmid, M. Buhner, R. Klein, A. Schneider, A. Kurz, and R. Perneczky. 2011. "Patient Participation in Medical and Social Decisions in Alzheimer's Disease." *Journal of the American Geriatrics Society* 59 (11):2045–2052. doi: 10.1111/j.1532-5415.2011.03661.x.

Hammes, B. J., and T. D. Harter. 2015. "Philosophisch-ethische Gründe für Advance Care Planning." In *Advance Care Planning*, edited by M. Coors, R. J. Jox, and J. in der Schmitten, 95–108. Stuttgart: Kohlhammer.

Hammes, B. J., and B. L. Rooney. 1998. "Death and End-of-Life Planning in One Midwestern Community." *Archives of Internal Medicine* 158 (4):383–390. doi: 10.1001/archinte.158.4.383.

Hammes, B. J., B. L. Rooney, and J. D. Gundrum. 2010. "A Comparative, Retrospective, Observational Study of the Prevalence, Availability, and Specificity of Advance Care Plans in a County That Implemented an Advance Care Planning Microsystem." *Journal of the American Geriatrics Society* 58 (7):1249–1255. doi: 10.1111/j.1532-5415.2010.02956.x.

Henderson, C., J. W. Swanson, G. Szmukler, G. Thornicroft, and M. Zinkler. 2008. "A Typology of Advance Statements in Mental Health Care." *Psychiatrics Services* 59 (1):63–71. doi: 10.1176/appi.ps.59.1.63.

Ho, G. W., L. Skaggs, G. Yenokyan, A. Kellogg, J. A. Johnson, M. C. Lee, K. Heinze, M. T. Hughes, D. P. Sulmasy, J. Kub, P. B. Terry, A. B. Astrow, J. Zheng, L. S. Lehmann, and M. T. Nolan. 2016. "Patient and Caregiver Characteristics Related to Completion of Advance Directives in Terminally Ill Patients." *Palliative & Supportive Care* 15(1):1–8. doi: 10.1017/s147895151600016x.

Houben, C. H., M. A. Spruit, M. T. Groenen, E. F. Wouters, and D. J. Janssen. 2014. "Efficacy of Advance Care Planning: A Systematic Review and Meta-Analysis." *Journal of the American Medical Directors Association* 15 (7):477–489. doi: 10.1016/j.jamda.2014.01.008.

In der Schmitten, J., R. J. Jox, S. Rixen, and G. Marckmann. 2015. "Vorausplanung für nicht-einwilligungsfähige Personen – 'Vertreterverfügungen'." In *Advance Care Planning*, edited by M. Coors, R. J. Jox, and J. in der Schmitten, 119–140. Stuttgart: Kohlhammer.

In der Schmitten, J., K. Lex, C. Mellert, S. Rotharmel, K. Wegscheider, and G. Marckmann. 2014. "Implementing an Advance Care Planning Program in German Nursing Homes: Results of an Inter-Regionally Controlled Intervention Trial." *Deutsches Ärzteblatt International* 111 (4):50–57. doi: 10.3238/arztebl.2014.0050.

In der Schmitten, J., and G. Marckmann. 2015. "Was ist Advance Care Planning? Internationale Bestandsaufnahme und Plädoyer für eine transparente, zielorientierte Definition." In *Advance Care Planning*, edited by M. Coors, R. J. Jox, and J. in der Schmitten, 75–94. Stuttgart: Kohlhammer.

In der Schmitten, J., S. Rotharmel, C. Mellert, S. Rixen, B. J. Hammes, L. Briggs, K. Wegscheider, and G. Marckmann. 2011. "A Complex Regional Intervention to Implement Advance Care Planning in One Town's Nursing Homes: Protocol of a Controlled Inter-Regional Study." *BMC Health Services Research* 11:14. doi: 10.1186/1472-6963-11-14.

Institute of Medicine. 2015. *Dying in America: Improving Quality and Honoring Individual Preferences near the End of Life*. Washington, DC: National Academies Press.

Jox, R. J. 2014. "Revocation of Advance Directives." In *Advance Directives*, edited by P. Lack, N. Biller-Andorno, and S. Brauer, 73–89. Dordrecht: Springer Netherlands.

Jox, R. J. 2016. "Lost decisional capacity, lost chance of advance care planning?" *Bioethica Forum* 9 (3):109–110.

Khandelwal, N., E. K. Kross, R. A. Engelberg, N. B. Coe, A. C. Long, and J. R. Curtis. 2015. "Estimating the Effect of Palliative Care Interventions and Advance Care Planning on ICU Utilization: A Systematic Review." *Critical Care Medicine* 43 (5):1102–1111. doi: 10.1097/ccm.0000000000000852.

Kirchhoff, K. T., B. J. Hammes, K. A. Kehl, L. A. Briggs, and R. L. Brown. 2012. "Effect of a Disease-Specific Advance Care Planning Intervention on End-of-Life Care." *Journal of the American Geriatrics Society* 60 (5):946–950. doi: 10.1111/j.1532-5415.2012.03917.x.

Klingler, C., J. in der Schmitten, and G. Marckmann. 2015. "Does Facilitated Advance Care Planning Reduce the Costs of Care near the End of Life? Systematic Review and Ethical Considerations." *Palliative Medicine* 30 (5):423–433. doi: 10.1177/0269216315601346.

Knaus, W. A., and The SUPPORT Principles Investigators. 1995. "A Controlled Trial to Improve Care for Seriously Ill Hospitalized Patients: The Study to Understand Prognoses and Preferences for Outcomes and Risks of Treatments (SUPPORT)." *The Journal of the American Medical Association* 274 (20):1591–1598.

Korfage, I. J., J. A. Rietjens, A. Overbeek, L. J. Jabbarian, P. Billekens, B. J. Hammes, E. Hansen-van der Meer, S. Polinder, J. Severijnen, S. J. Swart, F. E. Witkamp, and A. van der Heide. 2015. "A Cluster Randomized Controlled Trial on the Effects and Costs of Advance Care Planning in Elderly Care: Study Protocol." *BMC Geriatrics* 15:87. doi: 10.1186/s12877-015-0087-z.

Kutner, L. 1969. "Due Process of Euthanasia: The Living Will, a Proposal." *Indiana Law Journal* 44 (4):539–554.

Lack, P., N. Biller-Andorno, and S. Brauer, eds. 2013. *Advance Directives*. Dordrecht: Springer Netherlands.

Lenz, M., S. Buhse, J. Kasper, R. Kupfer, T. Richter, and I. Muhlhauser. 2012. "Decision Aids for Patients." *Deutsches Ärzteblatt International* 109 (22–23):401–408. doi: 10.3238/arztebl.2012.0401.

Martin, R. S., B. Hayes, K. Gregorevic, and W. K. Lim. 2016. "The Effects of Advance Care Planning Interventions on Nursing Home Residents: A Systematic Review." *Journal of the American Medical Directors Association* 17 (4):284–293. doi: 10.1016/j.jamda.2015.12.017.

Murray, S. A., M. Kendall, K. Boyd, and A. Sheikh. 2005. "Illness Trajectories and Palliative Care." *British Medical Journal* 330 (7498):1007–1011. doi: 10.1136/bmj.330.7498.1007.

Nauck, F., M. Becker, C. King, L. Radbruch, R. Voltz, and B. Jaspers. 2014. "To What Extent Are the Wishes of a Signatory Reflected in Their Advance Directive: A Qualitative Analysis." *BMC Medical Ethics* 15 (1):52. doi: 10.1186/1472-6939-15-52.

Pellegrino, E. D. 1999. "The Origins and Evolution of Bioethics: Some Personal Reflections." *Kennedy Institute of Ethics Journal* 9 (1):73–88. doi: 10.1353/ken.1999.0006.

Petri, S., and G. Marckmann. 2016. "Advance Directive Consultations: A Study of Selected Consultation Services in the Munich Region." *Deutsche Medizinische Wochenschrift* 141 (9):e80–e86. doi: 10.1055/s-0041-108100.

Rao, J. K., L. A. Anderson, F. C. Lin, and J. P. Laux. 2014. "Completion of Advance Directives among U.S. Consumers." *American Journal of Preventive Medicine* 46 (1):65–70. doi: 10.1016/j.amepre.2013.09.008.

Rietjens, J. A. C., I. J. Korfage, D. J. A. Janssen, R. J. Jox, M. Drickamer, J. Seymour, and R. L. Sudore. 2015. "Oral Abstracts: O-120 White Paper Defining Optimal Advance Care Planning." *BMJ Supportive & Palliative Care* 5:A41. doi: 10.1136/bmjspcare-2015-000978.126.

Slote, M. 2007. *The Ethics of Care and Empathy*. New York: Routledge.

Teno, J. M., S. Licks, J. Lynn, N. Wenger, A. F. Connors Jr., R. S. Phillips, M. A. O'Connor, D. P. Murphy, W. J. Fulkerson, N. Desbiens, and W. A. Knaus. 1997a. "Do Advance Directives Provide Instructions That Direct Care? SUPPORT Investigators. Study to Understand Prognoses and Preferences for Outcomes and Risks of Treatment." *Journal of the American Geriatrics Society* 45 (4):508–512.

Teno, J. M., J. Lynn, N. Wenger, R. S. Phillips, D. P. Murphy, A. F. Connors Jr., N. Desbiens, W. Fulkerson, P. Bellamy, and W. A. Knaus. 1997b. "Advance Directives for Seriously Ill Hospitalized Patients: Effectiveness with the Patient Self-Determination Act and the SUPPORT Intervention. SUPPORT Investigators. Study to Understand Prognoses and Preferences for Outcomes and Risks of Treatment." *Journal of the American Geriatrics Society* 45 (4):500–507.

Tong, R., and N. Williams. 2014. "Feminist Ethics." In *The Stanford Encyclopedia of Philosophy* (Fall 2014 edition, online), edited by E. N. Zalta. https://plato.stanford.edu/entries/feminism-ethics.

Tronto, J. 2005. "An Ethic of Care." In *Feminist Theory: A Philosophical Anthology*, edited by A. E. Cudd and R. O. Andreasen, 251–263. Oxford, UK/Malden, MA: Blackwell Publishing.

Van der Heide, A., L. Deliens, K. Faisst, T. Nilstun, M. Norup, E. Paci, G. van der Wal, and P. J. van der Maas. 2003. "End-of-Life Decision-Making in Six European Countries: Descriptive Study." *The Lancet* 362 (9381):345–350. doi: 10.1016/S0140-6736(03)14019-6.

Volicer, L., M. D. Cantor, A. R. Derse, D. M. Edwards, A. M. Prudhomme, D. C. Gregory, J. E. Reagan, J. A. Tulsky, and E. Fox. 2002. "Advance Care Planning by Proxy for Residents of Long-Term Care Facilities Who Lack Decision-Making Capacity." *Journal of the American Geriatrics Society* 50 (4):761–767. doi: 10.1046/j.1532-5415.2002.50175.x.

Wilson, D. M., D. Houttekier, S. A. Kunju, S. Birch, J. Cohen, R. MacLeod, and J. A. Hewitt. 2013. "A Population-Based Study on Advance Directive Completion and Completion Intention among Citizens of the Western Canadian Province of Alberta." *Journal of Palliative Care* 29 (1):5–12.

12 Articulating the case for the Longevity Dividend

S. Jay Olshansky

Introduction[1]

The rise in human longevity and the increase in our healthy lifespan are two of humanity's greatest achievements. In the developed world, and now even among growing subgroups in developing nations, increasingly larger segments of the population have gained access to one of the most precious of all commodities: the opportunity to live a long life. In developed nations, about 85 percent of everyone born today will live to at least their 65th birthday, and over 42 percent will live past their 85th birthday – a privilege that has been denied to most people throughout history (Human Mortality Database 2016). However, the price to pay for common access to older ages is the opportunity to witness the ageing of our bodies and the fatal and disabling diseases that accompany extended survival.

The trade-off of chronic degenerative diseases for decades of life that was accomplished during the 20th century has undeniably been worth it, but humanity now faces a rather daunting health and economic dilemma. The combination of additional life extension with a forthcoming rapid upward shift in age structure (population ageing) will lead to a dramatic increase in the prevalence of the fatal and disabling diseases common among people who live to older ages, producing a major challenge to healthcare systems and age-entitlement programs. The National Institutes of Health, World Health Organization, United Nations, World Economic Forum, MacArthur Foundation, and other organizations have appropriately acknowledged that ageing and life extension also offer an equal measure of opportunity (for example, see Beard et al. 2011; Rowe 2015, special issue of *Daedalus*; Olshansky, Beard, and Borsch-Supan 2012), but the rising prevalence of costly diseases is an inevitable by-product of our success.

The usual approach to combating the diseases of old age has been to lower the behavioral risk factors that influence their expression, to delay their appearance through earlier detection, and to use medical technology to extend survival for those whose bodies are already diseased. This approach has been successful in the past, but there is a growing body of evidence to suggest that continuing down this path will lead to diminishing gains in life extension (Dong, Milholland, and Vijg 2016) and, more importantly, the possibility (perhaps likelihood) that the historic rise in healthspan may come to a halt – leaving future older cohorts the prospect of rising frailty and disability in later ages (Butler et al. 2008; Olshansky et al. 2006). The fact is, the longer we live, the more the biological ageing of our bodies influences the fatal and disabling diseases that emerge (Miller 2012; Olshansky, Martin, and Kirkland 2015).

Recognizing the important linkage between the biological ageing of our bodies and disease expression, an exciting line of scientific research has emerged that offers us an opportunity to extend our healthy years further (Kirkland 2013; Miller 2002; Olshansky, Martin, and Kirkland 2015; Sierra et al. 2009). The health and economic benefits that would accrue to individuals and nations if this approach is successful has been documented (Goldman et al. 2013). As a result, a consortium of scientists has formed with the purpose of developing a new way to extend healthspan, combat the diseases of ageing, compress mortality, morbidity, and disability, and ameliorate the economic challenges of an anticipated rising prevalence of late-onset diseases. Numerous experimental animal studies have now demonstrated that interventions that ameliorate multiple fatal and disabling maladies of ageing are possible and will likely transform human health if brought to fruition. A large-scale, concerted, and coordinated effort is now underway to develop, test, and then push the translation of these findings into real-world clinical investigation, with the goal of developing therapeutic interventions. Referred to as the Longevity Dividend Initiative Consortium (LDIC) or Geroscience (Sierra 2015), it aims to accelerate the pace of translation from the basic biology of ageing into clinical interventions that will improve quality of life at all ages, but especially for people reaching older ages. The LDIC's goals are ambitious because they address needs in several scientific domains: basic biology, genetics, pre-clinical and clinical research, and population-level modeling. This chapter provides the rationale behind the LDIC and begins outlining the scientific pathways that researchers are pursuing to this end.

Healthy life extension

The most precious of all commodities is life itself, and if there is one attribute most of us share, it is the desire to remain alive. The yearning for healthy life is equally important, perhaps more so – especially for those struggling to regain health that has been lost. One would think, therefore, that making the case for the development of new, more effective methods of extending our healthy years would be universally accepted and easy to make, regardless of how it is achieved. Sadly, this is not the case.

In public health, interventions that in the past had a profound influence on the length and quality of life include the development and dissemination of clean water, sanitation, indoor living and working environments, and refrigeration. During the last century, epidemiologists made the public aware of the life-shortening effects of smoking and other harmful risk factors, as well as the life-extending effects of proper diet and exercise, among others. In the modern world of medicine and medical technology, a trip to the doctor, dentist, or other health professional is justified as a form of primary prevention. When a health issue arises, such as a serious infection, cancer, or heart disease, it is now routine to seek out and trust modern medical treatment as the best approach to regaining one's health. In fact, a strong endorsement for the efficacy of medicine's ability to extend healthy life comes from its validation by the insurance industry.

These three pillars of healthy life extension have earned our trust, and deservedly so, but now concerns are being raised about how much more healthy life can be manufactured using these approaches (Olshansky 2015). The reason is the biological ageing of our bodies. Public health can manufacture only so much survival time through lifestyle modification, after which medical technology has an important life-extending impact, but even these methods of life extension eventually lead the survivors to face the increased and accelerated ravages of the biological ageing of our bodies.

Think of the effect of ageing on the body as the same as the effect of miles on your car. Very few things go wrong with most cars during the first three years and 36,000 miles, and for some automobiles, the warranty period has been extended to ten years and 100,000 miles. Operate these cars beyond their warranty period, and a cluster of problems emerges. These problems are an inevitable by-product of the passage of time and the accumulation of damage that arises from operating the machine – they are not programmed to occur at a set time by the auto manufacturers. While planned obsolescence is part of the manufacturing ethos for some manufacturers of certain products, a programmed 'death time' is not built into a car.

The same principles hold true for human bodies. Once we operate our bodies beyond the equivalent of their biological warranty period, a large number of health issues begin to emerge and cluster tightly into later regions of the lifespan. Among scientists who track these events, this is known as 'competing causes,' which is another way of saying that a large number of lethal and disabling conditions accumulate in ageing bodies. Ameliorating any one lethal condition independent of all others leaves the person with a remaining high risk from all other remaining conditions. With time (and age), the treatments devised through medicine (which tend to focus on one disease at a time) and risk-factor modification then become progressively less effective as survivors move further into older age windows where ageing-related diseases cluster ever more tightly together. Keep in mind that just like automobiles, our bodies are not programmed with ageing or death genes that are set off at a predetermined age. Ageing is best thought of as an inadvertent by-product of fixed genetic programs that evolved under the direct force of natural selection for early life developmental events – ageing is a product of evolutionary neglect, not evolutionary intent.

Recognizing the fact that competing causes place a damper on the future effectiveness of medical interventions that are disease-oriented, scientists in the field of ageing have proposed that the next big step in public health and healthy life extension is to attack the seeds of ageing rather than just its consequences as we do now. The idea is to slow the ageing of our bodies such that one year of clock time is matched by less than one year of biological time. In this way, we would retain our youthful vigor for a longer time and, if delayed ageing interventions work the way we hope they will, experience a compression of the infirmities of old age into a shorter time frame at the end of life. Delaying the biological ageing of our bodies is the only viable approach to addressing the increasing importance of competing causes and the rise of ageing as an ever more important risk factor for disease.

'Anti-ageing' charlatanry

It is at this juncture where one of the main problems occurs. The contemporary proposal to slow ageing as a means to extend healthy life has historical links to medical deception, charlatanism, and greed (Gruman 1966). Historically, the quest for immortality was couched within a 'prolongevity' message suggesting that ingesting or injecting substances with alleged 'anti-ageing' properties could enable people to recapture their lost youth. One of the most famous among these is the alchemist's dream to transmute lead into gold, which at the time of its origin was thought to confer properties of immortality to those who ingested minute quantities.

In the late 19th century, the French physiologist Charles-Edouard Brown-Sequard claimed to have discovered the secret to rejuvenation. Brown-Sequard crushed the testicles of domesticated animals, extracted 'vital' substances from them, and then inoculated older people against the 'ageing disease.' Modern versions of these ancient 'anti-ageing' potions were described by the US Government Accounting Office as posing the "potential for physical and economic harm" (General Accounting Office 2001).

Finally, some scientists in the field of ageing have formed companies designed to attract investors interested in cashing in on a possible breakthrough in the field of ageing (Anton 2013). Although this approach enables some ageing science that would not otherwise be funded, it can lead and has led to exaggerated claims and unproven interventions that reach the marketplace before they are fully evaluated using the tools of science. This, too, creates suspicion among the public, who already have a difficult time distinguishing between medical fraud and genuine public-health interventions.

Taken together, these historical and contemporary roadblocks to legitimacy have delayed the entrance of ageing science into the realm of accepted discourse as a legitimate and, quite frankly, valuable and needed public-health intervention. However, these are not the only roadblocks.

Religious arguments

Religious objections are sometimes posed in response to proposals to enhance public health by modulation of ageing. The objection usually starts from the assertion that tampering with ageing is equivalent to tampering with God's plan for us – an effort that should not be pursued. However, this argument loses its power when those proposing it admit that both they and their children have been vaccinated against lethal childhood diseases. It is hard to imagine that God's plan is to kill most children from communicable diseases before the age of ten, but up until the 19th century, that was humanity's fate. Most people who make this argument also admit that they would seek medical attention if they (or their loved ones) experienced heart disease or cancer. Why is one form of disease prevention acceptable while another is not?

Population growth

When delayed ageing was first proposed as a public-health intervention in the 1950s, rapid population growth was a concern because the growth rate in the post-World War II era (between 1946 and 1964) was about 3 percent. To place this growth rate into perspective, at that rate it takes the population only 26 years to double in size. Thus, there was reason to be concerned about the population-growth rate during most of the second half of the 20th century – this was alarming to both demographers and environmentalists. Although the rate of population growth has attenuated considerably since 1950, the momentum for population growth will remain with us through the middle of this century. However, environmental concerns have escalated considerably. Population growth and resource depletion should be on our minds, and these are issues that are appropriate to raise when having a discussion about healthy life extension.

The thing is, those making this argument believe that delayed ageing will dramatically accelerate population growth, wipe out the reductions in the growth rate achieved in recent decades, further challenge resource depletion, and generate a new set of population and environmental headaches. As it turns out, none of these concerns are valid.

With regard to population growth, I have estimated how the growth rate (GR) would change with the hypothetical extreme scenario of immortality (i.e., no more deaths) (Olshansky 2013, Table 1). Under the extreme scenario of immortality, the GR would be about 1.5 percent (i.e., the GR would be defined by the birth rate, since the death rate would be zero) – which is three times as high as the current GR of about 0.5 percent. However, longer lives tend to be accompanied by lower fertility, so I estimate a GR under conditions of hypothetical immortality of about 0.9 percent – still twice the current GR. Since immortality is not likely to happen any time soon, and since delayed ageing would yield only marginal increases in life expectancy, the actual population GR would only rise slightly if the Longevity Dividend is achieved.

In fact, the population GR would also rise marginally with a cure for cancer or heart disease. I have yet to hear anyone argue that cures for these diseases should not be pursued for the reason that success would be accompanied by accelerated population growth and resource depletion. The bottom line is that the Longevity Dividend Initiative will have a negligible effect on population growth and the environment, but it will have a dramatically positive impact on work, retirement, healthcare financing and costs, and physical and psychological well-being (Goldman et al. 2013).

Delayed ageing means increased infirmity

Perhaps the most common misconception and fear about ageing science and the Longevity Dividend Initiative is the belief that delayed ageing will extend the period of infirmity at the end of life – the fear that most people have as they approach older ages. There is an irony to this view, because while there may be disagreement among scientists exactly how to accomplish the goals that have been set, the one thing we all have in common is the final and most important goal of extending the period of healthy life. An intervention that does not meet the test of extending the health and functionality of both body and mind together would not be pursued – in fact, such an intervention would be seen as harmful.

Emerging evidence indicating that delayed ageing is a plausible target

Numerous studies have been published recently suggesting that delayed ageing is a plausible target as a new public-health paradigm (Kennedy and Pennypacker 2014; Olshansky, Martin, and Kirkland 2015). But when a medical intervention such as this arises, what might it look like? Details of potential therapeutic interventions can be found in a chapter written by Kirkland (2015). To summarize briefly, maximum lifespan and age-related diseases have already been delayed in some species using a single-gene mutation (Bartke 2011). Centenarians have been documented to experience delayed onset of all fatal and disabling conditions with its attendant compression of morbidity and disability (Lipton et al. 2010), leading researchers to conclude that long-lived people (and their offspring) are likely to be senescing more slowly than the rest of the population. Because delayed ageing is likely to be a heritable trait, identifying the genes and related proteins that might be contributing to this phenomenon is a potential therapeutic pathway. Caloric restriction appears to be a viable method of extending healthy life in mammals (Anderson and Weindruch 2012); the removal of senescent cells appears to reduce chronic inflammation and promote reductions in numerous fatal and disabling conditions (Kirkland and Tchkonia 2014); and a broad range of research studies suggest that compounds such as rapamycin, metformin, flavonoids, and many others, could have therapeutic effects resulting in a systemic deceleration in the rate of biological ageing (for example, see Bannister et al. 2014). No one can know with certainty at this time which of the many research pathways now ongoing in the field are going to lead to a breakthrough in ageing science, but the fact that there are so many promising opportunities means that a breakthrough coming online in enough time to influence most people alive today is likely.

Rationale for the Longevity Dividend

The case for the Longevity Dividend is compelling and in theory should be easy to make to funders, public-health professionals, and the general public. Here is the line of reasoning:

(1) Treating diseases worked well in the past to extend healthy life, but in long-lived populations ageing has emerged as the primary risk factor for the most common fatal and disabling diseases.
(2) The longer we live, the greater the influence of ageing on disease expression.

(3) Ageing science offers medicine and public health a new and potentially far more effective weapon for delaying disease in the form of primary prevention, extending healthy life, compressing morbidity, and altogether avoiding many of the infirmities associated with old age (Butler et al. 2008; Goldman et al. 2013).
(4) Failing to take this new approach could leave people who reach old age in the future even more vulnerable to rising disability than they are now.
(5) Ageing science represents a new paradigm of primary prevention in public health that will lead to more effective methods of delaying most fatal and disabling diseases; extending healthy life; and reducing the prevalence of infirmities more commonly experienced at older ages.

(Kirkland 2013; Sierra et al. 2009; Tchkonia et al. 2013)

Language used to describe the Longevity Dividend must be unambiguous. Much as with the introduction of antibiotics in the mid-20th century and the broad dissemination of basic measures of public health a century ago, humanity is once again fortunate enough to witness the rise of a new public-health paradigm. Ageing science has successfully turned the spotlight on the origins of our ageing bodies and minds and disabling diseases that accompany us in our later years. What the scientific study of ageing reveals shakes up a long-held assumption that ageing is an inevitable and immutable by-product of the passage of time (Miller 2002), and these new discoveries fundamentally challenge the fatalist view that ageing and death are nature's way of removing the old to make way for the young.

Science has now demonstrated that ageing is inherently modifiable; most fatal and disabling diseases are amenable to delay through a single intervention; and morbidity and disability can be compressed into a shorter duration of time at the end of life. Furthermore, there is reason to believe that ageing science can be translated into new medical and public-health interventions that will be able to combat fatal and disabling diseases far more effectively than any intervention available today – yielding an extension of the period of healthy life in ways that could not even be conceived of just a few years ago.

Although people who benefit from advances in ageing science will probably live longer, it is the extension of healthy life that is the primary goal, along with reductions in the infirmities of old age and increased economic value to individuals and societies that would accrue from the extension of healthy life.

Conclusions

The ethical and political implications of the interventions proposed under the LDIC have been addressed extensively in the recent book by Olshansky, Martin, and Kirkland (2015). Suffice it to say that two ethical conditions should be considered at once. The first is "What could happen if the current medical model continues on with no significant effort or breakthrough in the field of ageing in this century?" What we are likely to witness is not just an increase in the prevalence of conditions of frailty as case-fatality rates from major fatal diseases continue to decline under the light of advances of the biomedical sciences; we may also witness a significant worsening of frailty and disability as survivors live longer into their frail years. The result could be an extension of the period of old age and its attendant harmful disease states – with Alzheimer's disease and other neurological conditions flaring up and out of control. Without any change in the rate of ageing, further life extension much beyond where we are today could be harmful.

The second ethical consideration is "What would happen if we succeed with the LDIC?" There is little doubt that a major breakthrough would initially be inequitably distributed. After all, there is not a single precious resource today that is humanely and universally available to everyone. Has inequality stopped humanity from inventing and disseminating vaccines, pursuing clean air and water, or creating temperature-controlled indoor living and working environments? Of course not. We seek to improve life at the same time as we try to reduce disparities. Success with the LDIC will also yield an increase in the size of the older population throughout most of this century, and most of those additional years of life are expected to be healthy. There would be challenges to age-entitlement programs to be sure, but these same challenges would arise with a cure for cancer. Given the alternative of curing a single disease and possibly extending frailty and disability because ageing marches on unaltered, or delaying ageing and simultaneously postponing the onset and progression of all fatal and disabling diseases at once and experiencing morbidity and disability compression – the choice is clear. We choose healthy life, and we believe that humanity would be far better off as a result.

It is only a matter of time before ageing science acquires the same level of prestige and confidence that medicine and public health now enjoy, and when that time comes, a new era in human health will emerge. There is an abundance of formidable obstacles standing in the way, including strongly held views on how to proceed, a history of association with dubious ageing interventions, and misconceptions about the goals in mind and the impact of success on population growth and the environment. Once the air clears and ageing science is translated into effective and safe interventions that can be measured and documented to extend our healthy years, the 21st century will bear witness to one of the most important developments in the history of medicine.

Note

1 Acknowledgments: The MacArthur Foundation Research Network on an Aging Society supported this work. Earlier versions of this manuscript were published in *Public Policy & Aging Report* (Goldman and Olshansky 2013; Olshansky 2013).

References

Anderson, R. M., and R. Weindruch. 2012. "The Caloric Restriction Paradigm: Implications for Healthy Human Aging." *American Journal of Human Biology* 24 (2):101–106. doi: 10.1002/ajhb.22243.

Anton, T. 2013. *The Longevity Seekers: Science, Business, and the Fountain of Youth.* Chicago: The University of Chicago Press.

Bannister, C. A., S. E. Holden, S. Jenkins-Jones, C. L. Morgan, J. P. Halcox, G. Schernthaner, J. Mukherjee, and C. J. Currie. 2014. "Can People with Type 2 Diabetes Live Longer Than Those Without? A Comparison of Mortality in People Initiated with Metformin or Sulphonylurea Monotherapy and Matched, Non-Diabetic Controls." *Diabetes Obesity and Metabolism* 16 (11):1165–1173. doi: 10.1111/dom.12354.

Bartke, A. 2011. "Single-Gene Mutations and Healthy Ageing in Mammals." *Philosophical Transactions of the Royal Society of London, Series B: Biological Sciences* 366 (1561):28–34. doi: 10.1098/rstb.2010.0281.

Beard, J. R., S. Biggs, D. E. Bloom, L. P. Fried, P. Hogan, A. Kalache, and S. J. Olshansky, eds. 2011. *Global Population Ageing: Peril or Promise?* Geneva: World Economic Forum.

Butler, R. N., R. A. Miller, D. Perry, B. A. Carnes, T. F. Williams, C. Cassel, J. Brody, M. A. Bernard, L. Partridge, T. Kirkwood, G. M. Martin, and S. J. Olshansky. 2008. "New Model of Health Promotion and Disease Prevention for the 21st Century." *British Medical Journal* 337 (7662):149–150. doi: 10.1136/bmj.a399.

Dong, X., B. Milholland, and J. Vijg. 2016. "Evidence for a Limit to Human Lifespan." *Nature* 538:257–259.

General Accounting Office. 2001. *Health Products for Seniors: "Anti-Aging" Products Pose Potential for Physical and Economic Harm.* GAO-01–1129.

Goldman, D. P., D. Cutler, J. W. Rowe, P. C. Michaud, J. Sullivan, D. Peneva, and S. J. Olshansky. 2013. "Substantial Health and Economic Returns from Delayed Aging May Warrant a New Focus for Medical Research." *Health Affairs* 32 (10):1698–1705. doi: 10.1377/hlthaff.2013.0052.

Goldman, D. P., and S. J. Olshansky. 2013. "Delayed Aging versus Delayed Disease: A New Paradigm for Public Health." *Public Policy & Aging Report* 23 (4):16–18. doi: 10.1093/ppar/23.4.16.

Gruman, G. 1966. "A History of Ideas about the Prolongation of Life." *Transactions of the American Philosophical Society* 56 (9):1–102. doi: 10.2307/1006096.

Human Mortality Database. Accessed October 25, 2016. www.mortality.org/.

Kennedy, B. K., and J. K. Pennypacker. 2014. "Drugs That Modulate Aging: The Promising Yet Difficult Path Ahead." *Translational Research* 163 (5):456–465. doi: 10.1016/j.trsl.2013.11.007.

Kirkland, J. L. 2013. "Translating Advances from the Basic Biology of Aging into Clinical Application." *Experimental Gerontology* 48 (1):1–5. doi: 10.1016/j.exger.2012.11.014.

Kirkland, J. L. 2015. "Translating the Science of Aging into Therapeutic Interventions." In *Aging: The Longevity Dividend*, edited by S. J. Olshansky, G. M. Martin, and J. L. Kirkland, 121–134. Cold Spring Harbor: Cold Spring Harbor Laboratory Press.

Kirkland, J. L., and T. Tchkonia. 2014. "Clinical Strategies and Animal Models for Developing Senolytic Agents." *Experimental Gerontology* 68:19–25. doi: 10.1016/j.exger.2014.10.012.

Lipton, R. B., J. Hirsch, M. Katz, C. Wang, A. E. Sanders, J. Verghese, N. Barzilai, and C. Derby. 2010. "Exceptional Parental Longevity Associated with Lower Risk of Alzheimer's Disease and Memory Decline." *Journal of the American Geriatrics Society* 58 (6):1043–1049. doi: 10.1111/j.1532-5415.2010.02868.x.

Miller, R. 2002. "Scientific Prospects and Political Obstacles." *The Milbank Quarterly* 80 (1):155–174. doi: 10.1111/1468-0009.00006.

Miller, R. 2012. "Genes against Aging." *The Journals of Gerontology, Series A: Biological Sciences and Medical Sciences* 67 (5):495–502. doi: 10.1093/gerona/gls082.

Olshansky, S. J. 2013. "Articulating the Case for the Longevity Dividend." *Public Policy & Aging Report* 23 (4):3–6. doi: 10.1093/ppar/23.4.3.

Olshansky, S. J. 2015. "Has the Rate of Human Aging Already Been Modified?" In *Aging: The Longevity Dividend*, edited by S. J. Olshansky, G. M. Martin, and J. L. Kirkland, 221–238. Cold Spring Harbor: Cold Spring Harbor Laboratory Press.

Olshansky, S. J., J. R. Beard, and A. Borsch-Supan. 2012. "The Longevity Dividend: Health as an Investment." In *Global Population Ageing: Peril or Promise?* edited by J. R. Beard, S. Biggs, D. E. Bloom, L. P. Fried, P. Hogan, A. Kalache, and S. J. Olshansky, 57–60. Geneva: World Economic Forum.

Olshansky, S. J., G. M. Martin, and J. L. Kirkland, eds. 2015. *Aging: The Longevity Dividend.* Cold Spring Harbor: Cold Spring Harbor Laboratory Press.

Olshansky, S. J., D. Perry, R. A. Miller, and R. N. Butler. 2006. "In Pursuit of the Longevity Dividend." *The Scientist* 20 (3):28–36. doi: 10.1196/annals.1396.050.

Rowe, J. W. 2015. "Successful Aging of Societies." *Daedalus* 144 (2):5–12.

Sierra, F. 2015. "The Emergence of Geroscience as an Interdisciplinary Approach to the Enhancement of Health Span and Life Span." In *Aging: The Longevity Dividend*, edited by S. J. Olshansky, G. M. Martin, and J. L. Kirkland, 1–14. Cold Spring Harbor: Cold Spring Harbor Laboratory Press.

Sierra, F., E. Hadley, R. Suzman, and R. Hodes. 2009. "Prospects for Life Span Extension." *Annual Review of Medicine* 60:457–469. doi: 10.1146/annurev.med.60.061607.220533.

Tchkonia, T., Y. Zhu, J. van Deursen, J. Campisi, and J. L. Kirkland. 2013. "Cellular Senescence and the Senescent Secretory Phenotype: Therapeutic Opportunities." *The Journal of Clinical Investigation* 123 (3):966–972. doi: 10.1172/JCI64098.

13 Paradoxes of planning later life

Anti-ageing practices and the lived body

Larissa Pfaller and Frank Adloff

Introduction

"Google Invests in Immortality"[1] is just one of the big headlines that has found its way into international news since 2013 – the year Google launched the research company Calico (short for California Life Company). Calico sees its mission as "tackling ageing, one of life's greatest mysteries".[2] It wants to investigate the very nature of biological ageing processes in order to develop interventions in age-related diseases and prolong human life. Implementing findings from genetic research, Human Longevity Inc. (HLI) – founded by Craig Venter, one of the pioneers of the human genome project – is also pursuing the early treatment of age-related diseases and conditions.

In contrast to these high-tech and sophisticated ventures, the actual anti-ageing interventions offered by commercial industry and in medical offices seem quite old-fashioned: They mostly comprise conventional medical provisions and therapies simply repackaged with the attractive 'anti-ageing' label, or booklets and magazines that offer guidelines for a long and healthy life. Thus, instead of advanced and innovative inventions, commonsense lifestyle advice is provided – for example, to engage in sports and maintain good nutrition. Moreover, the evidence related to more advanced biomedical anti-ageing technologies is highly controversial.

In German anti-ageing medicine, risk is the major category for thinking about ageing. Ageing is understood as the essential risk factor for age-related diseases, placing anti-ageing practices on the level of preventive medicine. In the inner logic of prevention, insecurities and dangers are transformed into risks, which can be calculated and thus controlled with regard to the future (Beck 1992). At the same time, individuals are held responsible for making decisions concerning later life based on future scenarios and relying on probabilities. In this logic, future ageing processes can be shaped by making the right medical decisions now. Thus, people are supposed to show responsibility not only for their current conduct but also for their future medical fate. As a consequence, everyday certainties concerning biological life are transformed into matters of malleability. The underlying scientific prevention models statistically derive from populations and can be communicated only in terms of probabilities. In everyday life, however, people reflect on their preventive behavior individually and in the light of their personal experience.

The chapter takes this contradiction seriously. In contrast to the cultural construction of anti-ageing as a genuinely medical project, it aims to understand the symbolic value of everyday anti-ageing practices, which transcends questions of scientific evidence and medical efficacy. Thus, we trace the attraction of anti-ageing to a symbolic power extending far beyond a mere medical effect. For this purpose, we take a close cultural-sociological look at those who are engaged in anti-ageing practices in everyday life in order to reduce the symptoms of ageing, to prevent or repair the functional ailments and diseases of old age, or even to prolong their own life. In doing so, we rely on qualitative interviews and focus groups, highlighting the central role of the lived body: While anti-ageing medicine is associated with future risk and uncertainty, and the inner logic of prevention can lead to a rat race of 'never having done enough,' everyday anti-ageing practices carried out in a self-caring way create a focus on the present, a positive bodily experience, and thus provide emotional security.

Background: anti-ageing in Germany

'Anti-ageing' is primarily used as a promotionally effective label for a wide range of commercial health, beauty and care products, and wellness treatments. Nevertheless, the relevance of anti-ageing medicine should not be underestimated (Stuckelberger 2008). Since the founding of the American Academy of Anti-Ageing Medicine (A4M) in the early 1990s[3] – when the term 'anti-ageing' was coined (Spindler 2014) – anti-ageing medicine has established itself as a discrete discipline. The A4M considers anti-ageing as the implementation of medical and biogerontological methods and findings:

> The phrase 'anti-ageing,' as such, relates to the application of advanced biomedical technologies focused on the early detection, prevention, and treatment of ageing-related disease. Anti-ageing medicine complements regenerative medicine, as both specialties embrace cutting-edge biomedical technologies aimed at achieving benefits for both the quality and quantity of the human lifespan.
>
> (www.worldhealth.net)

In particular, the A4M emphasizes the potential of innovative technologies, such as stem-cell therapy, therapeutic cloning, genetic engineering and genomics, and nanotechnology, for fighting the symptoms of ageing – that is, preventing or repairing the functional ailments and diseases of old age and prolonging the health span, life expectancy, or maximum lifespan in humans. The A4M's concept of ageing as a treatable meta-disease and the associated "war on ageing" (de Grey 2004) primarily influence anti-ageing medicine in the United States. But anti-ageing medicine has also been established in Europe. Thus, the German Society of Anti-Ageing Medicine (GSAAM) was founded in 1999. In German, the society's name also includes the word 'prevention' in order to show its focus on medical provision and – after the official separation of the GSAAM from its US umbrella organization (Spindler 2014, 19) – to distance itself from the A4M and its (in the German perception) overly commercialized and optimistic claims. In German anti-ageing medicine, biological ageing is seen as more a risk factor than a disease, as the GSAAM's president, Prof. Dr. Bernd Kleine-Gunk, explains: "Ageing is the process that most affects the probability of becoming sick and of dying. We want to do something about this biological process."[4] Kleine-Gunk also refers to the fact that in German everyday language, the term 'anti-ageing' is primarily associated with cosmetic products unless the word 'medicine' is added:[5] "For many people, 'anti-ageing' refers primarily to cosmetics or aesthetics – think of Botox. The GSAAM and I understand anti-ageing medicine as a kind of preventive medicine, which focuses on ageing-related diseases, such as osteoporosis, arteriosclerosis, degenerative arthropathy, or Alzheimer's disease" (expert interview).

With this focus on prevention and preventive medicine, the GSAAM also addresses younger people. Under the paradigm of prevention, ageing is not just an issue in later life but transforms into the ultimate (medical) risk factor. Thus, anti-ageing medicine becomes the means of controlling the problems associated with ageing. German anti-ageing medicine mainly uses conventional treatments, although with prior individual risk diagnosis (Spindler 2014, 198 ff.), not least due to the more restrictive German healthcare laws. In contrast to treatments that become necessary on medical grounds, the cost of anti-ageing products and practices is usually not covered by German public health-insurance companies. Thus, anti-ageing measures seem to be something special and – given the fact that health insurers are thought to accept only costs for effective medical treatment – appear somewhat dubious (Schweda, Herrmann, and Marckmann 2011). As a result, in Germany, anti-ageing medicine is not considered an alternative to conventional medicine (Watts-Roy 2009) and cannot be understood as a "patient-practitioner movement" (Mykytyn 2006a) – as is the case in the US.

Notwithstanding the heterogeneous and controversial use of the term in different national, socio-political, cultural, and practical contexts (Mykytyn 2006b; Spindler 2009), as well as in biogerontological and social-science debates (Spindler 2014, 29 ff.; Vincent 2006), we reconstructed three distinct basic objectives that proponents of anti-ageing practices – be they scientists, practitioners, or users – pursue: (a) the aesthetic correction of visual signs and symptoms of ageing; (b) the prevention or treatment of age-related functional failure, ailments, and diseases; and (c) the prolongation of human life (elaborated in Pfaller and Schweda 2017). Within these objectives, anti-ageing practices comprise cosmetic interventions, such as the application of crèmes, Botox, or filler injections (e.g., hyaluronic acid, collagen, body fat) to relieve wrinkles, laser therapy or chemical peeling to remove age spots; surgical interventions, such as face-lifts, to tighten the skin; and lifestyle interventions (e.g., avoiding alcohol and smoking, maintaining a healthy weight, and having regular preventive check-ups) as well as nutrition (e.g., caloric restriction and sports). There is also a range of dietary supplements (e.g., vitamins, antioxidants, functional food) and pharmaceutical interventions (e.g., hormone-replacement therapies using human growth hormone (HGH) or dehydroepiandrosterone (DHEA) to sustain muscle mass and bone density, statins or chelation therapy to prevent arteriosclerosis or cancer, or Viagra™ to repair erectile dysfunction). Life extension can aim at prolonging both individual life expectancy and biological lifespan. Visions of radical life extension or biological immortality focus on methods for slowing down, stopping, or reversing biological senescence (de Grey and Rae 2007).

Methods

The research presented in this chapter was part of the project "Biomedical Life Plans for Ageing" funded by the Germany Federal Ministry of Education and Research.[6] In this project, 12 focus groups and 20 narrative interviews (with a total of 96 participants) were conducted with persons engaged in anti-ageing practices and interested laypersons. Our interpretation is also based on expert interviews, observations of conferences and events, and document analysis.

All of the interviewees and participants in the focus groups were recruited through flyers, as well as advertisements in specialized online forums, snowball sampling, and relevant public events. Recruitment took place in accordance with the Grounded Theory approach of theoretical sampling, in which the search for minimal and maximal contrasts serves as a leading principle (Glaser and Strauss 2009). Similar and diverse cases were sampled to reconstruct the smaller sections of the field and to understand the entire spectrum of cases. Thus, the overall sample was developed in a step-by-step mode, iteratively referring back to the ongoing data analysis until empirical saturation was reached. During the recruiting process, all the respondents were informed about the consultation method, data protection, and incentives.

In the selection of participants and the composition of the focus groups, we aimed for a balance of both age and gender. The selected participants signed an informed-consent sheet that explained the project's aims and setting in detail. Before the study was launched, it was approved by the institutional review board (IRB) of the University Medical Center Göttingen. The interviews and focus groups were conducted in different German cities (Erlangen, Göttingen, Berlin, Rostock, Nürnberg, München, Leipzig) in 2011 and 2012. The focus groups were moderated by two facilitators using a semi-structured questionnaire comprised of questions on the practice and importance of anti-ageing and preventive-health provisions, as well as scenarios on the chances and risks of life extension. The discussions and interviews were audiotaped and the recordings were transcribed. The respondents were given pseudonyms, preserving only information on their gender (Ms./Mr.) and age (in parentheses behind the pseudonyms' initials). The final sample comprised a broad socio-demographic variety, allowing us to explore lay perspectives on anti-ageing in Germany across a wide range of individual viewpoints, situations, and backgrounds. The participants' ages ranged from 20 to 85, with an average of 56 and a median of 61. They represented a great diversity of educational, professional, and socio-economic backgrounds from western, eastern, northern, and southern regions of Germany, rural as well as urban. The gender ratio (36 male, 60 female) appeared acceptable given both the well-known gender bias in the willingness to participate in a focus group and the interest in the topic of prevention.

In the interpretation, we followed the documentary method (Bohnsack 2010) and thus a reconstructive paradigm. Taking into account that meaning is always created in the course of a concrete sequence of speech acts, both the focus groups and the interviews were analyzed using a sequential analysis (Nohl 2009), and individual statements could be interpreted as 'documents' of overarching individual orientations.

Paradoxes in planning and prevention

In general, our study uncovers a broad spectrum of attitudes toward anti-ageing medicine among German users and interested laypersons – from total rejection to active and ardent pursuit and promotion (for details, see Schweda and Pfaller 2014). In the following sections, we take a close look at the role of the experience of the lived body in dealing with uncertainties regarding preventive anti-ageing measures.

Anti-ageing medicine as prevention is generally directed toward the future. At the same time, the future is conceptualized not only as uncertain, but also as threatening. Especially in German anti-ageing medicine, ageing is understood in terms of risk and probability statements. The following quote from Prof. Dr. Kleine-Gunk can be interpreted along this line of thought:

> Many people ask: 'What should I take?' My reply is always: 'That's the wrong question. You should start by asking yourself what you should do.' Currently, therapeutic anti-ageing is mainly a lifestyle program . . . . Eighty percent of all diseases are not fate, but are due to lifestyle, wrong nutrition, or environmental influences and thus they can be prevented.
>
> (Expert interview)

In short, when ageing is understood as a statistical risk factor, the individual body is identified as the origin of these risks. The ageing person carries individually detectable risk factors, which are located in the ageing body as a biological disposition. Hence, for users of anti-ageing medicine, one's own body is not only permanently threatened by the risks of ageing, but also threatening in itself:

> What I deeply hope is really to live as long as possible, perhaps also to overwrite my genetic program a bit.
>
> – Mr. I. (32), interview

The use of anti-ageing medicine here involves a kind of bet on the future, and the knowledge regarding biomedical genetics is found interwoven with the everyday-life principle of hope (for the entanglement of 'regimes of truth' and 'regimes of hope' in anti-ageing medicine, see Schweda and Pfaller 2017).

At first glance, the attraction of anti-ageing practices can be described as a paradoxical attraction, because the effects of anti-ageing interventions as preventive and directed to the future cannot be perceived or measured by the users themselves – except in the case of direct cosmetic interventions, such as surgery or Botox. The benefits of anti-ageing measures in terms of the creation or maintenance of health, beauty, or longevity, as promised by medicine or industry, take effect in the future – if at all. And even then, it cannot be proven beyond doubt that the effects are due to one's past behavior:

> Of course, it is in your hands. . . . But you never know how much it actually brings about . . . . Just to live maybe a year longer. And you never know if it really accounts for that one year.
>
> – Ms. T. (52), focus group

As anti-aging practices are basically directed toward ageing and later life, we can follow Lengwiler and Madarász in their description of two essential paradoxes of preventive practices. First, they find a basic contradiction between scientific preventive claims and preventive practices in everyday life, a kind of socio-cultural dissonance in preventive ideas of experts and laypersons. Scientific prevention models are rational, derive from collectives and populations, and can be communicated only in terms of probabilities. In everyday life, however, people consider their preventive behavior individually and in light of their own experience (Lengwiler and Madarász 2010, 16). The second paradox in preventive logic relates to the non-intended increase of uncertainty. Following preventive imperatives, formerly harmless practices – such as eating, drinking, or sports – appear to become medical risks (Lengwiler and Madarász 2010, 17). In the case of anti-ageing practices, we can even speak of a double insecurity, given that these interventions are controversially discussed in view of their scientific evidence base, medical efficacy, and risks – particularly with regard to attempts to delay ageing or extend life (Binstock 2004; Butler 2001; Butler et al. 2002; Ehni 2013; Olshansky, Hayflick, and Carnes 2002a, 2002b; Olshansky, Hayflick, and Perls 2004a, 2004b).[7] Anti-ageing practitioners still use mainstream medical interventions, although individually designed for each patient under the anti-ageing label (Fishman, Settersten, and Flatt 2010). Against this background, the promises of anti-ageing medicine seem rather suspect. Olshansky, Hayflick, and Carnes (2002b) even state that "anyone purporting to offer an anti-ageing product today is either mistaken or lying" (Olshansky, Hayflick, and Carnes 2002b, 92).

It stands to reason that anti-ageing practices not only can be seen as attractive offers to reduce the signs of ageing, but also create further uncertainties. Moreover, even the users of anti-ageing practices declare that they do not fully believe in their effects. Therefore, anti-ageing practices should actually be plunged into a legitimation crisis, because there is neither scientific proof nor – despite plentiful sources of information – well-founded directives for everyday life.

The rat race of anti-ageing practices

From the perspective of prevention, the body seems to be degenerative, threatened by the procession of time, and never perfect. The very wording found in anti-ageing medicine – for example, 'hormone replacement' or 'supplementation' – classifies ageing bodies as mainly lacking (of hormones or vitamins) and therefore as degenerative and deficient (see also Pfaller and Adloff 2017). In the 'war against ageing,' prevention does not aim to create something new or better; rather, it seeks to avoid the occurrence of something worse, such as disease or death. Users describe dealing with ageing processes using metaphors of fight and defense, which are directed against visible symptoms interpreted as caused by ageing:

> Certainly, I want to control and also slow down the symptoms of ageing that will inevitably occur . . . . And there are things that can be kept under control by lifestyle or healthy diet, but there are also changes like wrinkles that you have to fight against with interventions like Botox or fillers.
>
> – Ms. D. (56), interview

The symptoms occur "inevitably"; they can be delayed but never entirely prevented. Thus, as a matter of principle, this project of prevention can never be finished; it is always possible to do more (Bröckling 2008). Hence, the goal is a kind of optimum, yet it can never be reached. At the same time, one's body is seen not only in relation to a possible future body, but also in relation to an imagined ideal:

> I thought a person always has to present an ideal, and what I had was not enough . . . . I have already had injections below the skin, in my lips, and my nasolabial fold. Not to change my face but to make it ideal again, to cover the tracks . . . . First, one has to try to make the body fit, so eating as healthily as possible, exercising a lot – so that one stays in a healthy frame, or first of all discovering sports, with which one can optimally keep in shape. So, how do I keep myself fittest? And how do I feel most comfortable? And that also contributes to my health.
>
> – Ms. A. (29), interview

Consequently, anti-ageing practices create a body suspended in an everlasting state of comparison. First, there is an imagined ideal that can never be reached, because its construction fundamentally includes elusiveness; the aim of prevention, as the example illustrates, is not a condition of being fit, being healthy, or being well, but perpetual optimization without a defined endpoint ("as healthy as possible," "fittest," "most comfortable"). Second, there is a future body that cannot be perceived and is present only in the imagination.

However, if we connect these imaginings with the intention to realize them, the result is an overt action. During the planning phase, the action is rehearsed as a fantasy. Following Alfred Schütz (1932), it can be said that planning action means anticipating the results of the action in the future tense II – that is, the future perfect simple. I imagine a future in which something *will have been done* (I look at the future in *modo futuri exacti*). The action can be seen as a completed act. At a later time, I will be able to reflect on my act and evaluate it based on how far the past anticipations have become real. Thus, current action cannot be reviewed with regard to the intended and anticipated results, only the completed – and therefore past – act (see Brauer in this volume).

Prevention, however, is a mode of action that can never be reviewed from the future point of view, because it is always an ongoing action and never a completed act. Therefore, we can never really know whether prevention succeeds. It has a hypothetical implication that can never be reviewed; it is a kind of safety measure that we think will be of relevance. The aiming points are always shifted and deferred into the future; the moving target of successful prevention is thus never reached. The situation becomes worse through medical progress: Time and again, medicine propagates new means and new goals for anti-ageing measures and prevention.

Anti-ageing practices have led to an unsatisfying rat race: If they follow only the inner logic of prevention, they can never come to an end. There can never be enough prevention. In the following section, we describe the role of the body as a lived body in overcoming this logic and transforming anti-ageing practices from a high-strung rat race into a meaningful and fulfilling part of everyday life.

The lived body in discipline and self-care: overcoming the paradoxes and leaving the rat race

As we have seen, in understanding ageing as a risk factor, the body is threatened and threatening at the same time because it is exposed to inherent risks. Therefore, it is necessary to observe and control it; as a result, anti-ageing practices become a war against one's own body with its dispositions and changes. The body is thus seen as something problematic that needs to be controlled, shaped, and transformed. Anti-ageing interventions are often linked with practices that are experienced in everyday life as stressful and costly. And thus users say that they have to discipline themselves to carry them out regularly:

> Regular exercise, you really have to get over yourself for that . . . that's discipline for me, getting up and going out, year after year, at six o'clock in the morning, when it's raining, in the dark, in the winter, or when it's cold . . . . Of course, after a certain age you're fighting weight problems . . . and here exercise helps to keep it more or less under control. And this takes us to the next discipline: diet. For example, I've stopped eating white bread, actually I eat very little bread in general.
>
> – Ms. D. (56), interview

Here, anti-ageing measures involve self-discipline, which is also documented in the metaphor of the struggle ("fighting") against changes in the body. Under the control of self-discipline, the body seems to be permanently objectified and instrumentalized.

But as the philosophical anthropology of Helmuth Plessner (1975) has pointed out, we can always have two different attitudes toward the body. On one hand, we can have the perspective that the body is an objective fact, an instrument of our will, an object and a resource that may decline as people grow old. Thus, we have a body that we can control and use as an instrument. On the other hand, we *are* our body. There is no self that can be totally dissociated from the body. The self and the body are the same in most situations. Thereby, humans *have* bodies as objective bodies and humans *are* bodies as lived bodies.[8]

In the rat race of prevention, anti-ageing practices focus on the aspect of having a body and objectifying it, being able to shape it, and comparing it with other bodies. However, in everyday life, humans always have to balance the two aspects of having a body and being a body. A resolution of the difference is impossible: We can never stop being a lived body, and we need to objectify the body. If we only had an objectifying and reflexive attitude toward the body, our ontological security – which relies on the certainties of the lived body – would become precarious. For persons engaged in anti-ageing practices, these practices also involve experiences of being conscious and living in the present, 'listening' to one's own body, and taking good care of it:

> And that is this listening to my body. I did not do this before, because I ignored everything. Okay, maybe it is because now I simply have more time to perceive myself and my body . . . . Clearly, there are many people who burn the candle at both ends. But as I said, that rests on the individual. In my opinion, everyone is responsible for him- or herself, and takes care of themselves, no matter what the context.
>
> – Ms. C. (56), interview

In consciously dealing with oneself and one's own body ("perceive" as opposed to "ignored," "takes care of themselves" as opposed to "burn the candle at both ends"), the body appears precious and worth protecting in the implementation of anti-ageing practices. This self-caring and intensive preoccupation with the self, listening to and feeling the body, relates to basic everyday activities such as eating and drinking:

> I always ask myself: What's the reason? Why am I not balanced? Then we come to the questions of how I feel about my body, how I perceive myself, and how much I take care of myself . . . . Do I drink enough? Does my body have enough water? Do I eat well-balanced meals? How do I feel, how do I look?
>
> – Ms. A. (29), interview

In addition, using anti-ageing practices as self-care can contribute to personal identity. Thus, if Ms. C. "listens to her body" and "takes care of herself," she can dissociate herself from those who overexploit their bodies. Here, self-care is framed as part of a call for personal responsibility ("everyone is responsible for him- or herself"), yet this involves not only a positive orientation toward the self, but also a negative one:

> Life is price and profit. And people, or human beings, only want the profit, but have never learned to pay the price and are also not ready to do so. Yes, if I want something, I have to be ready to pay for it, in whatever form. And if I smoke, if I drink alcohol excessively, if I take drugs, if I do something else to botch my life – fine, I can do it, but then I also have to accept the consequences.
>
> – Ms. E. (66), interview

The logic of ownership, here metaphorically framed as "price and profit," aims in two directions: On one hand, if a person would like to stay healthy and live long, something has to be done for this ("one has to pay for it"). On the other hand, the consequences of a failure or negative behavior must be borne, because this is defined as "botching" an individual life – or as Mr. K. puts it, "wasting" one's life. Moreover, self-care can be achieved only if one's own self is sensed and perceived. One should therefore "consciously do what is good for the body and the spirit" (Mr. K., 66, interview). This conscious treatment of the body should be described as care and looking after oneself, rather than merely observing, controlling, and disciplining. In this dialectic of self-discipline and self-care, the feeling and bodily sensing of the here and now becomes an important facet of anti-ageing practices. The self-discipline required for the implementation of many anti-ageing practices is not just experienced as a constraint; it provides structure and orientation in everyday life, thus assuming a stabilizing and safeguarding function.

As a consequence, in performing daily practices that may be difficult and exhausting but are routinized and ritualized, those engaged in anti-ageing practices reach a kind of lived presence, practical certainty, and thus ontological security. If daily anti-ageing practices can be integrated into the habits of the lived body, the users can profit – whether or not the effects of these practices are actually realized in the future. By performing anti-ageing practices, they are able to dissociate themselves from lifestyles experienced as negative and to position themselves as self-caring and rational actors.

Discussion and conclusion

In the 'age of prevention' (Bröckling 2008, 40), modern society not only takes up the cause of a healthy population, but also induces an altered self-relation of its members. Because modern preventive medicine presents the individual lifestyle as a precondition for healthy life and ageing, the responsibility for health issues is assigned to individuals and becomes a relevant reference in their everyday life. Thus, the paradigm of prevention becomes a political program as well as a template for our daily life, while the 'preventive self' (Lengwiler and Madarász 2010) becomes a modern social figure.

In the case of anti-ageing medicine, the logic of prevention is based on the socially imagined possibility of successful, young, or active ageing. Anti-ageing medicine considers the individual body as a shapeable and improvable object. At the same time, it appears as corporal capital (an instrument and resource) that is lost with old age (Schroeter 2009). In this objectifying attitude, the Janus-faced character of human existence as having a body and being a body is systematically ignored (Plessner 1975).

The ageing body seems to be an inadequate means for expressing a self that is experienced as younger than one's chronological age (Featherstone and Hepworth 1991). Hence rejuvenation appears necessary in order to establish a coherent relationship to one's body. Nevertheless, we always feel and empathize with our ageing body and consider it a part of ourselves. This physical sense, and the corporeality and presence experienced in everyday life, constitute limits to a strictly objective optimization of the human body and at the same time introduce a degree of freedom regarding the requirements of anti-ageing medicine.

Our empirical analysis has attempted to state how this process may transpire. At the same time, these findings raise further questions for sociological research: The popularity of the semantics of 'mindfulness' toward one's own body indicates, for example, that the experience of corporeality is not simply a 'natural fact' (Nehring and Ernst 2013). The body is neither given without socio-cultural presuppositions nor completely constructed. Therefore, in the analysis, it has to be considered as a dimension of and participant in practices. The vocabulary of mindfulness is not only used in everyday language, but also rooted in the felt corporeality that unfolds a disproportionately greater cultural power – and this makes it tangible for sociology. In this sense, our contribution underlines that sociological analysis has to take the interaction of body, corporeality, and cultural imagination seriously and systematically include it in the reconstruction of practices. Only in this manner can we grasp the full scope of a practice such as anti-ageing.

Along these lines, our considerations indicate that engaging in anti-ageing practices is not merely an effect of general social developments. Rather, the users themselves produce and reproduce the significance of anti-ageing practices in their concrete everyday life. Therefore, anti-ageing must also be reconstructed from the perspective of those who, for example, buy anti-ageing products, use services in anti-ageing practices, follow a radical calorie restriction, or take hormones and dietary supplements in order to live longer and healthier (Pfaller 2016; Watts-Roy 2008, 2009). In this vein, our considerations contribute to the broader field of "cultural gerontology" (Twigg and Martin 2015), because the fact that the appeal and success of anti-ageing practices cannot be credited to actual medical effects does not necessarily mean that its users fall for the 'false promises' of the anti-ageing industry. The empirical material in no way suggests that users are grasping at straws in the sense of the "Dorian Gray Syndrome,"[9] a desperate and frantic clinging to youth, or that the measures and related promises of anti-ageing are completely far-fetched. The appeal of anti-ageing practices can be understood by analyzing these practices as concretely embodied in everyday life. Thus, our results point to the symbolic and performative potential of anti-ageing, which goes beyond the mere medical or cosmetic effect of a product. This potential can be adequately exposed only by reconstructing the everyday life of the relevant actors: Anti-ageing practices offer an ideal platform for people to present modern knowledge and value orientations, to act as rational actors and self-caring and independent subjects. These practices can help orient individuals and provide them with concrete ways of structuring their everyday life. Through the meanings involved in engaging in anti-ageing practices, the paradoxes of prevention are countered with practical certainty, thus creating an emotional security based on positive physical experience rather than medical evidence.

Notes

1 Ronald Bailey, "Google Invests in Immortality," Reason.com, https://reason.com/blog/2015/03/10/google-invests-in-immortality.
2 Calico LLC, "Calico," www.calicolabs.com/.
3 For the A4M, different founding dates can be found: On www.worldhealth.net/about-a4m/, the year is 1991. On www.a4m.com/about-a4m-overview.html, 1992 is mentioned. On Wikipedia, 1993 is mentioned.
4 Quotes from expert interviews, individual interviews, and focus groups were translated into English.
5 In the Anglo-American world, 'anti-ageing' is associated more with anti-ageing medicine and, in particular, with hormonal therapy. In Germany, 'anti-ageing' is primarily associated with cosmetic measures or products and hardly with genuine medical interventions. In the recruitment process and in the interviews and group discussions that provide the data basis for this article, this fact was taken into account by always explicitly speaking of 'preventive medical measures.' However, the more intensively users deal with anti-ageing practices and, for example, use medical and pharmaceutical services, the more likely they will associate the concept with the field of medicine.
6 The aim of the interdisciplinary joint project of medical ethics at the University Medical Center Göttingen and Sociology at Friedrich Alexander University Erlangen-Nürnberg was to better understand the importance of biomedicine for life planning with regard to aging and dying. Two practices – the living will and preventive/anti-ageing medicine – were considered. In addition to the analysis of users' everyday lives relevant for this article, the expert discourse and the institutional framing of the practices were also reconstructed (document analysis, expert interviews, observations at congresses and events). Taking part in the project were Silke Schicktanz, Frank Adloff, Mark Schweda, Larissa Pfaller, and Kai Brauer. 2010–2014, Project No. 01GP1004. See also www.biomedizinische-lebensplanung.uni-goettingen.de.
7 Stuckelberger (2008) seems to be optimistic with regard to the development of effective anti-ageing measures but pleads for strict quality and safety testing.
8 In German, this is the distinction between 'Körper' and 'Leib.'
9 "Das Dorian-Gray-Syndrom als psychoanalytisches Konzept," http://dorian-gray-syndrom.org.

References

Beck, U. 1992. *Risk Society: Towards a New Modernity*. London: Sage.
Binstock, R. H. 2004. "Anti-Aging Medicine: The History: Anti-Aging Medicine and Research: A Realm of Conflict and Profound Societal Implications." *The Journals of*

Gerontology, Series A: Biological Sciences and Medical Sciences 59 (6):523–533. doi: 10.1093/gerona/59.6.B523.

Bohnsack, R. 2010. "Documentary Method and Group Discussions." In *Qualitative Analysis and Documentary Method in International Educational Research*, edited by R. Bohnsack, N. Pfaff, and W. Weller, 99–124. Opladen: Barbara Budrich.

Bröckling, U. 2008. "Vorbeugen ist besser . . . Zur Soziologie der Prävention." *Behemoth: A Journal on Civilisation* 1 (1):38–48. doi: http://dx.doi.org/10.1524/behe.2008.0005.

Butler, R. N. 2001. "Is There an 'Anti-Aging' Medicine?" *Generations* 25 (4):63–65.

Butler, R. N., M. Fossel, S. M. Harman, C. B. Heward, S. J. Olshansky, T. T. Perls, D. J. Rothman, S. M. Rothman, H. R. Warner, M. D. West, and W. E. Wright. 2002. "Is There an Antiaging Medicine?" *The Journals of Gerontology, Series A: Biological Sciences and Medical Sciences* 57 (9):B333–B338. doi: 10.1093/gerona/57.9.B333.

Dyk, S. van. 2009. "'Junge Alte' im Spannungsfeld von liberaler Aktivierung, Ageism und Anti-ageing-Strategien." In *Die jungen Alten. Analysen einer neuen Sozialfigur*, edited by S. van Dyk and S. Lessenich, 316–339. Frankfurt am Main: Campus.

Ehni, H.-J. 2013. *Ethik der Biogerontologie*. Wiesbaden: VS Verlag für Sozialwissenschaften.

Featherstone, M., and M. Hepworth. 1991. "The Mask of Ageing and the Postmodern Life Course." In *The Body: Social Process and Cultural Theory*, edited by M. Featherstone, M. Hepworth, and B. S. Turner, 371–389. London: Sage.

Fishman, J. R., R. A. J. Settersten, and M. A. Flatt. 2010. "In the Vanguard of Biomedicine? The Curious and Contradictory Case of Anti-Ageing Medicine." *Sociology of Health & Illness* 32 (2):197–210. doi: 10.1111/j.1467-9566.2009.01212.x.

Glaser, B. G., and A. L. Strauss. 2009. *The Discovery of Grounded Theory: Strategies for Qualitative Research*. New Brunswick/London: Transaction Publishers.

Grey, A. D. N. J. de. 2004. "The War on Aging." In *The Scientific Conquest of Death: Essays on Infinite Lifespans*, edited by Immortality Institute, 29–46. Buenos Aires: LibrosEnRed.

Grey, A. D. N. J. de, and M. Rae. 2007. *Ending Aging: The Rejuvenation Breakthroughs That Could Reverse Human Aging in Our Lifetime*. New York: St. Martin's Press.

Lengwiler, M., and J. Madarász. 2010. "Präventionsgeschichte als Kulturgeschichte der Gesundheitspolitik." In *Das Präventive Selbst. Eine Kulturgeschichte moderner Gesundheitspolitik*, edited by M. Lengwiler and J. Madarász, 11–28. Bielefeld: Transcript.

Mykytyn, C. E. 2006a. "Anti-Aging Medicine: A Patient/Practitioner Movement to Redefine Aging." *Social Science & Medicine* 62 (3):643–653. doi: 10.1016/j.socscimed.2005.06.021.

Mykytyn, C. E. 2006b. "Contentious Terminology and Complicated Cartography of Anti-Aging Medicine." *Biogerontology* 7 (4):279–285. doi: 10.1007/s10522-006-9016-z.

Nehring, A., and C. Ernst. 2013. "Populäre Achtsamkeit. Kulturelle Aspekte einer Meditationspraxis zwischen Präsenzerfahrung und implizitem Wissen." In *Präsenz und implizites Wissen. Zur Interdependenz zweier Schlüsselbegriffe der Kultur- und Sozialwissenschaften*, edited by C. Ernst and H. Paul, 373–401. Bielefeld: Transcript.

Nohl, A.-M. 2009. *Interview und dokumentarische Methode. Anleitungen für die Forschungspraxis*. Wiesbaden: VS Verlag für Sozialwissenschaften.

Olshansky, S. J., L. Hayflick, and B. A. Carnes. 2002a. "Position Statement on Human Aging." *The Journals of Gerontology, Series A: Biological Sciences and Medical Sciences* 57 (8):B292–B297. doi: 10.1093/gerona/57.8.B292.

Olshansky, S. J., L. Hayflick, and B. A. Carnes. 2002b. "No Truth to the Fountain of Youth." *Scientific American* 286 (6):92–95.

Olshansky, S. J., L. Hayflick, and T. T. Perls. 2004a. "Anti-Aging Medicine: The Hype and the Reality: Part I." *The Journals of Gerontology, Series A: Biological Sciences and Medical Sciences* 59 (6):B513–B514.

Olshansky, S. J., L. Hayflick, and T. T. Perls. 2004b. "Anti-Aging Medicine: The Hype and the Reality: Part II." *The Journals of Gerontology, Series A: Biological Sciences and Medical Sciences* 59 (7):B649–B651. doi: 10.1093/gerona/59.7.B649.

Pfaller, L. 2016. *Anti-aging als Form der Lebensführung*. Wiesbaden: VS Verlag für Sozialwissenschaften.

Pfaller, L., and F. Adloff. 2017. "'Mein Leben ist ein Fortfahren von Eigenreparatur' – der Körper im Zeichen des Anti-Aging." In *Alter(n) und vergängliche Körper*, edited by R. Keller and M. Meuser, 91–107. Wiesbaden: VS Verlag für Sozialwissenschaften.

Pfaller, L., and M. Schweda. 2017. "Altern zwischen Medikalisierung und reflexiver Praxis: Der Alltag im Zeichen des Anti-Aging." In *Alter(n) als soziale und kulturelle Praxis: Ordnungen – Beziehungen – Materialitäten*, edited by C. Endter and S. Kienitz, 155–176. Bielefeld: transcript.

Plessner, H. 1975. *Die Stufen des Organischen und der Mensch. Einleitung in die philosophische Anthropologie*. Berlin: De Gruyter.

Schroeter, K. R. 2009. "Die Normierung alternder Körper – gouvernementale Aspekte des doing age." In *Die jungen Alten. Analysen einer neuen Sozialfigur*, edited by S. van Dyk and S. Lessenich, 359–379. Frankfurt am Main: Campus.

Schütz, A. 1932. *Der sinnhafte Aufbau der sozialen Welt. Eine Einleitung in die verstehende Soziologie*. Wien: Springer.

Schweda, M., B. Herrmann, and G. Marckmann. 2011. "Anti-Aging-Medizin in der gesetzlichen Krankenversicherung? Sozialrechtliche Entscheidungspraxis und gerechtigkeitsethische Reflexion." In *Altwerden ohne alt zu sein. Ethische Grenzen der Anti-Aging-Medizin*, edited by G. Maio, 172–193. Freiburg: Karl Alber.

Schweda, M., and L. Pfaller. 2014. "Colonization of Later Life? Laypersons' and Users' Agency Regarding Anti-Aging Medicine in Germany." *Social Science & Medicine* 118:159–165. doi: 10.1016/j.socscimed.2014.07.064.

Schweda, M., and L. Pfaller. 2017. "'Regimes of Hope' in Planning Later Life: Medical Optimism in the Field of Anti-Aging Medicine." In *Framing Age: Contested Knowledge in Science and Politics*, edited by I. Loffeier, B. Majerus, and T. Moulaert, 60–75. Abingdon, New York: Routledge.

Spindler, M. 2009. "Natürlich alt? Zur Neuerfindung der Natur des Alter(n)s in der Anti-Ageing-Medizin und der Sozialgerontologie." In *Die jungen Alten. Analysen einer neuen Sozialfigur*, edited by S. van Dyk and S. Lessenich, 380–402. Frankfurt am Main: Campus.

Spindler, M. 2014. *"Altern ja – aber gesundes Altern." Die Neubegründung der Anti-Aging-Medizin in Deutschland*. Wiesbaden: VS Verlag für Sozialwissenschaften.

Stuckelberger, A. 2008. *Anti-Ageing Medicine: Myths and Chances*. Zürich: vdf.

Twigg, J., and W. Martin, eds. 2015. *Routledge Handbook of Cultural Gerontology*. London/New York: Routledge.

Vincent, J. A. 2006. "Ageing Contested: Anti-Ageing Science and the Cultural Construction of Old Age." *Sociology* 40 (4):681–698. doi: 10.1177/0038038506065154.

Watts-Roy, D. M. 2008. *Delaying Aging and Extending Life: An Ancient Dream Revisited: Using Body Regimens as a Window to Reflect on Aging, Identity, and the Body*. http://hdl.handle.net/2345/1370.

Watts-Roy, D. M. 2009. "A Protest Vote? Users of Anti-Ageing Medicine Talk Back." *Health Sociology Review* 18 (4):434–445. doi: 10.5172/hesr.2009.18.4.434.

14 The visionary shaping of dementia research

Imaginations and scenarios in biopolitical narratives and ethical reflections

Silke Schicktanz

Introduction

"The past lies in the future": This motto can be referred to the special attention given to memory and memory loss in dementia which also is applied in the movie *Rise of the Planet of the Apes* directed by Rupert Watt.[1] In this 2011 prequel, fans of the original late 1960s sci-fi movie *The Planet of the Apes* not only learn how the apes became so intelligent that they managed to rule and even domesticate humans, but also how important today's Alzheimer's dementia research is. Dementia, a condition mainly neglected in the collective memory of public health until the end of the 20th century, has now gained so much popular attention that some even speak of a "cultural dementia boom" (Swinnen and Schweda 2015, 10).

In the 2011 movie *Rise of the Planet of the Apes*, in present days a new (somatic) gene therapy targeted at dementia and applied in nonhuman-primate experiments significantly boosts the primates' social and cognitive intelligence. The movie's story relies on the scientific idea that increased cognitive resources are the silver bullet against the illness of 'forgetting.' Feeling inspired by the outstanding intelligence performances of the tested chimpanzees, the young leading researcher (here rather a failed hero than a mad scientist) is tempted to apply the new drug to his demented father. He does so, bypassing common professional ethics of informed consent of his father or any review-board assessment, justifying his actions as a case of 'ultimate ratio' and by his passionate love for his father.

Although the movie, overall, presents more fiction than science, there are allusions to some historical scientific facts. For example, in the movie the success of the illicit treatment for the demented father is brief and unsustainable; this is reminiscent of the famous story of *Awakenings*, a 1990 movie based on neurologist Oliver Sacks's (1973) published memories of the first treatment of neurological patients with encephalitis lethargica where the application of L-DOPA revealed the still complex feelings and intentions of patients but did not lead to a healing or long-term treatment. Both movies' lesson for research ethics is that some problems or side effects are often unforeseen in modern research. In *Rise of the Planet of the Apes*, the somatic gene therapy of a pregnant chimpanzee leads to a transfection to her offspring by inserting the 'new genes' into the gene pool of the fetus. Hence, this baby chimp develops, after being saved during a laboratory accident and then raised by the young researchers and his demented father, into a cognitively and socially perfectly equipped 'human ape' – later becoming the leader of the new race of apes.

Apart from the many interesting ethical provocations this pop-cultural account offers – including themes such as animal minds being similar to human minds, the criteria for achieving (or losing) personhood status, and the possibility of 'enhancing' species by transgressing common boundaries of clinical research – the aim of finding a 'silver bullet' against dementia seems morally unrevoked.

There is a common sense that any healing or efficient treatment for dementia would be a noble thing, but it still remains fiction rather than science. Apart from the Hollywood-blockbuster strategies of oversimplification and of using stereotypes, *Rise of the Planet of the Apes* illustrates to a great extent many critical, interlinked issues within the broader debate on dementia research[2] and how we address to various types of future anticipations for developing an individual as well as a collective perspective about dementia in general and dementia research in particular.

In the following, I will discuss the critical issues and open questions and related phenomena from a normative point of view in three main steps. First, I will critically analyze how imaginations and worst-case scenarios are used in the biopolitics of dementia. I use the term 'biopolitics' here in regard to publicly made claims or accounts about the value of life sciences or healthcare by representatives of institutions or politically active actors, in situations in which the normative agenda is often rather hidden. Second, I will highlight specifically how different cultural resources of images or worst-case scenarios are activated by various stakeholders to argue in favor of or against dementia research. I will focus on political, administrative stakeholders and then on patient advocates or patient organizations and show how "neurocultures" (Williams, Higgs, and Katz 2012) frame such biopolitical endeavors. Third, I will elicit from a more general moral point of view the use of imaginations, scenarios, and later-life planning to guide individual and collective decisions. For this, I will expand the scope and explore some essential aspects of how anticipation guides our long-term decision-making by taking psychological and decision-theoretical insights into account. In this way, I will examine how negative anticipations of future events can particularly influence our planning, and therefore our dealing with and developing of such negative anticipations requires special normative attention.

So, overall, I will not argue for eliminating or deleting imaginations and scenarios from our discourse but make a case for a more reflective and norm-grounded use of such anticipations in the public and expert debate on dementia and ageing. I will illustrate how bioethics should always be understood as culturally embedded. Reflecting on these cultural perspectives as a positive source and provocation of bioethical content relies on a dialectic nature of reasoning.

The biopolitical doubling effect of anticipation: from dementia care to risk prediction

Dementia is understood as a syndrome of progressive or chronic nature that impairs a person's cognitive functions, including his/her memory, orientation, planning and learning abilities, comprehension, language, and judgment. In its advanced stage, it includes serious motor and sensory impairments. Alzheimer's disease (AD), one of the most common forms of dementia, dominates the public's perception of this sydrome. Several therapies are being tested, but a cure is still not available. Thus, existing medication only moderates symptoms for some AD patients. According to current theories, a major reason for this is that AD is a form of slowly progressing dementia with a long pre-clinical phase that starts with an asymptomatic stage and transforms into a symptomatic stage involving subjective or mild cognitive impairment (SCI/MCI); AD eventually develops into a clinical syndromal disease with an already advanced pathology (Hampel et al. 2014). Current research in diagnosis and treatment targets this so-called prodromal stage of AD. Predictive biomarkers are currently used in different types of (primary and secondary) prevention trials, involving the long-term hope that this can delay or even prevent the onset of dementia in the future (Sperling, Karlawish, and Johnson 2013; Le Couteur et al. 2013). The term 'biomarker' includes "clinical, cognitive, imaging, genetic and biochemical" (Weiner et al. 2010) approaches. Biomarkers are used "to determine the likelihood of cognitive and functional progression that will occur within a defined period" (Albert et al. 2011, 5). The effective use of such biomarkers in the clinical field will require the ability to predict a probability of decline or progression of dementia in an individual person for a specific time interval with a single biomarker or multiple ones. The MCI stage seems especially useful as a baseline for further predictive biomarker research and prevention trials, as it is much better validated now. Although earlier attempts at using genetic testing for AD (APOE in particular) are no longer recommended due to a very low predictive value, various biomarkers are currently being developed.[3] These are examined in various international multicenter studies, to test and compare their clinical predictive validity through prospective longitudinal research (Vellas et al. 2011). This research aims at defining scores and standardized, reproducible protocols. This is an ongoing research-validation process, as a current study by Vos et al. (2015) has revealed variance and different predictive values of existing protocols for MCI due to AD. In light of this variance, the challenges of risk communication become evident: It will be difficult to provide information on not only whether there is a higher risk, but also which probability or test validity this assessment of risk is based on.

These new forms of risk prediction indicate that research is shifting from a focus on care and living with dementia to the aim of prevention and/or curing of dementia.[4] Overall, this seems to be a legitimate goal. However, what we are observing here is what I call the 'doubling effect' of dementia anticipation. First, there is the mostly unavoidable individualized anticipation every affected person has to struggle with in the case of an early diagnosis of dementia. This can already be classified as 'passage' into a new illness identity (Glaser and Strauss 1971; Orona 1990). From an everyday-life perspective, it entails not only adjusting to limited physical or cognitive resources and to social stigma, for example, but also anticipating, making, or delegating decisions concerning care, driving, financial issues, housing, exercise, eating or drinking habits, and so on.

However, the new paradigm of dementia as a continuum and the current focus on prediction or identification of at-risk persons adds another layer to this individual, ordinary issue of anticipation. What is needed in addition is a collective form of anticipation encompassing what to do when with whom in which stage of at-risk, prodromal, early, or late dementia. The concept of prediction not only creates a new group of affected persons (Schicktanz 2015; Schicktanz, Schweda, and Franzen 2008) but also involves a collective perspective entering all individual questions on a socio-political side: When and how do we need to 'inform' or confront people with such predictions? Does a risk of dementia mean we should prepone basic decisions about financial, care, or end-of-life issues? How do public or healthcare institutions foster the idea that making decisions under risk prediction or uncertainty is better than just surrendering to fate (Schicktanz et al. 2014)?

Various authors have pointed to conceptual problems of prodromal dementia and MCI (e.g., Mukadam et al. 2015; Werner and Korczyn 2008), as there is a complicated entanglement of pathological and normal cognitive decline in ageing (Lock 2013; see Werner and Schicktanz in this volume).

However, these important debates are unlikely to hinder the broad implementation of biomarkers in clinical practice in the not-too-distant future. This can be assumed by the success story of genetic testing for non-treatable or late-onset diseases. Because despite the questionable necessity of assessing risk for certain diseases, despite ethical concerns, and despite legal loopholes (see below), biological predictors of disease hold a general fascination for some people, and for them it remains relevant to obtain visions of their future, as they want to plan ahead.

Moral framing of predictive testing as knowing or not knowing the future

The prevailing question in genetic testing is whether we *want* to know or rather not. Following from here, one can ask how the ethical and legal approaches that have been developed along the lines of a 'right to know' as well as a 'right not to know' (including the emerging 'duties to know' in the field of genetics) can be applied to the predictive application of other biomarkers for diagnosing prodromal dementia (Beck and Schicktanz 2016). The leading consequential question of which psychological and social risks may arise from such early knowledge is prevalent in the medical-professional context, for good reason: It corresponds with the professional duty to promote well-being and avoid harm by disclosing or not disclosing the results of a predictive test. Especially in cases of late-onset diseases, such as dementia, one can critically question whether there is any benefit, from an individual or a social point of view. The medical profession has a gatekeeper function and responsibility to foresee effects (such as psychosocial ones) of how the affected person will cope with this information. The dilemma of predictive medicine has led to numerous national genetic testing laws and international guidelines around the 'right to know' for those who want to be tested, enabling them to have access to results of genetic testing, but also 'the right not know' for those who do not want to know. Both combined rights were introduced in 1997 by the Council of Europe's *Convention of Human Rights and Biomedicine*, and they represent the practical-ethical and legal standard for protection of the individual right to self-determination in the context of predictive medicine (Andorno 2004). A paradigmatic case is genetic testing for Huntington's disease (HD), a late-onset, non-treatable neuroprogressive disease. Current standards for genetic counselling in the case of HD require intensive pre-test genetic and psychosocial counselling. Professionals have to stress the fact that testing is voluntary and provide comprehensive post-counselling about the scientific meaning of being 'at risk,' including likelihood, penetrance, and variations, even if HD counts as a case with a relatively high level of prediction. Moreover, all affected persons should receive sufficient information about social, economic, and psychological effects once the diagnosis is disclosed. Finally, there are requests for providing sufficient time for decision-making (MacLeod et al. 2013). These rules are defeated in cases of diseases for which no efficient treatment is available, and therefore the main value of such disclosure can be seen in the relief or personal value of knowing. In this sense, the debate has tried to fix the dilemma of predicting late-onset diseases by focusing on the professional duties of proper information and well-reasoned communication. Overall, we can learn from the ethical debate of genetic testing for late-onset, untreatable diseases and assess how professional standards of counselling should also be applied to predictive dementia testing (Beck and Schicktanz 2016). However, from a moral point of view, the question of whether professionals should respect the right to know (or the right not to know) is not the only relevant one. In addition, we need a change of perspective: We need to put ourselves in the shoes of those to be tested. Morally, it is a crucial question of personal wisdom and individual responsibility whether we would like to know how we will age. Do we really want to know which age-related disease we might have to face in the next 10, 20, or 30 years, and, if so, what will we do with such information? As in the case of dementia prediction, current risk prediction is even vaguer than in cases of, for example, HD; therefore the value of the knowledge of risk can be critically questioned.

One way to deal with this question is to reject any deterministic insight into our fate by assuming that our ignorance of tragic events such as the hour of our death or major calamities ensures true freedom concerning our actions and agency. Apart from the convincing refusal of such tragic and radical information, one can still believe that some information in one's own biography or in that of a closely related person is a meaningful 'project' of life conception inevitably related to late modernity. Since the 20th century, increasing knowledge about how social, medical, or economic factors shape individual biographies (Giddens 1991) has permeated our daily lives; thus, it seems not only rational but also reasonable to search for and consider such information for the planning of our later life. With the shift in understanding one's biography as one's own project, each of us is responsible for it (unless the social system does not hinder us) instead of understanding the life course and one's biography as solely ruled by the Gods or stars (see also Schweda in this volume).

However, the increasing interest in our future relies not only on individual preferences but also on collective expectations, which are often intermingled; both individual preferences and collective expectations are highly dependent on humans' ability to form imaginations and scenarios (Taylor 1989). These imaginations and scenarios often implicitly and sometimes explicitly play a role concerning whether a person decides for or against the disclosure of predictive information. For example, some people may believe that dementia is so horrible that they do not want to know whether they are at risk, because they fear psycho-social effects such as depression or stigmatization before the onset. Other people may believe that dementia is just another inevitable form of ageing and therefore cheerfully embrace such changes.

How is the spectrum of our imaginations framed by existing socio-cultural images of ageing and diseases such as dementia? This descriptive question is of utmost relevance for further socio-ethical considerations, concerning how we and others shape the current discourse – which imaginations, visions, and scenarios do we spread, develop, or assess?

The current professional paradigm of counselling and respecting the right to know/not to know, as introduced on page 208, suggests that individual preferences are mainly or even exclusively influenced by the professionals' input. For very rare diseases, such as HD, which are rarely publicly discussed and unknown to most laypersons this might be very plausible. But still, family experience (McAllister 2003) is an additional, possibly highly important, source of information that influence the individual's anticipation what a prognosis can entail. This is particularly true for dominant hereditary diseases, while for recessive, rare diseases family experience does not exist that can be referred to.

In contrast, age-related syndromes such as 'dementia' differ significantly with regard to their popularization. While most laypersons still have no idea what HD implies physically and psychologically for those affected, everybody *seems* to know what 'dementia' means to themselves and to the social environment. This observation is based on two facts. First, the higher prevalence of dementia (or specific forms such as AD) due to demographic ageing statistically increases the possibility that more people share family experience. Many have their own family story about living with dementia. Grandparents, aunts, uncles, or parents who in one way or another suffer from memory loss, forgetfulness, or loss of social functioning during their process of ageing serve as examples and as a projection screen for one's own expectations.

However, these experiences are not isolated but embedded in a cultural framework. Accordingly, a second source of information about dementia are publicly and culturally shared narratives and images – in the following summarized as anticipations (how dementia is or will be) – popularized through movies, newspaper reports, and literature, as well as dominant biopolitical voices.

Therefore, when reflecting on the dilemma of 'to know versus not to know our later fate,' we are well advised to include a thorough understanding of the social framing of these underlying, often implicitly culturally embedded anticipations.

In the following, I will therefore differentiate between types of content of anticipation, especially when it comes to dementia research, and afterward discuss the procedure of decision-making and how this helps ethically reflect life plans according to predictive dementia information.

Anticipation of future dementia: dominant imaginations and scenarios in the biopolitical discourse

Overall, I understand anticipation as our human ability to project ideas into a prospective timeframe. While our memory builds the capacity to explore the retrospective timeframe, it often serves as a reservoir of analogies for future anticipation. Fantasy and creativity can provide us with "day dreams and utopias," as Ernst Bloch (1985) called them. In the context of public discourses and sociocultural framing, two main types of anticipation prevail: imaginations and the 'scenario.'

Imaginations are visually formed thoughts. Imaginations are powerful in their spatial-visual concreteness, framed by canonical presentations and stereotypes.[5] The often even iconic presentations are internalized social constructs that pretend to present social reality. As such, they can be understood as an in-between, a third complementation to be added to the two main forms of 'Anschauung.' Immanuel Kant (1974) epistemologically differentiated 'empirical perceptions' (sensibility) and 'true ideas' (understanding) such as time and space, both essential to our ability of reasoning. The third form of 'Anschauung' is in Kant's terminology the "facultas imaginandi" – a human faculty for imagination and fantasy relevant for art and creativity (see also Brook 2013). In the following, I am mainly interested in how such imaginations are used in an anticipatory way, presenting a vision of future comings or developments.

The 'scenario' is often used in technology assessment and future studies (Chermack, Lynham, and Ruona 2001; Tran and Daim 2008; Van Den Ende et al. 1998). A scenario can be understood as a temporal narration, in which we anticipate individual, social, or technical development over time. The scenario – whether considered worst or best case – is rather generalized and less concrete than many imaginations. However, it consists of elements that can more easily be identified as morally loaded in a negative as well as positive sense.

The use of scenarios – mainly worst-case scenarios – currently dominates public-policy debates in most Western industrialized countries (OECD 2015; World Health Organization 2012). During the 2013 G8 summit, UK prime minister David Cameron and his advisers embedded their call for intensified research, bio-banking, and biotech-industry involvement to 'fight dementia,' and by equating dementia with diseases such as cancer, HIV, or malaria, the media echoed dementia as 'a 21st century plague.'[6] However, the use of military metaphors of war, such as 'the fight' or 'combat,' (George, Whitehouse, and Whitehouse 2016) is common when discussing dementia in public-policy contexts: In the European parliament, the disease was framed as an upcoming invasion ("this number is estimated to nearly double every 20 years, possibly reaching 65.7 million in 2030"), followed by several economic prognoses (worst-case scenario) that "the total direct medical and social care costs of Alzheimer's disease in Europe amount to USD 135.04 billion" (European Parliament 2011).

In a similar manner, the Obama administration and US government communiqués have adopted such worst-case scenarios.[7] These *typical* worst-case scenarios always consist of four main elements:

1 the prospected timeline: the first half of the 21st century;
2 demographic developments: the sheer number of people with dementia (fully stripped of any relations or comparison to other collectives);
3 accumulated estimated cost development: 'many billions,' without any comparison to other estimated costs for socially challenging issues, such as military technologies or electronic waste disposal; and
4 a moral claim pro research, as it will 'automatically' provide prevention and the diagnostics of pre-dementia would solve the problem.

As typical for such a simplified scenario-drawing is the dramatization of some factors (costs, demographic development) in a time period that spans over our/the average reader's generation and lifespan. Therefore, it creates a personal affect by means of an emotional identification (not necessarily as a causal relationship; see for these differences Schicktanz, Schweda, and Franzen 2008). However, the promised solution 'research' is objectively unlinked to the major driving factors of the problem (demographic development/costs).

In a similar fashion, Annette Leibing (2015) argued that the analysis of public media such as newspapers indicates a less empathic picture. For a long time, dementia and demented people were presented as 'victims.' The new predictive paradigm, which frequently occurs in newspaper reports, does not change the overall impression but adds an impression of 'agency' and thus responsibility: If with preventive and pre-emptive agency it is possible to avoid dementia, those who still develop dementia are perceived no longer simply as victims but as careless or failing to some extent. Hence, we need to be aware that this paradigm change can cause a new wave of blaming and stigmatization for dementia patients. Once we understand dementia not as an involuntary, inevitable illness but as the result of careless behavior – irresponsible neglect of predictions and preventive measures – it is very likely that patients will be blamed or stigmatized in a new dimension. Other illnesses, such as obesity, lung cancer, and HIV, serve as examples for such societal developments.

Another relevant, but often less recognized, source of important biopolitical arguments in academic debate are patient organizations and their campaigns (Schicktanz 2015; Schicktanz and Jordan 2013). In the following, I summarize results of multi-sited research conducted between 2011 and 2015 comparing views and visions of the major leading US and German patient organizations (PO) for Alzheimer's disease.[8] The comparison of the US and German context will reveal the cultural framing and embedding of such biopolitical images and scenarios. The differences not only illuminate the complexity of bioethical and biopolitical argumentation embedded in historical contexts and current healthcare policies, but also contribute to a more differentiated picture of the assumed 'Western, industrialized' discourse.

The US Alzheimer's Association (which I will abbreviate as US ALZ) is the world's largest patient-advocacy group, providing support for affected people by means of local support groups, state chapter associations, telephone hotlines, and online material. Founded in 1980, the Alzheimer's Association (according to its own statement) is the largest private funder of research for Alzheimer's disease in the world (in 2011, US$13 million; in 2015, US$17 million). The implementation of a US federal act covering Alzheimer's disease in 2010 was a major result of the Alzheimer's Association advocacy campaign.[9] The German Alzheimer's Society (Deutsche Alzheimer Gesellschaft, which I will abbreviate as GER ALZ), founded in 1989, is the largest German AD-related advocacy group, also providing a help line, online materials, and research funding (max. €200,000 per year since 2011). It actively pursues political lobbying and is a member of the patient groups represented in the Federal Joint Committee – the highest decision-making body of the joint self-government of physicians, dentists, hospitals, and health-insurance funds in Germany.

In comparing the major slogans and statements on their respective websites, we discovered an interesting difference:[10] While US ALZ used slogans such as "Fighting a crisis" and "End Alzheimer's," the GER ALZ proposed "Ageing with dignity" or just positively framed "Living with AD." The content of their websites offers insight into different underlying worst-case scenarios. For US ALZ, an ageing society will suffer from economic and cultural costs of care for AD. Alzheimer's disease was portrayed according to its serious effects on family members and caregivers. US ALZ stressed the fact that the progressive nature of the disease worsens all situations and that patients lose their ability to make sense of the world.[11] In contrast, GER ALZ rather proposed the position that current science and society tend to discriminate and single out human beings with AD. They therefore stated that "disability and chronic disease should be regarded as part of being a human being" and propose "avoidance of singling out or manipulation." Their guiding principle was that the dignity and value of life of people with AD should not be questioned.[12]

The two advocacy groups also promoted different aims regarding research. For US ALZ, biomedical research was key to prevention and treatment.[13] The website said the organization funded multi-targeted research and had initiated so-called roundtables between experts, the pharma industry, and affected persons.[14] Further, US ALZ was searching for "volunteers for clinical trials" and was offering a "trial match" databank, where affected persons or their relatives could check for ongoing pharmaceutical or neuroimaging clinical research for the purpose of enrolling these patients as research participants.[15] While GER ALZ also supported research, most of it rather focused on how to improve medical care or explored new forms of communicative or social-care strategies for particular subgroups (such as people living in rural areas or diverse ethnic groups).[16] GER ALZ also explicitly objected to third-party beneficial research with incompetent patients. US ALZ was directly involved in current biomarker research of various types. It is worthwhile to note that the US health-insurance system, with its out-of-pocket coverage for long-term healthcare, does not provide a guarantee that people identified as being at a higher risk of dementia will not encounter disadvantages in the future (Zick et al. 2005). GER ALZ rejected any research or application of genetic tests if this would lead to exclusion or disadvantages of demented persons[17] but offered links to some clinical-research sites.[18]

These general tendencies are substantiated with posters or visual social advertisement campaigns supported or provided by these organizations (see Figures 14.1 and 14.2).

The US campaigns tend to use phrases and topics that can be summarized under the motto of 'heroization in a crisis.' This is because they use slogans such as "Create a world without Alzheimer's disease" and "Be a hero: Join a clinical trial. Sign up for the Alzheimer's clinical trial match." This supports the overall mission of US ALZ to increase the priority setting for Alzheimer's research in the US national healthcare and research agenda by dramatizing the economic and social costs. Having said this, fighting stigmatization is not a neglected issue and is regularly mentioned by representatives of US ALZ. They try to give the affected persons (mainly selected advocate) or younger celebrities a 'voice' and 'face' in their campaigns. These persons are serving as testimonial for the serious necessity to fight the cause of the disease.

The German campaigns illustrate a rather different 'image' and imagination of dementia.[19] Here, happy or funny elderly persons are depicted, often in social interactions. Hence, there is a tendency to fight the stigma of dementia as eroding

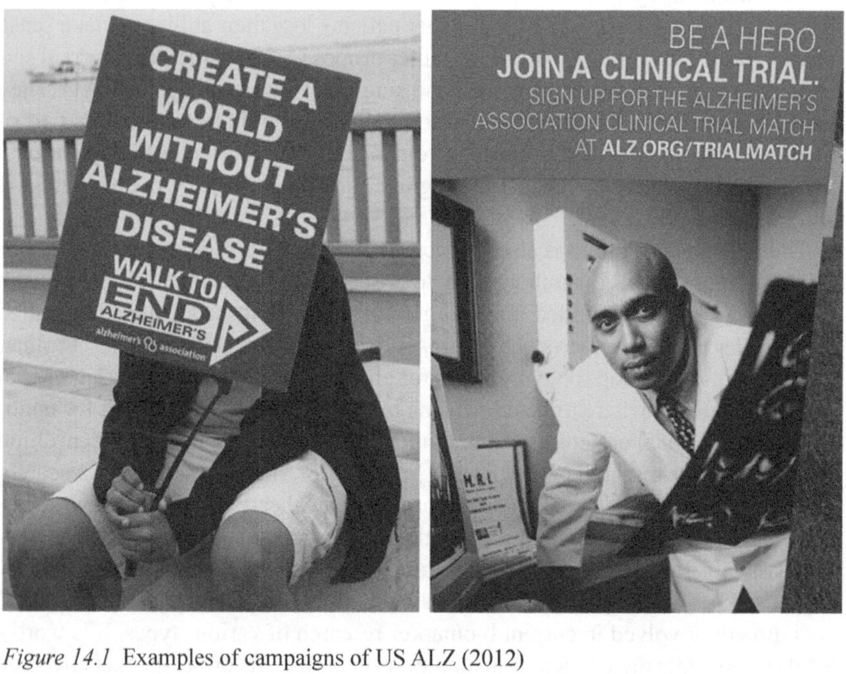

Figure 14.1 Examples of campaigns of US ALZ (2012)

Source: Pictures taken by the author during Alzheimer's Walk in San Francisco.

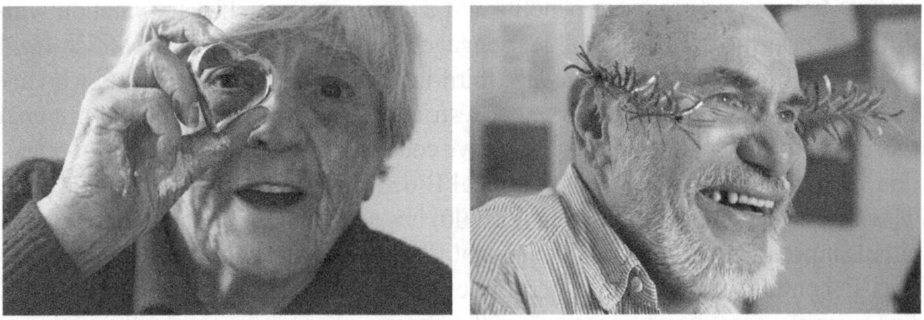

Figure 14.2 Examples of motifs from campaigns supported by GER ALZ

Note: On the left: "Active living with dementia"; and on the right: "Confetti in the mind."

Source: Johanniter – Birgit Betzelt / "Konfetti im Kopf" – Michael Hagedorn.

one's personality and quality of life. The campaigns propose a different image of dementia, in which persons with dementia are depictured in an undramatic or harmless stage of otherness.

Both, worst case scenarios and images provided in these different channels (Internet and poster campaigns) still offer a coherent but differing manner for dealing with dementia as PO. The coherence can be seen with regard to the overall position toward healthcare provision. That is, in Germany, it seems that the public is confident in or satisfied with the provision of public healthcare for the elderly.[20] This allows GER ALZ to take a position insisting on care and social solutions for dealing with dementia. In the US, as nursing homes and long-term care are not fully covered by Medicare or Obamacare, a feeling of distrust prevails in public healthcare. Therefore, solutions beyond care, such as prevention or healing treatments, are the logical consequence.

Patient advocacy in Germany tends to stress the vulnerability of demented patients and their need for protection not only in the context of research, but also generally; this strategy risks impeding the empowerment of affected persons. On the other hand, the US has quite strong procedural and relational tools to empower patient autonomy, including the very strong, highly politically active US ALZ. The systematic involvement of patient representatives in the current National Institute for Ageing (NIA)'s initiatives and their continuous exchange with researchers in closed workshops shows the impact of patient advocacy on policymaking. However, there is a risk of instrumentalizing demented patients by overstressing self-determination or volunteering (in research) as a social duty.

The shaping of dementia research by these two patient organizations thus differs with regard to both the epistemic (what is the problem?) and ethical (how should we solve it?) dimensions of research. On one hand, they differ in their prioritization of the kind of research necessary to 'solve' the serious problems dementia causes for patients, their families, and societies. On the other hand, they have different opinions about whether involving patients with severe cognitive impairment in clinical, pharmaceutical, psychological, or even sociological research is ethically acceptable, as they balance risks against benefits and agency against self-determination with different priorities. This biopolitical engagement is embedded in a politico-legal and cultural framework.[21] In the US, third-interest research with patients who are cognitively impaired is allowed under restrictions for proxy consent and minimal risk or if a legally authorized representative consents and there are no signs of objection by the incompetent person (National Bioethics Advisory Commission 1998). The American College of Physicians (2000) has added that if research participation entails more than minimal risk, a national IRB should review the research application. In contrast, the German expert discourse on ethics and law is less permissive. For example, Germany has not signed the Oviedo *Convention for the Protection of Human Rights and Dignity of the Human Being with Regard to the Application of Biology and Medicine: Convention on Human Rights and Biomedicine* developed by the Council of Europe (1997), because the convention does allow third-interest research with cognitively impaired patients. In Germany, there is no consensus about how to deal with this problem; the Central Ethics Board of German Chamber of Physicians (1997) suggests allowing such research, but only if there is a minimal burden, consent by a legal representative, and no opposing behavior of the patient. Others suggest that it should be allowed only if consented to in an advanced research directive (ARD) (Honnefelder in Hirnliga e.V. 1995, 49f.; Jongsma and van de Vathorst 2015), but the instrument of ARD is yet not common in Germany. Patient representatives have contrarily stated that there are no acceptable conditions and they would reject any proxy consent even if there were only minimal burden because they address the risk of instrumentalization by referring to historical experience of Nazi medicine (Helmchen 1999; Hirnliga e.V. 1995). In the summer of 2016, a draft for reforming a set of regulations for pharmaceutical testing in accordance with EU regulations fired up the dispute in Germany over whether third-party research with demented persons should be allowed. In November 2016 a bill was finally adopted in which the concept of ARD was introduced for allowing research with demented participants. Whether this compromise will practical work is unclear, as the composing of ARD for dementia research is very new and might poses new ethical problems.

Thus, the differences between the US and German patient organizations might be explained not only by different biocultural and health-political frameworks but also by how historical experience serves as a cultural resource in the creation of scenarios. In Germany, the historical experience of Nazi medicine, with its practice of singling out and discriminating against patients with mental illness and those counted as 'economically valueless' (such as elderly people), remains an unspoken critical threshold for the 'common good.' Such historical legacy is not as relevant in the US.[22]

Strategies for making life plans and long-term decisions: some general considerations

As already mentioned, I am ethically interested in the manner in which anticipations of the future guide our individual and collective (long-term) decision-making.

To understand the critique of current anticipations of dementia in biopolitics from a normative point of view, we first need to clarify how these anticipations *can or even do influence decisions.* Often, we *assume* that there is an interaction – but what kind is rarely spelled out. In the following, I therefore back up some of these assumptions by exploring in more detail what I mean by 'life planning' or 'long-term decision making.'

Planning our own biography in advance can be considered part of modern identity concepts (Giddens 1991). Whether such life plans are still in line with social expectations related to gender, class, or ethnic belonging or are less socially predictable, more fractured, and highly individualized can be disputed – and definitely varies by culture. Some might object to the idea that our human capacity to anticipate the future is very well established. Neither the oracle of Delphi nor mentalists or fortune-tellers can count as trustworthy sources for exactly predicting future events – even if their popularity seems unbroken until today. And academic areas such as foresight (future) studies also do not count to the most established scientific fields. In contrast, foresight studies are often rather used in political contexts for determining particular interests or for justifying new trends in technology policy.[23] Also, proponents of postmodernity draw a picture of us as fractured, fluid, hybrid selves, living in multiple worlds, focusing on the here and now. While this may be true for some in our late-modern times, we can hardly adopt this as a general rule from a perspective that tolerates pluralism in lifestyles – and, as such, we need to consider both extremes as ends of a spectrum, the socially conforming and the hybrid self.[24]

Theories of strategic thinking in modern psychology provide an interesting alternative approach to these extreme endpoints. They have increasingly contributed to our understanding of how complex but also anthropologically manifested the idea of anticipation and planning is. Modern psychology classifies this as decision-making or planning under uncertainty – or under risk if there are probabilities available for future events (e.g., Kahneman 2011; Kahneman, Slovic, and Tversky 1982). The phenomena of short-term decision-making and long-term decision-making are not always sufficiently distinct in our debates. Thus, it is clear that our capacities of assessment differ according to our time awareness, the cultural resources (i.e., stability), or our fantasy. Moral philosophers rarely directly address the time dimension when postulating general moral commitments – whether our actions will kill somebody today or in ten years seems irrelevant from a deontological perspective, as killing is morally wrong (whether we do it by stabbing someone with a knife or by secretly administering arsenic). However, in a positive sense, moral orientation sometimes differs radically whether we provide moral orientation for this or the next generation (i.e., in evaluating the environmental impacts of our actions) or whether we propose responsible actions for the coming weeks or years (Schicktanz 2016; Schicktanz and Schweda 2012).

Many modern political ethical theories rely on the assumption that planning and thinking ahead is a human prerequisite for our moral thinking of universality and justice (Immanuel Kant or John Stuart Mill), for the concept of social responsibility in a globalized world (Iris Young) or for building fair and just social relationships in a concrete political system (John Rawls). In this sense, reformistic political ethical theories have a vision of a just and fair system in the not-too-far but also not immediate future. In order to achieve this vision, we need to deliberate and implement moral, political, and legal norms. But what remains very vague is the manner in which we use different strategies for anticipating such long-term explorations: What time and social dimension do we take into account? What kind of statistics or heuristics do we incorporate into our assessment of future events (Gigerenzer 2003; Kahneman, Slovic, and Tversky 1982)? How do we balance different outcomes, their moral and emotional evaluations, and how do we value potential outcomes by satisfaction or regret (Zeelenberg 1999, 2015)?

In the following, I mainly focus on the socio-cultural anticipations and how they may impact our rational decision-making. This is also inspired by some findings of current decision theory in psychology and behavioral economy. According to Zeelenberg (2015), current decision theory is much beyond the traditional concept of rational choice, as emotions and/or values are now included for elaborating 'wise judgments.' Instead of economic maximization of outcome, now wise judgments are the hallmarks of 'rationality.' Those wise judgments may not be appropriate for discussing our choices between chocolate and strawberry ice-cream[25] but count in cases where we reason about decisions for important life choices. By life choices, I mean planning actions such as training for occupation A, marrying person B, having 0-n children, buying a house C, moving to city D, and so on (see also Schwartz 2015). This type of long-term decision-making is characterized by uncertainty or ambiguity, as all outcomes originate from multi-causality. Therefore, the standard expected utility calculation cannot be accomplished (as rationalists normally assume). We are aware of this, and still we try to achieve robust satisfaction with our decisions by applying different reasoning strategies (Zeelenberg 2015). Some strategies seem to anticipate most negative or most positive outcomes and assess them against each other in a pessimistic minimax or an optimistic maximax strategy (what would be the worst-case or what would be the best-case scenario). To give these scenarios flesh and blood, we allude to cultural and personal experiences of outcomes in similar situations. However, what complicates these decision-making procedures is that we assess not only the material outcome of our decisions, but also how that outcome may impact our identity and self. Satisfaction, regret, and other emotions therefore factor into important life decisions. Especially in cases where we will receive feedback of forgone alternatives, it seems that regret guides many choices (Zeelenberg 2015, 162).

Ethically speaking, planning is important for guaranteeing continuity and social safety but also for shaping personal and moral identity. Although planning helps us create a continuous identity (that we reconstruct by narration), it depends on some *external* continuity. The stability of social and legal frameworks and the reliability and authenticity of our personal preferences and desires are mainly constitutive and increase the chance that long-term decisions can be identified as such. It is important to stress again that the dimension of planning is relevant for most modern conceptions of individual and social moral life. For example, John Rawls (1971, chapters 6.3–6.4) already pointed to the necessity of planning as part of ethical self-deliberation – an important requirement for all rational-communicative ethics as well as for ethical approaches stressing the necessity for a qualitative conception of identity as a source for action. Finally, it is problematic to understand the wish for planning simply as narcissism. Planning is often socially motivated and can also be understood as part of our moral identity guiding our moral commitment. What type of person do I want to be: Do I want to care for others – if so, whom? Do I care about future generations or the environment – if so, what does this imply?

As argued on page 218, such planning of individual life takes place in a socially pre-structured context of time and space. It is no different in the case of planning medical decisions or making decisions in the context of predictive medicine. While many philosophers and political theorists focus on positive visions (as political ideals) for orientation, the interesting question for me remains how negative anticipations or dystopian views guide our planning. In current times of global and political crisis, such a perspective requires special attention.

As my former critique of the biopolitical discourse on dementia and dementia research has revealed, particular negative anticipations occupy our discourse. Therefore, I want to discuss the ethical dimension of those negative stereotypes, bad images, and worst-case scenarios and will hereby rely on the 'theory of regret' in decision theory and how it might be relevant for our ethical reflections.

The regret theory in decision psychology assumes that regret occurs in decisions in which persons compare outcomes to what they would have been had they chosen differently (Zeelenberg 2015, 162). For example, I decide to forgo surgery on my slightly impaired hip because I fear the risk of side effects and calamity of a hospital stay. Later on, I discover retrospectively that I would have preferred this operation, because the problem has worsened and now I need a hip replacement. We use this same cognitive process of comparing outcomes when weighing (anticipated) consequences of our actions as part of decision-making. Anticipated regret is, however, a counterfactual emotion and is linked to our understanding of responsibility. The more we feel responsible for the outcome produced by our own action (or inaction/omission), the more we regret the experience (Zeelenberg 1999, 327). Regret and anticipated regret are mainly relevant in cases in which we receive feedback later on that making a different choice would have had a better outcome, because regret stems from comparison. In many cases, we have even adopted complex behavior to avoid such feedback. For example, we might break contact with former partners because we do not want to know how happy they are with their new partner or family. This deliberate ignorance of potential alternative choices protects us from the regret that we would encounter when thinking about the happier, richer, or more interesting life we could have had. Similar considerations may justify our disinterest in former classmates and how they took alternative routes for their study or job training because we do not want to compare the 'outcome.' In this sense, ignorance can be a wise decision and increase one's satisfaction with one's own life (Hertwig and Engel 2016), and this might also apply to the medical context, which is nowadays presented with the 'right not to know.'

The theoretical considerations about decision-making have illustrated how complex the internal logic of particular strategies such as anticipated regret is.

This concept also serves as a major guide for decision-making in predictive medicine, as the medical system pretends to provide us with alternative outcomes. In the healthcare system, such comparisons are inevitable when it is argued that healthy outcomes are a result not of fate (e.g., 'good/bad genes') but of healthy lifestyle (in the case of primary prevention), taking the right medication early on (secondary prevention), or following rehabilitation guidelines (tertiary prevention). If we are considering declining testing, medications, or interventions, we anticipate regret in the case of a negative outcome because of our inaction concerning our own body.

Anticipation of a demented future and its impact on decision-making: some conclusions

A crucial question now is how to link the socio-cultural anticipations of dementia with wise decision-making strategies in the case of predictive medicine.

The predominantly negative scenarios and imaginations dominating the public discourse serve – that is my final consideration – as such comparative alternative outcomes and prime our personal anticipated regret. Dementia is mainly regarded as a negative 'outcome' of personal and social failures. Responsibilization can thereby address individuals who failed to pursue a *correct* lifestyle or early testing for taking up right counter-measures as well as the collective which is not able to address the 'overwhelming' problem. The current predictive and preventive paradigm might produce both: A particular assumption about anticipated regret and the understanding of individual accountability and prospective responsibility for future outcomes. The decision 'to know' means then I can or must adopt a healthy life style to reduce my risk for dementia, because if I do not behave according to these rules I am responsible for this bad outcome. Alternatively, if I avoid learning about my risk as this reduces my responsibility, still I might learn later that I have dementia and regret then that I did not want to know. So there occurs a 'responsibilization of knowing' which is a moralization of the epistemic practice of knowing/not knowing. The ethical problem relies hence on the double effect of anticipation: I assume that dementia is influenced by my own behavior, even if not fully, then partly; it undermines my solidarity with myself as a vulnerable person as well as with other persons and the choice is not an individual choice anymore because the biopolitical dramatization of dementia via worst-case scenarios and negative images impacts our anticipation of the outcome.

A better understanding of the underlying mechanisms and strategies might help us increasingly reflect about our interpretations of the past and the anticipated future and about which imaginations and scenarios are brought into existence. This social level of reflection needs to be accompanied by a critical examination of our own wishes and characters and of the reasons for adopting such anticipations in a particular way. The direction my argumentation has taken here is perhaps uncommon in the sense that I tried to link social and political discourses with individual decision-making strategies by not giving up the moral-cognitive paradigm of reflection. Classical biopolitical critique in a Foucauldian sense tends to imply a manner of internalization that rather resembles the 'black box' paradigm in behaviorism: We do not know (neither do we question) how we individually adopt or internalize such collective imaginations or norms – we just claim that we do so. This line of thought is not what I find constructive and meaningful for applied ethics. In contrast, the ethical reflection I am defending here is more than just a critical reflection or liberal defense of pluralism but a dialogical procedure of personal and public deliberation about the implications of social, political, and economic changes we currently observe – and are part of. But what I definitively share with the critical strands of thought is an interest in drawing a broader picture, where we can integrate individual and social procedures of decision-making beyond simplistic autonomy claims or traditional utility calculations.

Of course, this kind of critical assessment should also lead to a more publicly deliberated practice of particular stakeholders (professionals, but also advocacy groups). Their production of imaginations and scenarios has such a social impact that critical questioning is required. The dementia discourse illustrates – as only few other topics have before (e.g., HIV) – how current bioethical and biopolitical debates are historically evolving from a long-standing social practice of stigmatization, dramatization, and exclusion of the *Other*. Therefore, we need more reflective spaces considering the rights and duties of the professions not only in healthcare and life science research, but also in related fields of public communication and media.

Notes

1 For more details, see "Rise of the Planet of the Apes," Wikipedia, https://en.wikipedia.org/wiki/Rise_of_the_Planet_of_the_Apes, accessed September 17, 2016.

2 As most issues discussed here apply not only to Alzheimer's disease, but also to other forms of age-related dementia, I use the term 'dementia' as an umbrella term.

3 The spectrum of research on predictive dementia biomarkers is broad and will only be briefly summarized. Apart from genetic testing of APOE ε4 (Keage et al. 2010) and genetic testing of APP and PSEN1/2, which is recommended only for individuals with a strong family history of AD, biomarkers predominantly measure the level of amyloid plaques or neuronal injury (like the abnormal tau-protein) by neuroimaging technologies (Albert et al. 2011; Filippi et al. 2012; Hampel et al. 2014; Nordberg et al. 2013; Visser et al. 2009). However, current methods of testing are limited, as they are either invasive, time-consuming, expensive, or raise ethical issues (e.g., medical risks for patients in the case of CSF or PET). Hence, brief neuropsychological and cognitive tests (e.g., Mini-Mental State Examination (MMSE); Jessen et al. 2011) and blood tests (Mapstone et al. 2014) are being explored as low-cost/low-risk tests for future public screening.

4 This shift of focus is currently mitigated by the fact that most policy documents emphasize both cure and care. However, at the moment, the research focus of leading international research consortia rather lies on prediction – although its relevance for cure is yet not proven. Thus, one may worry that the relevance of care is diminished.

5 Here I suggest a slightly differentiated access to imaginations and metaphors starting from Draaisma's (2000) discussion of the main theories of metaphors, which refer to substitution, comparison, and interaction. As *substitutions*, metaphors serve as a form of decoration but have no original meaning and can be replaced by a literal expression. For example, a German metaphor for doctors is 'demigods in white,' alluding to their power position and white coats. Alternatively, we could say that doctors are expressing

their power and superiority by wearing their white coats. Such metaphors are pictorial. According to the *comparison* theory of metaphors, there is a similarity of main features, which can be expressed literally. Thus we say that 'time flows,' because we know that a river flows and time is similar to a river in the sense that we cannot stop it. According to Draaisma, neither substitution nor comparison works for psychological metaphors, because we want to express something 'new' – that is, ideas or theories we cannot yet describe in a literal way. Following an *interactive* theory, a metaphor evokes new epistemic insights about the phenomena we are interested in, and this will be more intense and subtle the more the association is evoked by the metaphor. Imaginations therefore often serve as metaphors, but some imaginations (such as the image of a wrinkly face with a bewildered gaze) in their concreteness also have a simplistic interactive and pejorative meaning, which is different from symbolic metaphors such as 'old age is the autumn of life.'

6 Cameron did not use the term 'plague' himself but drew parallels between dementia and other infectious diseases. See Department of Health, *Guidance: G8 Dementia Summit: Global Action against Dementia – 11 December 2013*, www.gov.uk/government/publications/g8-dementia-summit-global-action-against-dementia/g8-dementia-summit-global-action-against-dementia-11-december-2013, accessed August 3, 2016; Chris Smyth, "Crisis over '21st Century Plague' of Dementia," *The Times*, December 10, 2013, www.thetimes.co.uk/tto/health/news/article3944446.ece, accessed August 3, 2016.

7 See also Danny George, "The War (on Terror) on Alzheimer's," www.academia.edu/12629796/The_War_on_Terror_on_Alzheimer_s, accessed October 7, 2016.

8 I would like to thank Lisa Frebel, Isabella Jordan (IJ), Elisabeth Späth, and Karin Jongsma (KJ) for their support in data collection and preliminary analysis. For this purpose, our analysis included material from various sources (collected between 2011 and 2015): expert interviews with representatives of the US Alzheimer's Association (in Washington and in the California section (n = 4), conducted by the author) and of the German Alzheimer's Society (Deutsche Alzheimer Gesellschaft (n = 4), conducted by KJ and IJ). We further compared the content of the patient organizations' websites (Alzheimer Association, "About Us," www.alz.org/ and Deutsche Alzheimer Gesellschaft, "Willkommen bei der Deutschen Alzheimer Gesellschaft (DAlzG): Informationen, Tipps und Adressen – wir helfen!" www.deutsche-alzheimer.de/index.php?id=1; accessed October 7, 2016), and analyzed annual reports of both patient organizations (until 2015). The author translated the German statements for this article.

9 See U.S. Dept. of Health & Human Service: National Alzheimer' Project Act (NAPA) http://napa.alz.org/national-alzheimers-project-act-background, accessed October 7, 2016.

10 The content analysis was conducted for the first time in 2011 by comparing the websites of GER ALZ at www.deutsche-alzheimer.de/index.php?id=1 and US ALZ at www.alz.org/. Main differences described here can still be found in the current versions of these websites, but the wording may have changed.

11 Content on the US ALZ website: 'Intro,' 'Living with AD,' and 'Index.'

12 GER ALZ website: 'Leitsätze,' www.deutsche-alzheimer.de/fileadmin/alz/pdf/leitsaetze_ethik_dalzg.pdf, accessed October 10, 2016.

13 US ALZ website: 'About us, www.alz.org/about_us_about_us.asp, accessed October 10, 2016.

14 US ALZ website: 'Research'; see also www.alz.org/about_us_strategic_plan.asp, accessed October 10, 2016.

15 US ALZ website: 'Living with AD'; 'Research'; see also www.alz.org/research/overview.asp, accessed October 10, 2016.

16 GER ALZ website: 'Leitsätze'; 'Forschungsförderung'; see "Deutsche Alzheimer Gesellschaft e.V.: Leitsätze der Deutschen Alzheimer Gesellschaft zu ethischen Fragestellungen" at www.deutsche-alzheimer.de/fileadmin/alz/pdf/leitsaetze_ethik_dalzg.

pdf, accessed October 10, 2016, and www.deutsche-alzheimer.de/die-krankhe it/forschung/forschungsfoerderung-der-dalzg.html, accessed October 10, 2016.

17 GER ALZ website: 'Leitsätze.'

18 GER ALZ website: 'Forschung.'

19 See the campaign "Confetti in the mind" (in German: "Konfetti im Kopf") supported by GER ALZ: www.konfetti-im-kopf.de/konfetti-im-kopf/Aktivierungskampagne.html, accessed October 10, 2016.

20 Overall, it seems that citizens are significantly satisfied with the German healthcare system (Böcken, Braun, and Meierjürgen 2014).

21 There is no internationally accepted regulation for third-party beneficial research with patients with dementia (Kim et al. 2011).

22 I assume this would be different with all health issues pointing to racial issues – for example, differences in medical or social treatment regarding race, historical events such as the Tuskegee Study and, even more relevant, systematic racial discrimination and the history of slavery (Brandon, Isaac, and LaVeist 2005; Brandt 1978).

23 See, for example, EU research and innovation policy and how it justifies its setting by means of 'foresight studies' at European Commission, "What Is Foresight and Why Is It Useful?" https://ec.europa.eu/research/foresight/index.cfm, accessed September 26, 2016.

24 With Hazan (2015), I share some reservations concerning the appraisal of the hybrid as a post-modern ideal, because it produces new forms of injustice and vulnerabilities instead of overcoming them.

25 Perhaps they do for some people, but the example serves only to illustrate the fact that we all know distinct areas of serious and important versus arbitrary decision-making.

References

Albert, M. S., S. T. DeKosky, D. Dickson, B. Dubois, H. H. Feldman, N. C. Fox, A. Gamst, D. M. Holtzman, W. J. Jagust, R. C. Petersen, P. J. Snyder, M. C. Carrillo, B. Thies, and C. H. Phelps. 2011. "The Diagnosis of Mild Cognitive Impairment Due to Alzheimer's Disease: Recommendations from the National Institute on Aging – Alzheimer's Association Workgroups on Diagnostic Guidelines for Alzheimer's Disease." *Alzheimer's & Dementia* 7 (3):270–279. doi: 10.1016/j.jalz.2011.03.008.

American College of Physicians. 2000. "Position Paper: Cognitively Impaired Subjects." In *Medical Ethics: Codes, Opinions and Statements*, edited by B. A. Brody, L. B McCullough, M. A. Rothstein, and M. A. Bobinski, 788–793. Washington, DC: National Bureau of Affairs.

Andorno, R. 2004. "The Right Not to Know: An Autonomy Based Approach." *Journal of Medical Ethics* 30 (5):435–439. doi: 10.1136/jme.2002.001578.

Beck, S., and S. Schicktanz. 2016. "'Wer viel weiß, hat viel zu sorgen'? Zur Prädiktion von Altersdemenz mittels Biomarker: ethische und rechtliche Fragestellungen." *Jahrbuch Recht und Ethik* [*Annual Review of Law and Ethics*] 161–184.

Bloch, E. 1985. *Das Prinzip Hoffnung*. Frankfurt am Main: Suhrkamp.

Böcken, J., B. Braun, and R. Meierjürgen. 2014. "Gesundheitsmonitor 2014. Bürgerorientierung im Gesundheitswesen; Kooperationsprojekt der Bertelsmann Stiftung und der BARMER GEK." Accessed October 7, 2016. http://gesundheitsmonitor.de/uploads/tx_itaoarticles/2014-07-Beitrag.pdf.

Brandon, D. T., L. A. Isaac, and Th. A. LaVeist. 2005. "The Legacy of Tuskegee and Trust in Medical Care: Is Tuskegee Responsible for Race Differences in Mistrust of Medical Care?" *Journal of the National Medical Association* 97 (7):951–956.

Brandt, A. 1978. "Racism and Research: The Case of the Tuskegee Syphilis Study." *Hastings Center Report* 8 (6):21–29.
Brook, A. 2013. "Kant's View of the Mind and Consciousness of Self." *Stanford Encyclopedia of Philosophy*. Accessed October 7, 2016. http://plato.stanford.edu/entries/kant-mind/#3.2.
Central Ethics Board of German Chamber of Physicians (Zentrale Ethikkommission der Bundesärztekammer). 1997. "Zum Schutz nicht-einwilligungsfähiger Personen in der medizinischen Forschung." *Deutsches Ärzteblatt* 94 (15):A1011–A1012. www.zentrale-ethikkommission.de/downloads/Schutz1.pdf.
Chermack, T. J., S. A. Lynham, and W. E. A. Ruona. 2001. "A Review of Scenario Planning Literature." *Futures Research Quarterly* 17:7–31.
Council of Europe. 1997. *The Oviedo Convention: Protecting Human Rights in the Biomedical Field: The Convention for the Protection of Human Rights and Dignity of the Human Being with Regard to the Application of Biology and Medicine: Convention on Human Rights and Biomedicine*. Accessed October 7, 2016. www.coe.int/en/web/bioethics/oviedo-convention.
Draaisma, D. 2000. *Metaphors of Memory: A History of Ideas about the Mind*. Cambridge: Cambridge University Press.
European Parliament. 2011. "European Initiative on Alzheimer's Disease and Other Dementias." Accessed October 8, 2016. www.europarl.europa.eu/oeil/popups/ficheprocedure.do?lang=en&reference=2010/2084%28INI%29.
Filippi, M., F. Agosta, F. Barkhof, B. Dubois, N. C. Fox, G. B. Frisoni, C. R. Jack, P. Johannsen, B. L. Miller, P. J. Nestor, P. Scheltens, S. Sorbi, S. Teipel, P. M. Thompson, and L. O. Wahlund. 2012. "EFNS Task Force: The Use of Neuroimaging in the Diagnosis of Dementia." *European Journal of Neurology* 19 (12):1487–1501. doi: 10.1111/j.1468-1331.2012.03859.x.
George, D. R., E. R. Whitehouse, and P. J. Whitehouse. 2016. "Asking More of Our Metaphors: Narrative Strategies to End the 'War on Alzheimer's' and Humanize Cognitive Aging." *The American Journal of Bioethics* 16 (10):22–24. doi: 10.1080/15265161.2016.1214307.
Giddens, A. 1991. *Modernity and Self-Identity: Self and Society in the Late Modern Age*. Stanford: Stanford University Press.
Gigerenzer, G. 2003. *Reckoning with Risk: Learning to Live with Uncertainty*. London: Penguin.
Glaser, B., and A. Strauss. 1971. *Status Passage*. Chicago: Routledge & Kegan Paul.
Hampel, H., S. Lista, S. J. Teipel, F. Garaci, R. Nisticò, K. Blennow, H. Zetterberg, L. Bertram, C. Duyckaerts, H. Bakardjian, A. Drzezga, O. Colliot, S. Epelbaum, K. Broich, S. Lehéricy, A. Brice, Z. S. Khachaturian, P. S. Aisen, and B. Dubois. 2014. "Perspective on Future Role of Biological Markers in Clinical Therapy Trials of AD." *Biochemistry Pharmacology* 88 (4):426–449. doi: 10.1016/j.bcp.2013.11.009.
Hazan, H. 2015. *Against Hybridity*. Cambridge: Polity.
Helmchen, H. 1999. "Forschung mit nicht-einwilligungsfähigen Demenzkranken. Ein aktuelles Problem im Lichte der deutschen Geschichte." *Jahrbuch für Wissenschaft und Ethik* 4:127–142.
Hertwig, R., and C. Engel. 2016. "Homo Ignorans: Deliberately Choosing Not to Know." *Perspectives on Psychological Science* 11 (3):359–372. doi: 10.1177/1745691616635594.
Hirnliga e.V. 1995. *Am Beispiel Demenz und Schlaganfall: Forschung mit einwilligungsunfähigen Patienten. Anhörung der Hirnliga e.V. und Deutschen Alzheimer Gesellschaft e.V, am 27. November 1995*, Bonn.

Jessen, F., B. Wiese, H. Bickel, S. Eifflãnder-Gorfer, A. Fuchs, H. Kaduszkiewicz, M. Köhler, T. Luck, E. Mösch, M. Pentzek, S. G. Riedel-Heller, M. Wagner, S. Weyerer, W. Maier, and H. van den Bussche. 2011. "Prediction of Dementia in Primary Care Patients." *PLoS One* 6 (2):e16852. doi: 10.1371/journal.pone.0016852.

Jongsma, K. R., and S. van de Vathorst. 2015. "Dementia Research and Advance Consent: It Is Not about Critical Interest." *Journal of Medical Ethics* 41 (8):708–709. doi: 10.1136/medethics-2014-102024.

Kahneman, D. 2011. *Thinking, Fast and Slow*. New York: Farrar, Straus and Giroux.

Kahneman, D., P. Slovic, and A. Tversky. 1982. *Judgment under Uncertainty: Heuristics and Biases*. New York: Cambridge University Press.

Kant, I. 1974. "Kritik der Urteilskraft." In *Werkausgabe*, Vol. 10, edited by W. Weischedel, Frankfurt am Main: Suhrkamp.

Keage, H. A. D., F. E. Matthews, A. Yip, L. Gao, C. McCracken, I. G. McKeith, D. C. Rubinsztein, C. Brayne, and MRC Cognitive Function and Ageing Study. 2010. "APOE and ACE Polymorphisms and Dementia Risk in the Older Population over Prolonged Follow-Up: 10 Years of Incidence in the MRC CFA Study." *Age and Ageing* 39 (1):104–111. doi: 10.1093/ageing/afp210.

Kim, S. Y. H., J. H. Karlawish, H. M. Kim, I. F. Wall, A. C. Bozoki, and P. S. Appelbaum. 2011. "Preservation of the Capacity to Appoint a Proxy Decision Maker: Implications for Dementia Research." *Archives of General Psychiatry* 68 (2):214–219. doi: 10.1001/archgenpsychiatry.2010.

Le Couteur, D. G., J. Doust, H. Creasey, and C. Brayne. 2013. "Political Drive to Screen for Pre-Dementia: Not Evidence Based and Ignores the Harms of Diagnosis." *British Medical Journal* 347:f5125. doi: 10.1136/bmj.f5125.

Leibing, A. 2015. "Dementia in the Making: Early Detection and the Body/Brain in Alzheimer's Disease." In *Popularizing Dementia: Public Expressions and Representations of Forgetfulness*, edited by A. Swinnen and M. Schweda, 275–294. Bielefeld: transcript.

Lock, M. 2013. *The Alzheimer Conundrum*. Princeton: Princeton University Press.

McAllister, M. 2003. "Personal Theories of Inheritance, Coping Strategies, Risk Perception and Engagement in Hereditary Non-Polyposis Colon Cancer Families Offered Genetic Testing." *Clinical Genetics* 64 (3):179–189. doi: 10.1034/j.1399-0004.2003.00133.x.

MacLeod, R., A. Tibben, M. Frontali, G. Evers-Kiebooms, A. Jones, A. Martinez-Descales, and R. A. Roos. 2013. "Recommendations for the Predictive Genetic Test in Huntington's Disease." *Clinical Genetics* 83 (3):221–231. doi: 10.1111/j.1399-0004.2012.01900.x.

Mapstone, M., A. K. Cheema, M. S. Fiandaca, X. Zhong, T. R. Mhyre, L. H. MacArthur, W. J. Hall, S. G. Fisher, D. R. Peterson, J. M. Haley, M. D. Nazar, S. A. Rich, D. J. Berlau, C. B. Peltz, M. T. Tan, C. H. Kawas, and H. J. Federoff. 2014. "Plasma Phospholipids Identify Antecedent Memory Impairment in Older Adults." *Nature Medicine* 20 (4):415–418. doi: 10.1038/nm.3466.

Mukadam, N., C. Cooper, N. Kherani, and G. Livingtone. 2015. "A Systematic Review of Interventions to Detect Dementia or Cognitive Impairment." *International Journal of Geriatric Psychiatry* 30 (1):32–45. doi: 10.1002/gps.4184.

National Bioethics Advisory Commission. 1998. "Report and Recommendations on Research Involving Persons with Mental Disorders That May Affect Decisionmaking Capacity." Accessed October 7, 2016. https://bioethicsarchive.georgetown.edu/nbac/capacity/TOC.htm.

Nordberg, A., S. F. Carter, J. Rinne, A. Drzezga, D. J. Brooks, R. Vandenberghe, D. Perani, A. Forsberg, B. Långström, N. Scheinin, M. Karrasch, K. Någren, T. Grimmer, I. Miederer, P. Edison, A. Okello, K. Van Laere, N. Nelissen, M. Vandenbulcke, V. Garibotto,

O. Almkvist, E. Kalbe, R. Hinz, and K. Herholz. 2013. "A European Multicentre PET Study of Fibrillar Amyloid in Alzheimer's Disease." *European Journal of Nuclear Medicine and Molecular Imaging* 40 (1):104–114. doi: 10.1007/s00259-012-2237-2.

OECD. 2015. *Addressing Dementia: The OECD Response*. Paris: OECD Publishing Paris. doi: http://dx.doi.org/10.1787/9789264231726-en.

Orona, C. J. 1990. "Temporality and Identity Loss Due to Alzheimer's Disease." *Social Science & Medicine* 30 (11):1247–1256. doi: 10.1016/0277-9536(90)90265-T.

Rawls, J. 1971. *A Theory of Justice*. Cambridge, MA: Harvard University Press.

Sacks, O. 1973. *Awakenings*. London: Duckworth & Co.

Schicktanz, S. 2015. "The Ethical Legitimacy of Patient Organizations' Involvement in Politics and Knowledge Production: Epistemic Justice as Conceptual Basis." In *The Public Shaping of Medical Research*, edited by P. Wehling, W. Viehöver, and S. Koenen, 246–265. London: Routledge.

Schicktanz, S. 2016. "Genetic Risk and Responsibility: Reflections on a Complex Relationship." *Journal of Risk Research* (published online Sep. 26). doi: 10.1080/13669877.2016.1223157.

Schicktanz, S., and I. Jordan. 2013. "Kollektive Patientenautonomie: Theorie und Praxis eines neuen bioethischen Konzepts." In *Patientenautonomie*, edited by A. Simon and C. Wiesemann, 287–302. Münster: Mentis.

Schicktanz, S., and M. Schweda. 2012. "The Diversity of Responsibility: The Value of Explication and Pluralization." *Medicine Studies* 3 (3):131–145. doi: 10.1007/s12376-011-0070-8.

Schicktanz, S., M. Schweda, J. F. Ballenger, P. J. Fox, J. Halpern, J. H. Kramer, G. Micco, S. G. Post, C. Thompson, R. T. Knight, and W. J. Jagust. 2014. "Before It Is Too Late: Professional Responsibilities in Late-Onset Alzheimer's Research and Pre-Symptomatic Prediction." *Frontiers in Human Neuroscience* 8:1–6. doi: 10.3389/fnhum.2014.00921.

Schicktanz, S., M. Schweda, and M. Franzen. 2008. "'In a Completely Different Light'?: The Role of Being Affected for Epistemic Perspectives and Moral Attitudes of Patients, Relatives and Lay People." *Medicine, Health Care, and Philosophy* 11 (1):57–72. doi: 10.1007/s11019-007-9074-2.

Schwartz, B. 2015. "What Does It Mean to Be a Rational Decision Maker?" *Journal of Marketing Behaviour* 1:113–145. doi: 10.1561/107.00000007.

Sperling, R. A., J. Karlawish, and K. A. Johnson. 2013. "Preclinical Alzheimer Disease: The Challenges Ahead." *Nature Reviews Neurology* 9 (1):54–58. doi: 10.1038/nrneurol.2012.241.

Swinnen, A., and M. Schweda, eds. 2015. *Popularizing Dementia: Public Expressions and Representations of Forgetfulness*. Bielefeld: transcript.

Taylor, C. 1989. *Sources of the Self: The Making of Modern Identity*. Cambridge, MA: Harvard University Press.

Tran, T. A., and T. Daim. 2008. "A Taxonomic Review of Methods and Tools Applied in Technology Assessment." *Technological Forecasting and Social Change* 75 (9):1396–1405. doi: 10.1016/j.techfore.2008.04.004.

Van Den Ende, J., K. Mulder, M. Knot, E. Moors, and P. Vergragt. 1998. "Traditional and Modern Technology Assessment: Toward a Toolkit." *Technological Forecasting and Social Change* 58 (1–2):5–21. doi: 10.1016/S0040-1625(97)00052-8.

Vellas, B., P. S. Aisen, C. Sampaio, M. Carrillo, P. Scheltens, B. Scherrer, G. B. Frisoni, M. Weiner, L. Schneider, S. Gauthier, C. C. Gispen-de Wied, S. Hendrix, H. Feldman, J. Cedarbaum, R. Petersen, E. Siemers, S. Andrieu, D. Prvulovic, J. Touchon, and H.

Hampel. 2011. "Prevention Trials in Alzheimer's Disease: An EU-US Task Force Report." *Progress in Neurobiology* 95 (4):594–600. doi: 10.1016/j.pneurobio.2011.08.014.

Visser, P. J., F. Verhey, D. L. Knol, P. Scheltens, L. O. Wahlund, Y. Freund-Levi, M. Tsolaki, L. Minthon, A. K. Wallin, H. Hampel, K. Bürger, T. Pirttila, H. Soininen, M. O. Rikkert, M. M. Verbeek, L. Spiru, and K. Blennow. 2009. "Prevalence and Prognostic Value of CSF Markers of Alzheimer's Disease Pathology in Patients with Subjective Cognitive Impairment or Mild Cognitive Impairment in the DESCRIPA Study: A Prospective Cohort Study." *The Lancet Neurology* 8 (7):619–627. doi: 10.1016/S1474-4422(09)70139-5.

Vos, S. J., F. Verhey, L. Frölich, J. Kornhuber, J. Wiltfang, W. Maier, O. Peters, E. Rüther, F. Nobili, S. Morbelli, G. B. Frisoni, A. Drzezga, M. Didic, B. N. van Berckel, A. Simmons, H. Soininen, I. Kłoszewska, P. Mecocci, M. Tsolaki, B. Vellas, S. Lovestone, C. Muscio, S. K. Herukka, E. Salmon, C. Bastin, A. Wallin, A. Nordlund, A. de Mendonça, D. Silva, I. Santana, R. Lemos, S. Engelborghs, S. Van der Mussele, Alzheimer's Disease Neuroimaging Initiative, Y. Freund-Levi, Å. K. Wallin, H. Hampel, W. van der Flier, P. Scheltens, and P. J. Visser. 2015. "Prevalence and Prognosis of Alzheimer's Disease at the Mild Cognitive Impairment Stage." *Brain* 138:1327–1338. doi: 10.1093/brain/awv029.

Weiner, M. W., P. S. Aisen, C. R. Jack Jr., W. J. Jagust, J. Q. Trojanowski, L. Shaw, A. J. Saykin, J. C. Morris, N. Cairns, L. A. Beckett, A. Toga, R. Green, S. Walter, H. Soares, P. Snyder, E. Siemers, W. Potter, P. E. Cole, and M. Schmidt. 2010. "The Alzheimer's Disease Neuroimaging Initiative: Progress Report and Future Plans." *Alzheimer's & Dementia* 6 (3):202–211. doi: 10.1016/j.jalz.2010.03.007.

Werner, P., and A. D. Korczyn. 2008. "Mild Cognitive Impairment: Conceptual, Assessment, Ethical and Social Issues." *Clinical Interventions in Aging* 3 (3):413–420.

Williams, S. J., P. Higgs, and S. Katz. 2012. "Neuroculture, Active Ageing and the 'Older Brain': Problems, Promises and Prospects." *Sociology of Health and Illness* 34 (1):64–78. doi: 10.1111/j.1467-9566.2011.01364.x.

World Health Organization. 2012. *Dementia: A Public Health Priority*. Geneva: World Health Organization.

Zeelenberg, M. 1999. "The Use of Crying over Spilled Milk: A Note on Rationality and Functionality of Regret." *Philosophical Psychology* 12 (3):325–340. doi: 10.1080/095150899105800.

Zeelenberg, M. 2015. "Robust Satisficing via Regret Minimization." *Journal of Marketing Behavior* 1 (2):157–166. doi: 10.1561/107.00000010.

Zick, C. D., C. Mathews, J. S. Roberts, R. Cook-Deegan, R. J. Pokorski, and R. C. Green. 2005. "Genetic Testing for Alzheimer's Disease and Its Impact on Insurance Purchasing." *Behavior Health Affairs* 24 (2):483–490. doi: 10.1377/hlthaff.24.2.483.

15 Solidarity and family care for an ageing population

Ruud ter Meulen

The increase in life expectancy in many countries over the world is leading to severe pressures on societal institutions and resources. One of the main concerns regards the systems of healthcare and social services, which are increasingly under pressure to deal with the medical and social needs of the ageing population. Although many older people are living in good health, there is an increased risk to be confronted with chronic, often debilitating diseases in later life. Many countries now have policies to enable access to care for people with long-term conditions, yet these policies are strained by a large number of older people needing care. In a number of European countries, access to care is based on the principle of solidarity, meaning that the stronger shoulders should bear the burden of the weaker members of society. However, the growing costs of care in combination with the rise of neoliberal and market-based policies have resulted in a rethinking of the principle of solidarity and a restriction of the thus far rather generous and 'universalist' policies with regard to access to care. Policies are moving toward more individual responsibility for healthcare and social services – in particular more financial responsibility, by means of requiring individual financial contributions or imposing limits on funding. In addition, there are increased efforts to involve families in the care for their dependent family members as a substitute for the care supplied by the state.

The shift in policies raises a number of ethical issues about the access to care and the quality of care, particularly for the ageing population. This chapter will analyze these issues from the perspective of solidarity, not only at the level of societal policies, but especially in the context of family caregiving. The stated developments will be illustrated with the case of long-term care reform in the Netherlands, where solidarity has been an important principle in healthcare and social services for a long time but is now being reconsidered in the face of pressures on the care system and a diminished role of the state. This analysis may contribute to a better understanding of the value of solidarity and its contribution to healthcare. The results apply not only in the Netherlands, but also in other European countries where solidarity has been an important moral principle whose limits are increasingly under debate.

The idea of solidarity

According to Bayertz (1999), the core meaning of solidarity is the perception of mutual obligations between the members of a community. This perception of mutual obligation can be considered from a sociological and from a moral point of view. In sociology, solidarity is a concept to describe the degree of social cohesion in a group or society – that is, the extent to which individuals are willing to serve and promote the collective interest of the group or of society, as well as their motivations to do so, compared to more individualistic motives. The sociological interpretation of solidarity does not consider the moral implications of this concept – that is, whether it is a *good* thing for individuals to contribute to the greater good and subordinate their own interests. The question of the moral importance of solidarity is answered in moral philosophy and practical ethics. In bioethics, there is an emergent interest in solidarity, mainly in response to the dominance of liberal and individualistic approaches to bioethical issues. A special issue of the journal *Bioethics* (2012) on the contribution of solidarity to bioethics – as well as the report *Solidarity* (Prainsack and Buyx 2011), published by the Nuffield Council on Bioethics – are signs of this emerging interest. In these approaches, solidarity is put forward as an alternative to an individualized concept of autonomy in which the individual is seen as a rational decision-maker mainly guided by enlightened self-interest. As opposed to this rather narrow view of the individual, a solidarity-based approach argues that human persons are shaped by their social relations. Thus, social and political arrangements should take social relations into account instead of merely focusing on individual interests (Prainsack and Buyx 2011, xi). A perspective of solidarity can foster a different view on the ethical and legal regulation of various areas in healthcare and research – for example, the management of biobanks and measures for public and global health (idem, xvii). In the context of healthcare policies and allocation of resources, the concept of solidarity can help justify access to care for vulnerable groups (ter Meulen 2011). This kind of solidarity-based approach would lead to different policies than those based on libertarian or liberal-egalitarian approaches only, such as the philosophy of justice of John Rawls, which emphasize the enlightened self-interest of individuals (Houtepen and ter Meulen 2001).

Due to its focus on the relatedness of individuals and their willingness to contribute to the needs of others, solidarity is often referred to as a 'European' value: It expresses a feeling of togetherness and commitment to the common good, which are supposedly typical for the 'old world.' This 'European' value is highlighted as different from and superior to the emphasis on individualism and free choice associated with the culture and liberal values of countries such as the United States, where millions of individuals have been excluded from access to appropriate health insurance and care for a long time (and still are).

Solidarity in healthcare and its limits

In healthcare and social-services systems, solidarity means that everyone is assumed to make a fair financial contribution to a collectively organized and compulsory insurance system that guarantees equal access to healthcare and social services for all members of society. Although prudence and self-interest are strong motivations in the acceptance of compulsory solidarity, there is also an understanding of solidarity as a feeling of responsibility and a motivation to support those who are in need of care but unable to pay for it (ter Meulen, Arts, and Muffels 2001, 1). The principle of solidarity is enforced by the state in a number of European countries by way of compulsory payments of an insurance premium in exchange for financial support in case of medical need or social distress. This system was first established by German chancellor Otto von Bismarck in the 1880s to compensate workers for the impact of old age, accidents, disability, and illness. Bismarck's approach was followed by other continental countries, where state-enforced solidarity replaced local initiatives of social security and medical support (Companje et al. 2009). In the decades after the Second World War, the solidarity-based approach was supported by the ruling Christian democratic and social democratic parties (Stjernø 2004) and led to generous support policies for a large range of social and medical needs. Solidarity became synonymous with unlimited collective responsibility, leading to a state-provided safety net for illness and disability, as well as for unemployment, work-related illness, and pensioning. However, since the 1990s, there has been increasing concern over whether such an unlimited and generous interpretation of solidarity is still feasible and sustainable.

First of all, there are concerns about the support for solidarity in modern society. Although solidarity is enforced by the state, it is based on individual motivations and voluntary decisions to obey the rule of the state (Durkheim 2014 [1893]). As individuals are becoming more autonomous while living in an ever more heterogeneous society, there is concern over whether they will maintain their willingness to share benefits and burdens, such as paying taxes for the common good and to support others (Lukes 2014, xxxv). In a society that may drift apart due to emphasis on individual autonomy and cultural heterogeneity, solidarity can become fragile and difficult to organize. In such situations, solidarity gets the connotation of 'interest solidarity,' meaning that individuals pay their premiums and taxes merely because they have an interest to do so. They expect a satisfactory return on their 'investments' in the healthcare system and do not accept rising premiums if, at the same time, they are faced with poor healthcare services (ter Meulen and Houtepen 2012). If the healthcare system is not able to deliver – for example, if waiting times are too long – the modern patient-consumer will withdraw his support and will try to find his own solutions to deal with the scarcity of available services.

A second threat to solidarity is the growing influence of neoliberal ideologies that emphasize the role of individual responsibility and regard the market as a superior way of organizing social institutions as opposed to 'big government' exercised by the state. Neoliberalism is strongly driven by conservative motives, as it endorses individual self-reliance over dependency on the state and state-supported institutions. According to the neoliberal view, individuals should take more initiative in organizing their life and should turn to their families and small civic societies, rather than to state welfare agencies, when in need of help; the 'minimal state' is the best way to generate social solidarity and to foster good character and personal virtues (Giddens 1998). The state is believed to be destructive to such virtues, but the markets are not, since they thrive on individual initiative (Giddens 1998). Markets should therefore be left alone not only at the national level, but also at the global level, where they will lead to universal prosperity. According to neoliberalism, social inequalities do not exist: There are only individuals who are trying to improve their life by working hard and striving to accomplish whatever lies within their capabilities. They do not need a generous welfare state, which is seen as disruptive to individual initiative.

A third development is the scarcity of resources. While the demand for care is growing, national governments are under pressure to preserve or to curtail the level of public spending via 'austerity' measures. As a result of these policies, there is a growing gap between the demand for and the supply of healthcare and social services, resulting in a shortage of care services and diminishing quality of care, particularly in the area of long-term care for the elderly.

One of the policy options to cope with the pressures on social solidarity is to increase individual financial responsibility for healthcare and social services. Financial contributions by individuals are seen as a way to cut costs and to reduce the role of collective responsibility and solidarity as embodied in the public healthcare system. Moreover, by increasing individuals' awareness of the costs of healthcare, private financial contributions could have an inhibiting effect on the use of healthcare services and thus reduce costs. However, such policies will have an impact on solidarity, since direct, non-income-related payments to insurers or care providers mean a greater burden for lower income groups (ter Meulen, Arts, and Muffels 2001, 4).

While solidarity has been a leading principle in the design of public healthcare systems in many European countries, the rising costs of healthcare, in combination with the rise of neoliberalism and individualizing tendencies, have resulted in a larger emphasis on individual responsibility in the financing and delivery of healthcare and social services. An important question is "What will be the impact of these developments on solidarity between the generations and the position of the elderly in our society?"

The ageing of the population

In 2013, life expectancy at birth in the EU-28 was estimated at 80.6 years, reaching 83.3 years for women and 77.8 years for men (Eurostat 2015). These figures mean that over the past 50 years, life expectancy at birth has increased by about ten years for both men and women in the EU-28 (Eurostat 2015), mainly owing to a reduction in mortality at older ages. However, due to an accompanying reduction in fertility rate, these developments have resulted in an increase in the relative number of aged persons in the total population of the EU-28. As of 2015, the percentage of people over 65 years of age in the 28 EU countries is 18.5 percent, a number that is expected to rise to nearly 28.4 percent in 2060 (Eurostat 2015). The percentage of people over 80 years is expected to increase from 5.1 percent of the total population to 11.8 percent in 2060. The old-age dependency ratio of 28.1 percent is projected to nearly double by 2080.

The rise in average life expectancy has some people wondering what it means for the health status and the burden of disease of the older population. Different scenarios have been envisioned with respect to the growing burden of disease. The pessimistic scenario argues that increased longevity has not resulted in an improvement in our health and that we will inevitably be living in decreased health for the final 20 or so years of our lives. This scenario is called the theory of expansion of disability; Gruenberg has called it the "failures of success" (Gruenberg 1977). A more optimistic scenario is based on the theory of "compression of morbidity" (Fries 1980, 2005). This theory argues that an improvement in therapy and prevention will lead to increased longevity as well as a shorter period of disability at the end of life. On the basis of a review of trends in disability in the ageing population of 12 OECD countries, Lafortune and Balestat (2007) argue that it is difficult to draw a conclusion about the direction of the trend in disability levels. There is clear evidence of a decline in disability among elderly people in 5 of the 12 countries (Denmark, Finland, Italy, the Netherlands, and the United States), but three countries (Belgium, Japan, and Sweden) witnessed an increasing rate of severe disability among people aged 65 and over during the past five to ten years, while two countries (Australia and Canada) report a stable rate. In France and the United Kingdom, data from different surveys show different trends in activities of daily living (ADL) disability rates among elderly people. Lafortune and Balestat argue that although disability prevalence rates have declined to some extent in some countries, "the ageing of the population and the greater longevity of individuals can be expected to lead to increasing numbers of people at older ages with a severe disability" (Lafortune and Balestat 2007, 4). The conclusion of the review is that due to the ageing of the population, "in most OECD countries there will be a need therefore to expand the capacity to respond to this growing need for long-term care" (Lafortune and Balestat 2007, 56). The need for care will be particularly high for those aged 80 years and above, who are at an increased risk of chronic and debilitating conditions such as arthritis, stroke, dementia, depression, and chronic heart disease.

The pressure on long-term care is further increasing due to a change in family structures and family obligations. Family caregiving is an essential part of long-term care, even when long-term care is provided by the public system. In southern Europe, family caregiving is dominant in so-called 'residual' care regimes, in which the state leaves much responsibility to families to care for their dependent family members (Pavolini and Ranci 2013). However, even in Scandinavia and in countries such as the Netherlands, where most of the care is delivered by 'universalist' healthcare systems financed and organized by the government, care by family members is still much needed. Long-term care includes a wide range of services such as help with bathing, eating, dressing, getting in and out of bed or chairs, moving around, and using the bathroom (OECD 2011). In many cases, family caregivers such as spouses or elder children are involved in such support. These caregivers are often women, who may be confronted with the responsibility to care for their elderly parents as well as for their children (that is, they are members of the 'sandwich generation'). Moreover, they are at an age at which they themselves increasingly face health problems.

Due to the pressure on the public systems of long-term care (nursing homes, daily care, home care, etc.), the pressure on families to deliver such support and other care is increasing. At the same time, the availability of family caregivers is decreasing, even in countries such as Italy, where family care has been dominant for a long time (Carrera et al. 2013). This demographic change has increased the reliance on public systems of long-term care and is leading to a further increase in costs.

The case of family care in the Netherlands

In some countries, the rising cost of long-term care has led to a revision of the universalistic policies regarding the access to care for older people (Pavolini and Ranci 2013). One of the policy changes is the shift of responsibilities from the state toward local government and more involvement of family caregivers. This shift is an expression of a more fundamental change in the expectations of governments regarding the contributions of individuals to the care of family members. The Dutch government has taken the stance that the pressure on solidarity has become too great and that solidarity can be preserved only if people take on more individual and social responsibility (Maarse and Jeurissen 2016). The expansion of long-term care on the basis of a generous public-funding scheme has created a system in which the citizens have become passive and dependent recipients of care. The assumption of the Dutch government is that there is a wide and unused potential of social and volunteer networks that can be tapped into when it comes to the delivery of social services. Although professional caregivers will still be around to deliver care for people in need, according to the government, a substantial part of social services can be delivered by family members, neighbors, and friends.

Critics argue that the government is too optimistic in its assessment of the potential for family care. Family members do not necessarily have harmonious relations; neither do potential family caregivers necessarily live close to their dependent family members or have the time to attend to them. Even though many families live in harmony with each other, they can fall apart due to divorce. Children move away from their parents to other parts of the country (or abroad) and may have their own families to take care of. They may have a more individualistic lifestyle, with norms and values that are different from those of their elderly parents. Moreover, an increasing part of the population is living in other arrangements than the traditional family. The willingness to provide informal care is additionally and prominently decreased by a decline in the number of children as well as by the emancipation of women, who have increasingly joined the workforce.

On these premises, delivering family care on a daily basis will prove difficult. Moreover, the willingness within families to provide care can be limited. In a Dutch study with almost 21,000 respondents, 50 percent of people surveyed said they were willing to supply care for somebody close to them (Maarse and Jeurissen 2016). However, although they were inclined to provide domestic support, many said they would have difficulty providing intimate care. A large majority of the respondents (80%) did not agree with the implementation of this kind of compulsory care for family members or other related persons. A study by the

Netherlands Institute for Social Research (SCP) reports that 33 percent of respondents agreed with the idea that the government is right to expect people to take care of individuals with chronic diseases or disabilities, while 35 percent did not agree (Putters 2014, 20).

Besides physical and psychological burdens, people who care for dependent family members are increasingly confronted with assessment procedures, such as 'kitchen-table discussions' in which municipal officials meet with the person in need of care and his family members to determine the availability of informal care within the family network. If the officials approve the supply of care, families still need to pay for it. Although there is a financial protection for the lower income groups, the middle and higher incomes have to pay a substantial amount per hour as a contribution for day care and support. As a result, many of them decline the support by the municipality due to the high costs. Moreover, 40 percent of the family caregivers experience an increase in the burden of care after the 'kitchen-table discussion' (Mezzo 2015).

The efforts to increase personal involvement in home care for family members or friends and neighbors is presented in policy documents as a way to promote the so-called participation society and to implement the principle of 'reciprocity' as a new type of solidarity in care relations (RVZ 2013). The 'participation society' means a society in which everybody who is able to do so takes responsibility for his own life and environment without support or facilitation by the government. This idea is supported by a recent report of the Council for Public Health and Health Care, according to which 'reciprocity' means that the burdens and benefits of social care are distributed fairly. In informal care, reciprocity means that the recipient and the giver work together in the caring process: "The person who helps and the person who is being helped work together and both are finding satisfaction in doing so. This stimulates the preparedness for mutual support and limits the demand for support, so that it will be relatively easier to deliver; it will then create more room to support people who are not physically or mentally capable of reciprocity" (RVZ 2013, 16).

According to the report, solidarity and reciprocity will create more unity and cohesiveness in society, whereas lack of reciprocity and overreliance on state support will lead to division and exclusion. In spite of the emancipatory potential of participation and reciprocity, the call for increased involvement of family members and volunteers has much to do with the need to reorganize the care system, which has become untenable because of its ever-growing need for care services (RVZ 2013, 17). There is a risk that such care will not be available or will be difficult to arrange due to high financial thresholds. As many individuals and their families will not be able to afford such help, the policy to promote more involvement of family members in family care may lead to an increased burden for families and older people themselves, as many of them lack financial resources to pay for professional support at home. Moreover, there is a risk that the emphasis on personal relations and flourishing of virtues reflects the conservatism of neoliberal approaches, in which families are seen as the main place for informal care and for development of individual character.

Substitution or communicating vessels?

Family solidarity is a type of solidarity that needs to be maintained and supported by professional help from nurses, paramedics, home helps, and day-care centers. This professional help is an important condition for informal caregivers to keep caring for their partners, parents, neighbors, and friends. Waiting lists, high financial contributions, and diminishing professional support will weaken this preparedness (van der Made, ter Meulen, and van den Burg 2001). Unfortunately, government policies are built on the belief that family care or informal care will be able to complement or substitute the withdrawal of professional care, the belief that families will step in when professional help becomes too expensive. However, instead of this 'substitution model,' family care or non-professional care should be considered from the idea of 'communicating vessels.' This idea sees the care system as an open system that is in frequent contact with the surrounding environment and that is heavily influenced by structural and contextual changes (Muffels and Verburg 2001).

The idea of communicating vessels implies that the supply of care may diminish or 'leak away' due to context changes as mentioned on page 232 (changing family networks, individualization, and increased participation of women in the labor force). It also implies that a low level of care in the "professional vessel" might correspond with a low level of care in the "family care vessel" (Muffels and Verburg 2001, 269). In view of reduced professional support, the changing family networks, reduced fertility, and rising labor market participation by potential caregivers, the "position of caregivers is obviously not a very attractive one" (Muffels and Verburg 2001, 269). Family care can only fulfill its role in the care system when it is seen not as a residual kind of support, but as an essential component that needs to be supported and recognized as a serious contribution to the supply of care for older and dependent persons (ter Meulen and Wright 2012).

The emphasis on individual responsibility will lead to an increase in private payments by individuals for personal care at home and for other care arrangements not supplied by the healthcare and social services systems. The reform of long-term care may lead to a two-tier system of healthcare, with a universally accessible basic tier of services and a 'luxury' tier of additional services for those who can afford them (ter Meulen 1995; ter Meulen and Maarse 2008). This policy might be considered to be in tension with the principles of solidarity and equal access to care that are considered fundamental ethical principles in the healthcare and social services systems of many countries in Europe. An important moral argument in defense of a two-tier system is that, provided society is supplying an adequate package of healthcare services to which all persons have equal access, persons who buy their own services exceeding this package do not offend any ethical principle in doing so (President's Commission 1983). However, there are some dangers to such a mixed system, particularly that services are moved from the basic tier into the private tier (financed by additional health-insurance packages or private payments). This is an attractive option for the government in case of shortage of collective funding (Maarse 2004, 195). However, it could overstrain individual responsibility and result in a system of basic services that is not adequate at all.

Because of the reduced funding for long-term care at home, it is increasingly difficult for individuals to get access to adequate care: Visits by home-care workers are very brief (15 minutes), and families must prove that they are not able to provide the support for their family members at home. Applications for home-care support are scrutinized by city councils or central agencies in order to determine whether families (particularly spouses) have the capacity to take care of their loved ones themselves and whether they are abusing the system. Care and home help are separated, with families held more accountable for household tasks. Similarly, access to long-term care facilities in nursing homes and other institutions is severely restricted, as admissions are based on a scrutiny of the potential within families to deliver care at home. Although this scrutiny is presented as fair and based on need, it comprises what Margalith (1996) has called *humiliating* procedures, in which individuals requesting help are evaluated as to whether they truly are unable to help themselves. According to Margalith, humiliating means injuring the self-respect of individuals, and individual self-respect is the basis of a just and decent society (Margalith 1996). It is not difficult to see that such a system, and the basic services it supplies in home and long-term care, cannot be called 'adequate' or 'decent' (ter Meulen 2011).

Conclusion

The ageing of the population is leading to increased problems for healthcare and social services systems in Europe, particularly in the area of long-term care. The higher incidence of chronic and debilitating diseases among the ageing population has resulted in a growing need for nursing-home care, home care, and geriatric services in hospitals. Although many countries in Europe have universally accessible long-term care policies, governments are now facing the need to cut services and to change legal entitlements in order to cope with the growing need for care. One of the options is to include family members more intensively in domestic services, but also personal support and care.

Such policies have important consequences for the role and meaning of solidarity as a principle in the organization of systems of healthcare and social services and other forms of social support. Solidarity basically means that everyone is assumed to make a fair financial contribution to a collectively organized and compulsory insurance system aimed at universal access to healthcare and social services. Although prudence and self-interest are strong motivations in the acceptance of compulsory solidarity, solidarity also includes a feeling of responsibility to organize care for those individuals who are in need of care but not able to pay for it. In view of the lack of resources and increasing premiums and other financial contributions, solidarity is narrowed down to so-called interest solidarity, in which individuals are supporting healthcare and social services arrangements predominantly because of their own interests rather than because of the needs of vulnerable others.

At the same time, as illustrated by the example of the Netherlands, access to home-care support becomes increasingly difficult: The supply of these services is devolved to local councils and stripped of substantial amounts of funding. Government policies are built on the belief that family care will be able to complement or substitute for professional care, which has become too expensive. However, many family members are not able or willing to supply this care because of changes in family structures, demographic changes, and dysfunctional family dynamics. Families have to undergo strict assessment procedures when they apply for care, and often they have to pay substantial amounts for professional support. As a result, professional support for home care is falling apart, resulting in increased burden for families with older and dependent family members.

However, family support would be much more widely available if family caregivers were supported by professional caregivers such as home-care nurses and district nurses. Instead of the 'substitution model,' government policies should be led by the 'communicating vessels model,' in which family care is seen as an open system: More professional support will stimulate the willingness of family members to supply care. Moreover, professional support will help family caregivers develop a caring relationship based on interpersonal solidarity and mutual recognition. The idea of solidarity as 'reciprocity' put forward by Dutch policymakers captures to some extent a wider meaning of solidarity than just the interest solidarity to support welfare and healthcare arrangements. The emphasis on individual responsibility, which is leading the idea of solidarity as reciprocity, can empower individuals to take care of their own needs and to arrange care services according to individual preferences. It can also promote care relations that are based on reciprocity and mutual recognition, as argued in some policy documents and reports. However, there is a risk that such reforms are supporting the neoliberal agenda of reducing the role of the state and leaving care for vulnerable people to individual initiative. Family support at the micro-level should not be accompanied by reduced support from governments, as this support is strongly dependent on support delivered by the healthcare and social services systems. Promoting individual responsibility without support from healthcare and social services comes down to irresponsible conservatism and unreflective cost-cutting that will lead to an increased care burden, humiliating procedures, and diminished quality of life for care recipients and their family members.

References

Bayertz, K. 1999. "Four Uses of 'Solidarity.'" In *Solidarity*, edited by K. Bayertz, 3–28. Dordrecht: Kluwer Academic Publishers.

Carrera, F., E. Pavolini, C. Ranci, and A. Sabatini. 2013. "Long-Term Care Systems in Comparative Perspective: Care Needs, Informal and Formal Coverage, and Social Impacts in European Countries." In *Reforms in Long-Term Care Policies in Europe: Investigating Institutional Changes and Social Impacts*, edited by C. Ranci and E. Pavolini, 23–52. New York: Springer.

Companje, K. P., R. H. M. Hendriks, K. F. E. Veraghtert, and B. E. M. Widdershoven. 2009. *Two Centuries of Solidarity: German, Belgian and Dutch Social Health Insurance 1770–2008*. Amsterdam: Aksant Academic Publishers.

Durkheim, E. 2014 [1893]. *The Division of Labor in Society*, edited by S. Lukes, translated by W. D. Hall. New York: Free Press.

Eurostat. 2015. *Key Figures on Europe*. Luxembourg: Publication Office of the European Union.

Fries, J. 1980. "Ageing, Natural Death and the Compression of Morbidity." *New England Journal of Medicine* 303 (3):130–135. doi: 10.1056/NEJM198007173030304.

Fries, J. 2005. "The Compression of Morbidity." *The Milbank Quarterly* 83 (4):801–823. doi: 10.1111/j.1468-0009.2005.00401.x.

Giddens, A. 1998. *The Third Way: The Renewal of Social Democracy*. Cambridge: Polity Press.

Gruenberg, E. M. 1977. "The Failures of Success." *The Milbank Memorial Fund Quarterly: Health and Society* 55 (1):3–24.

Houtepen, R., and R. H. J. ter Meulen. 2001. "Beyond Justice and Moralism: Modernity and Solidarity in the Health Care System." In *Solidarity in Health and Social Care in Europe*, edited by R. ter Meulen, W. Arts, and R. Muffels, 339–363. Dordrecht: Kluwer Academic Publishers.

Lafortune, G., and G. Balestat. 2007. "Trends in Severe Disability among Elderly People: Assessing the Evidence in 12 OECD Countries and the Future Implications." *OECD Health Working Papers* 26:81. doi: 10.1787/217072070078.

Lukes, S. 2014. "Introduction to This Edition." In *E. Durkheim: The Division of Labor in Society*, edited by S. Lukes, translated by W. D. Hall, 25–46. New York: Free Press.

Made, J. van der, R. ter Meulen, and M. van den Burg. 2001. "Solidarity and Care in the Netherlands." In *Solidarity in Health and Social Care in Europe*, edited by R. ter Meulen, W. Arts, and R. Muffels, 229–253. Dordecht: Kluwer Academic Publishers.

Maarse, H. 2004. "Towards a Comparative Analysis of Privatisation in European Health Care." In *Privatisation in European Health Care: A Comparative Analysis in Eight Countries*, edited by H. Maarse, 169–198. Maarssen: Elsevier.

Maarse, H., and P. Jeurissen. 2016. "The Policy and Politics of the 2015 Long-Term Care Reform in the Netherlands." *Health Policy* 120 (3):241–245. doi: 10.1016/j.healthpol.2016.01.014.

Margalith, A. 1996. *The Decent Society*. Cambridge, MA: Harvard University Press.

Meulen, R. H. J. ter. 1995. "Limiting Solidarity in the Netherlands: A Two-Tier System on the Way." *Journal of Medicine and Philosophy* 20 (6):607–616. doi: 10.1093/jmp/20.6.607.

Meulen, R. H. J. ter. 2011. "How 'Decent' Is a Decent Minimum of Health Care?" *Journal of Medicine and Philosophy* 36 (6):612–623. doi: 10.1093/jmp/jhr048.

Meulen, R. H. J. ter, W. Arts, and R. Muffels. 2001. "Solidarity, Health and Social Care in Europe: Introduction to the Volume." In *Solidarity in Health and Social Care in Europe*, edited by R. H. J. ter Meulen, W. Arts, and R. Muffels, 1–11. Dordrecht: Kluwer Academic Publishers.

Meulen, R. H. J. ter, and R. Houtepen. 2012. "Solidarity." In *Encyclopedia of Applied Philosophy*, edited by R. Chadwick, D. Callahan, and Peter Singer, 198–205. Oxford: Elsevier.

Meulen, R. H. J. ter, and H. Maarse. 2008. "Increasing Individual Responsibility in Dutch Health Care: Is Solidarity Losing Ground?" *Journal of Medicine and Philosophy* 33 (3):262–279. doi: 10.1093/jmp/jhn011.

Meulen, R. H. J. ter, and K. Wright. 2012. "Family Solidarity and Informal Care: The Case of Care for People with Dementia." *Bioethics* 26 (7):361–368. doi: 10.1111/j.1467-8519.2012.01992.x.

Mezzo. 2015. "Mantelzorger wel vaak gezien, maar niet gehoord." *Mezzo*, November 6, 2015. www.mezzo.nl/artikel/mantelzorger-wel-vaker-gezien-maar-niet-gehoord.

Muffels, R., and R. Verburg. 2001. "Reforms in Health and Social Care in Europe: The Challenge to Policy." In *Solidarity in Health and Social Care in Europe*, edited by R. H. J. ter Meulen, W. Arts, and R. Muffels, 255–276. Dordrecht: Kluwer Academic Publishers.

OECD. 2011. *Health at a Glance 2011: OECD Indicators*. Paris: OECD Publishing.

Pavolini, E., and C. Ranci. 2013. "Reforms in Long-Term Care Policies in Europe: An Introduction." In *Reforms in Long-Term Care Policies in Europe: Investigating Institutional Changes and Social Impacts*, edited by C. Ranci and E. Pavolini, 3–22. New York: Springer.

Prainsack, B., and A. Buyx. 2011. *Solidarity: Reflections on an Emerging Concept in Bioethics*. London: Nuffield Council on Bioethics.

President's Commission for the Study of Ethical Problems in Medicine and Biomedical and Behavioral Research. 1983. *Securing Access to Health Care: A Report on the Ethical Implications of Differences in the Availability of Health Services*. Washington, DC: US Government Printing Office.

Putters, K. 2014. *Rijk geschakeerd. Op weg naar de participatiesamenleving*. Den Haag: Sociaal en Cultureel Planbureau.

RVZ (Raad voor de Volksgezondheid en Zorg). 2013. *Het belang van wederkerigheid . . . solidariteit gaat niet van zelf.* Den Haag: Raad voor de Volksgezondheid en Zorg.

Stjernø, S. 2004. *Solidarity in Europe: The History of an Idea*. Cambridge: Cambridge University Press.

16 Legacies, generations, and ageing futures

The ethics of intergenerativity

Stephen Katz and Peter J. Whitehouse

This chapter moves through four connected parts to explore contemporary and emerging intergenerational ethics as a framework for anti-ageist practices and the future planning of ageing societies. We will focus on the relations between generations as a practical and conceptual area in which to pursue solutions to the ethical problems posed by medical, bioethical, and popular demographic discourses on ageing.

We will begin with bioethics, because it is the field under which ethical research issues of ageing and health are frequently overseen, yet mainstream biomedical ethics limits its scope to the concerns of the medical and other health professions while marginalizing the social, environmental, and long-term intergenerational dimensions of health.

Second, we will critique popular demographic 'apocalyptic' discourses that depict ageing populations as threats to the livelihood of younger groups and risks to the viability of state resources. Such discourses have created a powerful and unethical framework for understanding 'intergenerational injustice,' a framework that neglects the realities and continuities of intergenerational collaboration and intertwined life courses.

Third, we will revisit the concepts of 'population' and 'generation' in the context of ageing to deepen their historical and ethical value and counter their narrow bioethical and popular demographic formulations.

Fourth, we will summarize the exemplary context of The Intergenerational School (TIS) in Cleveland, Ohio, and its foundational ethic and learning model of 'intergenerativity' as one of intergenerational reciprocity and collaboration (George, Whitehouse, and Whitehouse 2011; Whitehouse et al. 2000). This final part provides a case study of how this bold school innovation suggests a way to expand the moral scope of ethical ageing that embraces public-health approaches, long-term legacies, the arts and humanities, and intergenerational mediations. At the conclusion, we will return to the importance of intergenerational relations as an ethical strategy for connecting generations and communities in planning for the future.

Ageing and the limited 'bio' of bioethics

Bioethics is an important entry point for this chapter because its practitioners claim to represent not only key issues in ageing, health, and welfare, but also the ethical interface between knowledge and humanity.

From its beginnings, bioethics had a bilocated, if not trilocated, birth (Reich 1994; Whitehouse 2003). Fritz Jahr was the first to use the term 'bioethics,' in the 1930s, but it was not adopted broadly (Beever and Whitehouse, in preparation; Whitehouse et al. 2015). In modern times, Van Rensselaer Potter reinvented the term in 1970, inspired by Aldo Leopold's environmentally oriented land ethic (Potter 1971). Potter probably influenced the Kennedy Institute for the Study of Human Reproduction and Bioethics, founded in 1971, to use the term as well (Beever and Whitehouse, in preparation; Whitehouse 2003). Potter's early intuition was that the scope of bioethics must extend to the full range of human relations, to the extent that bioethics includes concerns for ecosystems as a necessary condition for human health as well as concerns for the welfare of ecosystems themselves, both issues of intergenerational legacy as well. Potter and others also recognized that bioethics is an essentially political activity. Starting in the early 1970s, the ethical principles, conceptual frameworks, and empirical data sets were applied to particular problems in research. They were also applied to the practice of medicine, nursing, and other health practices, but not to public and environmental health.

Given this historical background, medical bioethics, the mainstream of professional bioethics, has focused primarily on evaluating biomedical solutions to human disease and suffering, thus cutting the bridge created by Potter to embrace a global 'bio' as an ethical domain. As such, medical bioethics has addressed human subjects' protection, researcher conduct, the potential power of genetic approaches to disease, and the use of neuroscience to explore the human mind and behavior. However, bioethics, while struggling with its own sense of professionalism, has too often served the goals of medicine rather than critically examining and, as necessary, contesting them in a complex and developing scientific landscape. For example, the National Human Genome Research Institute in the US is mandated to spend "not less than 5%" of the institute budget on Ethical, Legal, and Social Implications (ELSI) of genetic and genomic research – an indicator of the social and economic relevance of genetics for medical research (www.genome.gov/10001618/the-elsi-research-program/). This is a substantial funding opportunity for 'genethicists' that attracts the time and attention of bioethicists who work in the service of medical research. Given the excitement about progress in the brain sciences and the enormity of dementia issues and brain health in our ageing populations, neuroethics, like genethics, is almost a caricature of this celebratory mode of thinking about its root concern – clinical neuroscience. In this case, by asking questions that presume the power of scientific knowledge in neuroimaging, along with the potency of pharmacological and surgical interventions, neuroethicists often preclude or at least limit discussion of the merits of the science and its claims and the broader social implications of its impact (Whitehouse 2003). For example, should the ongoing exposure of children to lead and other environmental toxins in water supplies worldwide not really be a 'neuroethical' issue?

With this kind of thinking in mind, one of us (Peter J. Whitehouse) advocates at bioethics organizational meetings for the inclusion of intergenerative bioethics. The American Association of Bioethics and Humanities was created in 1998 by the American Association for Bioethics, Society for Bioethics Consultation, and

Society for Health and Human Values. The Ethics Section of the American Public Health Association is less than two years old. Other environmental ethics and philosophy groups, such as the International Association for Environmental Philosophy, are also relevant to our call for an integrated ethics. Whitehouse co-led the development and presentation of essentially the same panel program calling for an intergenerative bioethics at all 2015 meetings of these three groups (Beever and Whitehouse, in preparation; Whitehouse et al. 2015). Environmental, public health, and clinical bioethicists spoke about the necessary and important overlap of their fields. Whitehouse also spoke about the need for a new framing of ageing and age-related brain diseases as an example of the limited moral scope of current biomedical ethics and the need for a deeper and broader practice of ecoethics.

Thus, our argument here is that, because conventional bioethics is often seen as narrowly confined to professional and legalistic issues of medical research and practice, a critical revamping of bioethics is needed in order to imagine other kinds of 'bio' ethics. This may also help reduce the influence that hegemonic processes of medicalization of ageing and life in general currently has on bioethics in the United States and elsewhere. From microbial diversity to animal communities and agribusiness to environmental well-being and human health, the vast network of human relations to each other and to nature further problematizes the role and scope of bioethical inquiry. At the fundament of our thoughts about reinventing ageing ethics, as we will argue, fostering intergenerational learning organizations is one way that points to a more integrated and deeper global bioethics, perhaps also called an ecoethics, as an ethics of life itself that stretches from cellular communities to human populations and beyond.

In summary, bioethics started with Potter and Jahr attending broadly to values involving the relationships between humans and nature from an ecological stance. It then narrowed in the waning decades of the twentieth century to focus more on biomedical research and clinical issues, like informed consent and genetic testing. We are now suggesting a return to the historically more expansive global view mirroring the need to take a transdisciplinary systems perspective on the social and ecological determinants of health.

Apocalyptic ageism and intergenerational injustice

The narrowness and reductionism of mainstream biomedical ethics find parallels in popular demographic depictions of population ageing because both are based on crudely empirical, politically biased, and individualizing models of what it means to age. Yet, it would be rare to find an academic paper or book, popular media, or policy report that did not introduce the subject of ageing without a volley of rhetorically powerful statements about the size, growth, longevity, and risks characterizing our older populations and their supposed conflict with younger generations. Headlining such popular reports in the media are metaphors of 'the gray tsunami,' 'the silver tide,' and 'greedy geezers,' which further propagate the sense of threat to national prosperity posed by older people, who are often stereotyped as engaging in leisure activities funded by undeserved state provisions and pension rewards (Zeilig 2014). For example, an editorial in Canada's premier national newspaper, the Toronto *Globe and Mail*, states:

> Our biggest social problem is not how to redistribute more money to the needy old. It's how to protect everybody else from the tsunami of geezers that's about to crash on our shores and suck the wealth of future generations out to sea. The war against seniors' pension reforms is a war against the young. [. . .] With the geezer population set to double, their entitlements will double, too – pensions, health care and all the rest. But it's worse still because, thanks to modern medicine, people will live forever.
>
> (Wente 2012, A17)

If such statements were leveled against members of a particular racial, ethnic, or religious group, rather than those of a particular age group, we would be justifiably outraged. But we should be equally outraged at such discriminatory and negative victim-blaming images of old people and the ageist discourses that perpetuate them.

The unusually large 'boomer' generation, born between 1946 and 1964, has been particularly targeted as perpetrators of generational injustice and unethical self-enrichment (Bristow 2015; Moody 2008). They are lambasted in topical non-fiction books with sensationalist titles such as *Who Destroyed the Economy: The Case against Baby Boomers* (Tankersley 2012), *Baby Boomers Don't Care about Leaving Money to Their Kids, and Expect Their Kids to Be Poorer than They Are* (Goldman and Lubin 2011), and *The Pinch: How the Baby Boomers Took Their Children's Future – And Why They Should Give It Back* (Willetts 2011).

Shaped and shared through a discourse of demographic trends, the image of the ageing population is one of a social force set to transform the world's political economies. In demography, such trends are statistically aggregated into median ages, fertility and mortality rates, dependency ratios, migration patterns, and life expectancies. For example, statistical data on Canada (e.g., Statistics Canada 2011, 2012), the first author's country, reveal that in 2006, 13 percent of the Canadian population was over the age of 65, and by 2041, that figure is expected to almost double (to 24.5 percent), with 80 years and older being the fastest-growing age group. Median age calculations divide populations into younger and older halves so that a median age over 30 indicates a population that is 'older' rather than 'younger.' In Canada in 2011, the median age was 39.9, whereas Japan's median age was already over 40 in 2000. Predictions are that by 2050, in North American and Western European countries, as well as Japan and China, the median age will be between 40 and 50. Such trends influence government policymakers, healthcare-system planners, and financial planners, who hold the common view that as people live longer, they will also experience greater disability and dependency, which in turn will require more social services and healthcare resources. This view persists despite a multitude of policy research that demonstrates that healthcare costs are rising, particularly in the United States, due to the unregulated costs of drugs, overuse of technologies, insurance-company profits, malpractice-defense expenses, healthcare fraud and over-billing, and systematic waste and inefficiency, so that "contrary to popular belief, ageing of the population is not a major contributing factor to the overall growth in healthcare spending" (Rejda 2013, 171). In Canada, health costs have also risen because of government failures to shift funding from expensive hospital to less-expensive but needed community and home-care services (Carrière 2000).

Ageing demographic trends are also encapsulated in dependency ratios, which calculate the extent to which growing dependent populations rely on shrinking taxpaying working populations. For example, in Canada in 2006, the age-dependency ratio was 210 elders per 1,000 15-to-64-year-olds and 250 dependent youths per 1,000 15-to-64-year-olds. So the combined dependency ratio, old and young, was 460:1,000 or 46:100. That rate is expected to rise to 60:100 in the next couple of decades, and by 2056, the total ratio is predicted to be 84:100 (Wister and McPherson 2014). In addition, fertility rates are dropping. These trends are accelerating in Europe and parts of Southeast Asia even faster than in North America. It is expected that by 2050 Japan's and Russia's working-age populations will shrink 34 percent, Germany's will shrink 20 percent, France's will shrink 6 percent, and China's will shrink 3 percent (Haas 2007, 7). The social insecurities imagined to follow from such trends have also fired up the global political imagination. The American Central Intelligence Agency (CIA) produced a report in 2001 on the 'geopolitical landscape,' summarizing its major concerns about regional conflict and noting that those countries identified as poor, unstable, and "likely the most disruptive to US interests" – such as Afghanistan, Pakistan, Colombia, Iraq, and Gaza (Central Intelligence Agency 2001, 41) – also have large young populations. Here, the demographic divide between old and young is embedded in a militaristic vision of American surveillance over global 'hot spots' of political activism and terrorism, even if such surveillance is predicted to be beneficial and result in global 'geriatric peace' (Haas 2007).

Critics have consistently identified demographic statistical diagrams as well as their media sensationalizing as part of an age-blaming discourse of 'alarmist' (Katz 1992) or 'apocalyptic' (Gee and Gutman 2000) demography. They argue that dependency ratios misrepresent older people as being economically dependent just because of their age, as if retirement was synonymous with 'unproductivity.' In reality, people past retirement age perform essential work as volunteers, grandparents, domestic caregivers, and community mentors, even if such work is unpaid and undervalued. Most importantly, in the period between 1996 and 2041, the total combined dependency ratios have been and will continue to be relatively modest compared to the 1950s and 1960s, when the boom in fertility rates created large populations of children, who required family supplement support, new schools, and health programs. However, in the apocalyptic discourse children are a worthwhile investment, whereas support for older people is an expensive diversion of resources.

This is where popular apocalyptic demography intersects with the pernicious ideology of 'intergenerational injustice' and its implications of a war between the supposedly privileged old and the marginalized young. American gerontologist and activist Harry R. Moody (2007) attributes the idea of intergenerational injustice in the United States to the neo-liberal dismantling of the welfare state in the 1980s, along with increasingly conservative governments and groups such as Americans for Generational Equity (AGE) that pushed the idea of age-based rationing of healthcare resources. By the 1990s, the debates were further buoyed by 'positive' research that portrayed older people as healthier and wealthier than previously thought and chronological age itself as an outdated and ageist biomarker of questionable social significance. The critiques by Moody and his associates ring true for other countries that have recently used age-blaming to influence social policies – for example, Austria (Weicht 2013), Sweden (Jönson and Jönsson 2015), and Hong Kong (Kwok and Ku 2016).

Despite the assumptions that a self-empowered gerontocracy is impoverishing its own children and threatening economic sustainability and social democracy, critical research maintains that there is far more intergenerational interdependence and cooperation than antagonism (Kaplan and Liu 2004). Kemp (2005) argues that relationships between grandparents and grandchildren are important not only for family continuity and biographical sharing, but also for financial support and legacy investment, which help protect against economic risks and accumulated social disadvantages. Further, as Williamson, McNamara, and Howling (2003) note, many social policies that benefit older people also benefit younger people, and there is always a flow of goods and services between generations, substantiating a 'GI' (Generational Interdependence) rather than a 'GE' (Generational Equity) perspective, even if the latter has been more successful in framing policy debates (Williamson, McNamara, and Howling 2003, 10).

Revisiting population and generation

In the same way that the 'bio' of bioethics can be critically expanded to include far-reaching intergenerational relationships beyond medicine and health, the ethics of population ageing and generational reciprocity can be extended by revisiting 'population' and 'generation' as socio-historical ideas. As discussed elsewhere (Katz 1996, 2013), the accepted truth that older people constitute a 'population' is itself the result of a historical process, as are the statistical discourses that define them as such. Populations are not natural bodies, but socially organized and often problematized groupings made knowable for political reasons. The history of old age reveals that the 'ageing population' became a political product of 19th- and early 20th-century institutional and pension reform, new geriatric and gerontological sciences of ageing, and industrial labor models that included retirement. For example, one of the first surveys of the problem of 'old age dependency' in the United States was Lee Welling Squier's *Old Age Dependency in the United States: A Complete Survey of the Pension Movement* (1912), which states that "the American nation is face to face with a stupendous problem: Hundreds of thousands of working people already across the border into helpless and hopeless superannuation, tens and hundreds of thousands more now pressing the border line" (1912, 16). Although this negative portrayal was intended as political support for social-security planning, it created the image of older people as a special, age-graded population whose vulnerability was a national 'stupendous problem.' Differentiating 'the elderly' was also part of a deeper historical 'bio-power' insinuated within the modern state that governed the general population as a source of productivity, security, and national identity. This Foucauldian sense of government (Foucault 1980, 2004) remains highly relevant to understanding how ageing populations are organized as categories of persons in socially problematic ways (Moreira and Palladino 2011; Pickard 2013).

At the other end of the lifespan, youth and adolescence were similarly constructed as specific populations. American psychologist G. Stanley Hall, who coined the term 'adolescence,' left no doubt about its defining characteristics in his seminal two-volume book entitled *Adolescence – Its Psychology, Anthropology, Sociology, Sex, Crime, Religion and Education* (1904). The association of youth with delinquency and instability, as well as dependency, still mars younger cohorts as risk categories. However, as contemporary research illustrates, the real risks to young people are the result of the socially imposed pressures of ballooning student debt, poorly paid and unprotected jobs, stressful expectations for job-change 'flexibility,' financial constraints on starting a family and a career, dislocation of traditional places of residence, and environmental and urban degradation. As Settersten and Ray (2010) argue, young people today are actually more isolated and insecure than in the past, despite their unprecedented access to collective social-networking systems. "The number of young people nationally [United States] who are completely disconnected and on the brink of sinking before they even get started is alarming" (Settersten and Ray 2010, 74). And the racial division within the American population is also alarming, since "more than one-half of young black men ages sixteen through twenty-four are neither in school nor working" (Settersten and Ray 2010, 74), with an extraordinary number of those young black men having moved through the prison system. Life expectancy for younger generations may be expanding, but the security of their ageing is eroding because of the social forces aligned to the disruption of healthy and sustainable long-term and intergenerational lives.

If seeing ageing populations, both young and old, as biopolitical entities challenges their apocalyptic stereotypes, then we can similarly revisit the concept of 'generation' in a way that challenges the narratives of intergenerational injustice. Again, generations are neither naturalized age-determined groups nor self-determining identities. Generation is a social grouping and was introduced as such by Karl Mannheim in his essay 'The Problem of Generations' (1998 [1952]), which insightfully outlined how a generation is a congregation of identity, consciousness, class, history, and location. Mannheim wrote that only in a "utopian, imaginary society" could social life be envisioned as one generation living on forever, because in reality we live in a society where "the transition from generation to generation is a continuous process" (1998 [1952], 170). Each subsequent generation has "fresh contact" with the legacies left by previous generations, such that "generations are in a state of constant interaction" (1998 [1952], 180). Further, "whether a new *generation style* emerges every year, every thirty, every hundred years, or whether it emerges rhythmically at all, depends entirely on the trigger action of the social and cultural process" (1998 [1952], 191, emphasis in original). Mannheim's message was that there are no isolated generations, because age groups, their legacies, and their historical spaces are interlaced, co-constitutive, and transcendent of the limits imposed by any one generation upon others. Generations generate the transmission of culture itself (Burnett 2010; Edmunds and Turner 2002).

The historicity of populations and the transmissive power of generations undermine the static and ageist demographic diagrams that dominate public imagery about planning ageing and health futures. At the same time, they open new 'interethical' spaces of interdependence and intergenerativity that can undo the ways in which ageing has been compartmentalized into cohorts whose differences are posed as the bases for fear and competition. The ethical issues of care that follow from such compartmentalization have been many, the most prominent of which is a language of degeneration, dependency, suffering, and selfishness that affects how older people are treated in practice. The consideration of ageing concepts, such as 'population' and 'generation,' as fluid processes with positive tonality and shaped by historical and collective understanding is essential to imagining a shared future.

Intergenerativity and the Intergenerational School

In this final part of this chapter, we will look into how the ideas of 'intergenerativity' and intergenerational ethics about community, ageing, and generational bonding are practiced in the context of The Intergenerational School (TIS) in Cleveland, Ohio (see www.tisonline.org/).

TIS was founded in 2000 by Peter J. Whitehouse, his wife Catherine Whitehouse, and a team of others, as a place where inner-city students (of all ages) and volunteers could teach, study, and mentor together. The school's activities involve intergenerative programming in nature studies and sustainability, health and wellness, history and reading, and visits to long-term care facilities, museums, parks, and nature centers in order to create "shared spaces in which older persons can educate younger children about significant aspects of their life stories," which "fosters opportunities for increased senses of purpose and the furthering of legacies" (George, Whitehouse, and Whitehouse 2011, 401). The schools foster individual relationships between adults, including elders with cognitive impairment, and children, many of whom come from impoverished backgrounds. Mixed-methods research has demonstrated that older people with dementia benefit from participating in the school programs (George and Whitehouse 2010). The signature program is reading mentoring, in which pairs read books to each other or share stories from their own lives. TIS has received national and international awards for its impact on both children and elders, and the school has been highly rated for students' performance outcomes. The second author, Peter J. Whitehouse, is most familiar with this particular model but sees it as just one example of the intergenerative approach that can be adapted in conversation with local communities in the US, Canada, and abroad. Our position is that, while organizations such as the Alzheimer's Association may irresponsibly try to create fear and promote the risks of ageing in terms of loss in order to exaggerate the benefits of hypothetical medical treatments (Whitehouse and George 2008, 2015), TIS has demonstrated that the existence of older people in a community is an asset. Even elders with memory loss can play important roles in a community by serving as collective long-term memory and care enhancers, as well as reminders of the cognitive challenges we all face. In concept, TIS is part of a larger emphasis on intergenerational ethics taking place in academic circles in trans- and interdisciplinarity, transhumanism, and responsible innovation. Common to all these trends is a focus on connectedness, inclusiveness, future orientation, and a broad set of values. They are all, in the word we are promoting in this chapter, 'intergenerative.' They go 'between' to go 'beyond.'

The prefix 'inter-,' rather than 'multi-,' signifies a genuine conversation among fields of human endeavor, a conversation that can lead to cooperation – and, as needed, compromise – in service of a collaborative process that promises to be more effective at social reform than a simple co-presence of different knowledge-making silos. Think of a client-centered care plan constructed by a high-functioning, culturally sensitive, inter-professional team. And here we are confirming the conceptual and methodological importance of 'intergenerativity' as a new word with the potential to generate metaphors and narratives to temper the bioethical and apocalyptic demographic frameworks. 'Inter-' also signifies a space that is contingent upon the social structures that position generational and life-course differences, such that 'young' and 'old,' like 'population' and 'generation,' are recognized as flexible categories relative to each other, rather than as naturalized ahistorical age entities (see van Dyk 2014).

Thus, intergenerativity is the ethical foundation for TIS in Cleveland, which for 15 years has provided evidence and inspiration that seeking intergenerative solutions to social problems can lead to excellent results for both children and adults, even those with dementia (Whitehouse et al. 2000). Many citizens in the United States and other countries believe that public education is not only inadequate but failing. Recalcitrant teachers' unions and rigid administrative bureaucracies create, quite ironically, organizations that cannot learn and cannot change fast enough. In the United States, the public-charter-school model has been developed as an opportunity to foster innovation. In exchange for relaxing some of the bureaucratic regulations encumbering regular public schools, such schools are given the opportunity to demonstrate value in the form of better-educated students – for example, more college graduates. The results have been mixed, depending on the motivations and approaches of the educational reformers and the level of support and competence of the sponsors of the charter schools.

Social reformers are also looking for opportunities to take advantage of the national resource that elders represent. A variety of programs allow older adults to volunteer in schools, and for school students to visit elders in the community or long-term care residences. However, TIS was the first to design a learning organization from the bottom up that embraces lifelong learning and spirited citizenship for all learners, regardless of age. Because of the success of TIS in Cleveland (there are now three intergenerational schools throughout the city), the TIS team has founded Intergenerational Schools International (ISI) to disseminate the model in other national and cultural settings. Just as in the three schools in Cleveland, the pedagogical model is adapted to the community wishing to support such a school. Even in Cleveland, the schools are different, reflecting the ethnicities and values of the local communities. Nevertheless, the focus on learner-centered, intergenerational, and developmentally appropriate learning and the social construction of knowledge is promoted wherever the model is disseminated. Creating collective wisdom through story-sharing and relationship-building is highlighted as part of the core activities. Currently, the team is working in Asia, North America, and Europe to create intergenerational knowledge centers (which may or may not be based in an actual school) that respond to different community needs, such as private schools and after-school programs, rather than simply modeling schools closely after ours in Cleveland. The long-standing collaborative and sister program in Japan is such an after-school program. The team is also in the process of developing individual and organizational curricula that will allow people to develop their knowledge about intergenerative learning.

Not surprisingly, the first glocal (i.e., global thinking applied locally) project of ISI is The Intergenerativity Project (TIP). In recognition of the 15th anniversary of TIS, the team is collecting stories from students; teachers; staff members; administrators; community, national and international leaders; and others about their intergenerational learning experiences in the school or their hopes for the intergenerational schools. Under the direction of Richard Geer, founder of Community Performance International, the stories will be blended into a play performed by school and community members that will then be used to inform other organizations and individuals about TIS and its programs (Geer et al. 2012). It is hoped that what will emerge from the play and the associated international collaborations is a message not only about how we think and learn across generations, but also about how and what we value. The stories express the importance of fostering dignity for all individuals (regardless of ability), diversity, relationships, social justice, the arts and humanities, respect for nature, and solidarity across geographic and temporal distances.

Finally, legacy is a key focal point for ethical deliberations in this movement's intergenerational work. Legacy can be framed by key questions, such as "After your death, what is the narrative of your enduring impact on others in your family and community? How do you want to be remembered as others place you in the roster of departed ancestors?" Two specific intergenerative legacy projects illustrate the importance of mutual respect, dignity, diversity, and future-orientation to our moral compass. One is a book called *The Legacy of Clark Freeway Fighters* (Harris and Whitehouse 2011), based on stories our children collected from adults and elders, including some with dementia, about how they saved the community and its nature center (where our kids visit) from a corrupt politician who wanted to put a highway through it. The project inspired spirited citizenship and environmental activism (George, Whitehouse, and Harris 2012). TIS also participates with the Legacy Project in Canada on YOU 177 (Young Old United One World Seven Generations Seven Billion People; see www.legacyproject.org), a global effort to enhance long-term ecological thinking and valuing in community. Overall, the intergenerational-school movement is growing and demonstrates that the potent gathering of legacy, education, generation, and ethics around 'inter-' spaces, narratives, and practices provides an important direction to planning ageing futures. The principal lesson of this model is to foreground the experiences and capabilities of people at different points on life's journey. It is not about chronological age itself, but about the power of integrating knowledge from learners of very different backgrounds. A narrative ethic frames the creation of discourse spaces that release the human imagination to think about human diversity from a long-term perspective. Aiming for collective wisdom that informs spirited citizenship is the goal. Intergenerational schools are only one manifestation of this pedagogical and ethical approach (Kaplan and Sánchez 2014).

Conclusions

In *An Inconvenient Truth* (2006), Al Gore was correct to both employ the concept of 'intergenerational ethics' and claim that climate change is the biggest long-term issue we face. Indeed, the ecological, political, economic, health, and religious conflicts resulting from tensions around global inequalities are in some way counteracted by the long-term legacies of survival that pass from one generation to another. As Simon Biggs (2014) contends, successful cultural adaptation requires the "rediscovery of the importance of generational intelligence" that includes the "ability to negotiate between generational positions" (Biggs 2014, 14–15). Globally, rather than being a mega-problem, ageing, understood as a historical and social process, can be inverted to become a mega-solution because the transfer of human repositories of experience, stories, and wisdom is one way to deepen resistance to social instability, to say nothing of how ageing populations are influencing new transnational movements, identities, technologies, and forms of 'postnational' and cosmopolitan citizenship (Phillipson 2009). In this chapter, we have supported these claims in our critiques of bioethics, popular demography, population, and generation, and with the case study of TIS.

We believe that the overall discussion of ageing and ethics is key to planning the future of human relations, because ethics has always been an area of critical inquiry that bridges bio-, eco-, and socio-historical forces with the intergenerational dimensions of our humanity. How we age is essentially an ethical question and has been part of the planning of future life since well before the emergence of the medical and gerontological sciences. Ageing also offers us a magnifying lens – both a conceptual microscope and an imaginative telescope – to look deeply into ourselves and broadly across the distances we need to travel. In order to see ageing ethics in these ways, as this chapter has argued, we need to overturn the professional rigidities, cultural restrictions, dominant narratives, and public anxieties that isolate age groups and marginalize the power and creativity of the 'inter-' spaces between ages, dependencies, communities, and legacies that are germane to our ageing futures.

References

Beever, J., and P. J. Whitehouse, in preparation, "Ecology, Value and Health within Bioethics." *Public Health Ethics*.

Biggs, S. 2014. "Adapting to an Ageing Society: The Need for Cultural Change." *Policy Quarterly* 10 (3):12–16.

Bristow, J. 2015. *Baby Boomers and Generational Conflict*. Basingstoke: Palgrave Macmillan.

Burnett, J. 2010. *Generations: The Time Machine in Theory and Practice*. Farnham: Ashgate.

Carrière, Y. 2000. "The Impact of Population Aging and Hospital Days: Will There Be a Problem?" In *The Overselling of Population Aging: Apocalyptic Demography, Intergenerational Challenges and Social Policy*, edited by E. M. Gee and G. M. Gutman, 26–44. Toronto: Oxford University Press.

Central Intelligence Agency. 2001. *Long-Term Global Demographic Trends: Reshaping the Geopolitical Landscape*. Washington, DC: CIA Government Library Report.

Dyk, S. van. 2014. "The Appraisal of Difference: Critical Gerontology and the Active-Ageing Paradigm." *Journal of Aging Studies* 31:93–103. doi: 10.1016/j.jaging.2014.08.008.

Edmunds, J., and B. S. Turner. 2002. *Generations, Culture and Society*. Buckingham: Open University Press.

Foucault, M. 1980. *The History of Sexuality*. New York: Vintage.

Foucault, M. 2004. *The Birth of Biopolitics*. New York: Palgrave Macmillan.

Gee, E. M., and G. M. Gutman, eds. 2000. *The Overselling of Population Aging: Apocalyptic Demography, Intergenerational Challenges and Social Policy*. Toronto: Oxford University Press.

Geer, R. O., J. Corriere, N. Sylvia, M. Block, J. Brown, and D. Isaacs. 2012. *Story Bridge: From Alienation to Community Action*. Denver: Community Performance Press.

George, D. R., C. C. Whitehouse, and P. J. Whitehouse. 2011. "A Model of Intergenerativity: How the Intergenerational School Is Bringing the Generations Together to Foster Collective Wisdom and Community Health." *Journal of Intergenerational Relationships* 9 (4):389–404. doi: 10.1080/15350770.2011.619922.

George, D. R., and P. J. Whitehouse. 2010. "Intergenerational Volunteering and Quality of Life for Persons with Mild to Moderate Dementia: Results from a 5-Month Intervention Study in the United States." *Journal of the American Geriatrics Society* 58 (4):796–797. doi: 10.1111/j.1532-5415.2010.02790.x.

George, D. R., P. J. Whitehouse, and D. Harris. 2012. "'Occupy Nature': Passing Activism across Generations." *Journal of the American Geriatrics Society* 60 (9):1770–1771. doi: 10.1111/j.1532-5415.2012.04110.x.

Goldman, L., and G. Lubin. 2011. "Baby Boomers Don't Care about Leaving Money to Their Kids, and Expect Their Kids to Be Poorer Than They Are." *Business Insider*, April 20. www.businessinsider.com/baby-boomers-wont-leave-money-to-kids-2011-4.

Gore, Al. 2006. *An Inconvenient Truth: The Planetary Emergency of Global Warming and What We Can Do about It*. New York: Rodale.

Haas, M. L. 2007. "A Geriatric Peace? The Future of U.S. Power in a World of Aging Populations." *International Security* 32 (1):112–147.

Hall, G. S. 1904. *Adolescence*. New York: Appleton.

Harris, D., and P. J. Whitehouse. 2011. *The Legacy of the Clark Freeway Fighters*. Cleveland: Tec4Life.

Jönson, H., and A. Jönsson. 2015. "Baby Boomers as Future Care Users: An Analysis of Expectations in Print Media." *Journal of Aging Studies* 34:82–91. doi: 10.1016/j.jaging.2015.05.001.

Kaplan, M., and S. Liu. 2004. *Generations United for Environmental Awareness and Action*. Washington, DC: Generations United.

Kaplan, M., and M. Sánchez. 2014. "Intergenerational Programmes." In *International Handbook on Ageing and Public Policy*, edited by S. Harper, K. Hamblin, J. Hoffman, K. Howse, and G. Leeson, 367–383. Cheltenham: Edward Elgar.

Katz, S. 1992. "Alarmist Demography: Power, Knowledge and the Elderly Population." *Journal of Aging Studies* 6 (3):203–225. doi: 10.1016/0890-4065(92)90001-M.

Katz, S. 1996. *Disciplining Old Age: The Making of Gerontological Knowledge*. Charlottesville: The University Press of Virginia.

Katz, S. 2013. "Active and Successful Aging: Lifestyle as a Gerontological Idea." *Recherches sociologiques et anthropologiques* 44 (1):33–49. doi: 10.4000/rsa.910.

Kemp, C. L. 2005. "Dimensions of Grandparent-Adult Grandchild Relationships: From Family Ties to Intergenerational Friendships." *Canadian Journal on Aging* 24 (2):161–177. doi: 10.1353/cja.2005.0066.

Kwok, J. Y. C., and B. H. B. Ku. 2016. "Elderly People as 'Apocalyptic Demography'? A Study of the Life Stories of Older People in Hong Kong Born in the 1930s." *Journal of Aging Studies* 36:1–9. doi: 10.1016/j.jaging.2015.11.001.

Mannheim, K. 1998 [1952]. "The Sociological Problem of Generations." In *Essays on the Sociology of Knowledge*, edited by P. Kecskemeti, 163–195. London: Taylor & Francis.

Moody, H. R. 2007. "Justice between Generations: The Recent History of an Idea." In *Critical Perspectives on Ageing Societies*, edited by M. Bernard and T. Scharf, 125–137. Bristol: Policy Press.

Moody, H. R. 2008. "Aging America and the Boomer Wars." *The Gerontologist* 48 (6):839–844. doi: 10.1093/geront/48.6.839.

Moreira, T., and P. Palladino. 2011. "'Population Laboratories' or 'Laboratory Populations'? Making Sense of the Baltimore Longitudinal Study of Aging, 1965–1987." *Studies in the History and Philosophy of Biological and Biomedical Sciences* 42 (3):317–327. doi: 10.1016/j.shpsc.2011.05.001.

Phillipson, C. 2009. "Reconstructing Theories of Aging: The Impact of Globalisation on Critical Gerontology." In *Handbook of Theories of Aging* (2nd edition), edited by V. L. Bengtson, D. Gans, N. M. Putney, and M. Silverstein, 615–628. New York: Springer.

Pickard, S. 2013. "A New Political Anatomy of the Older Body? An Examination of Approaches to Illness in Old Age in Primary Care." *Ageing & Society* 33 (6):964–987. doi: http://dx.doi.org/10.1017/S0144686X12000293.

Potter, V. R. 1971. *Bioethics: Bridge to the Future*. Englewood Cliffs, New Jersey: Prentice-Hall.

Reich, W. T. 1994. "The Word 'Bioethics': Its Birth and the Legacies of Those Who Shaped It." *Kennedy Institute of Ethics Journal* 4 (4):319–335. doi: 10.1353/ken.0.0126.

Rejda, G. E. 2013. *Social Insurance and Economic Security*. New York: Routledge.

Settersten, R., and B. E. Ray. 2010. *Not Quite Adults*. New York: Bantam Books.

Squier, L. W. 1912. *Old Age Dependency in the United States: A Complete Survey of the Pension Movement*. New York: Macmillan.

Statistics Canada. 2011. *Life Expectancy at Birth, by Sex and by Province*. Ottawa: Statistics Canada.

Statistics Canada. 2012. *2011 Census of Population*. Ottawa: Statistics Canada.

Tankersley, J. 2012. "Who Destroyed the Economy? The Case against the Baby Boomers." *The Atlantic*, October 5. www.theatlantic.com/business/archive/2012/10/who-destroyed-the-economy-the-case-against-the-baby-boomers/263291.

Weicht, B. 2013. "The Making of the 'Elderly': Constructing the Subject of Care." *Journal of Aging Studies* 27 (2):188–197. doi: 10.1016/j.jaging.2013.03.001.

Wente, M. 2012. "The War against the Young." *The Globe and Mail*, February 2. www.theglobeandmail.com/opinion/the-war-against-the-young/article543236.

Whitehouse, P. J. 2003. "The Rebirth of Bioethics: Extending the Original Formulations of Van Rensselaer Potter." *The American Journal of Bioethics* 3 (4):26–31. doi: 10.1162/15265160332261475 1.

Whitehouse, P. J., J. Beever, B. Jennings, and L. Lee. 2015. *Bridging Bioethics: Historical and Contemporary Engagements*, symposium presented at the American Society for Bioethics and Humanities, Houston, TX.

Whitehouse, P. J., E. Bendezu, S. Fallcreek, and C. Whitehouse. 2000. "Intergenerational Community Schools: A New Practice for a New Time." *Educational Gerontology* 26 (8):761–770. doi: 10.1080/036012700300001412.

Whitehouse, P. J., and D. R. George. 2008. *The Myth of Alzheimer's: What You Aren't Being Told about Today's Most Dreaded Diagnosis*. New York: St. Martin's Press.

Whitehouse, P. J., and D. R. George. 2015. "A Tale of Two Reports: What Recent Publications from the Alzheimer's Association and Institute of Medicine Say about the State of the Field (Editorial)." *Journal of Alzheimer's Disease* 49 (1):21–25. doi: 10.3233/JAD-150663.

Willetts, D. 2011. *The Pinch: How the Baby Boomers Took Their Children's Future – and Why They Should Give It Back*. London: Atlantic Books.

Williamson, J. B., T. K. McNamara, and S. A. Howling. 2003. "Generational Equity, Generational Interdependence, and the Framing of the Debate over Social Security Reform." *The Journal of Sociology and Social Welfare* 30 (3):3–14.

Wister, A., and B. D. McPherson. 2014. *Aging as a Social Process: Canadian Perspectives*. Toronto: Oxford University Press.

Zeilig, H. 2014. "Dementia as a Cultural Metaphor." *The Gerontologist* 54 (2):258–267. doi: 10.1093/geront/gns203.

Index

Note: figures and tables are denoted with italicized page numbers. End note information is denoted with n and note number following the page number.